SCOPE 49
IPCS Joint Symposia 16
SGOMSEC 7

Methods to Assess Adverse Effects of Pesticides on Non-target Organisms

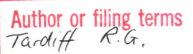

SCOPE 49
IPCS JOINT SYMPOSIA 16
SGOMSEC 7

Methods to Assess Adverse Effects of Pesticides on Non-target Organisms

Edited by
ROBERT G. TARDIFF
RiskFocus/VERSAR, Springfield, Virginia, USA

Prepared by
Scientific Group on Methodologies for the Safety Evaluation of Chemicals (SGOMSEC)

Published on behalf of the Scientific Committee on the Problems of the Environment (SCOPE) of the International Council of Scientific Unions (ICSU), and the International Program on Chemical Safety (IPCS) of the World Health Organization (WHO), the United Nations Environmental Program (UNEP) and the International Labour Organization (ILO)

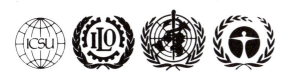

by
JOHN WILEY & SONS
Chichester · New York · Brisbane · Toronto · Singapore

Published by John Wiley & Sons Ltd.
          Baffins Lane,
          Chichester,
          West Sussex PO19 1UD, England

Other Wiley Editorial Offices

John Wiley & Sons, Inc., 605 Third Avenue,
New York, NY 10158-0012, USA

Jacaranda Wiley Ltd, G.P.O. Box 859, Brisbane,
Queensland 4001, Australia

John Wiley & Sons (Canada) Ltd, 22 Worcester Road,
Rexdale, M9W 1L1, Canada

John Wiley & Sons (SEA) Pte Ltd, 37 Jalan Pemimpin #05-04,
Block B, Union Industrial Building, Singapore 2057

Library of Congress Cataloging-in-Publication Data

Methods to assess adverse effects of pesticides / edited by Robert G. Tardiff ;
    prepared by Scientific Group on Methodologies for the Safety Evaluation of Chemicals
(SGOMSEC)
        p.   cm.—(SCOPE ; 49) (IPCS joint symposia ; 16) (SGOMSEC ; 7)
    'Published on behalf of the Scientific Committee on the Problems of the Environment
(SCOPE) of the International Council of Scientific Unions (ICSU), and the International
Program on Chemical Safety (IPCS) of the World Health Organization (WHO), the United
Nations Environmental Program (UNEP) and the International Labour Organization (ILO).'
    Includes bibliographical references and index.
    ISBN 0-471-93156-X
    1. Pesticides—Toxicology—Congresses. I. Tardiff, Robert G. II. Scientific Group
on Methodologies for the Safety Evaluation of Chemicals. III. International Council of
Scientific Unions. Scientific Committee on the Problems of the Environment.
IV. International Council of Scientific Unions. V. Series. VI. Series: SCOPE report ; 49
VII. Series: SGOMSEC (Series) ; 7. RA1270.P4M48   1991
668'.65'0289—dc20   91-27779
                                                                            CIP

British Library Cataloguing in Publication Data

A catalogue record for this book is available
from the British Library

ISBN 0 471 93156 X ✓

Typeset by Dobbie Typesetting Limited, Tavistock, Devon
Printed and bound in Great Britain by Courier International Ltd,
East Kilbride, Scotland

International Council of Scientific Unions (ICSU)
Scientific Committee on Problems of the Environment (SCOPE)

SCOPE is one of a number of committees established by the non-governmental group of scientific organizations, the International Council of Scientific Unions (ICSU). The membership of ICSU includes representatives from 75 National Academies of Science, 20 International Unions and 29 other bodies called Associates. To cover multidisciplinary activities which include the interests of several unions, ICSU has established 13 Scientific Committees, of which SCOPE is one. Currently representatives of 35 member countries and 21 Unions, Scientific Committees and Associates participate in the work of SCOPE, which directs particular attention to the needs of developing countries. SCOPE was established in 1969 in response to the environmental concerns emerging at the time: ICSU recognized that many of these concerns required scientific inputs spanning several disciplines and ICSU Unions. SCOPE's first task was to prepare a report on Global Environmental Monitoring (SCOPE 1, 1971) for the UN Stockholm Conference on the Human Environment.

The mandate of SCOPE is to assemble, review, and assess the information available on man-made environmental changes and the effects of these changes on man; to assess and evaluate the methodologies of measurement of environmental parameters; to provide an intelligence service on current research; and by the recruitment of the best available scientific information and constructive thinking to establish itself as a corpus of informed advice for the benefit of centres of fundamental research and of organizations and agencies operationally engaged in studies of the environment.

SCOPE is governed by a General Assembly, which meets every three years. Between such meetings its activities are directed by the Executive Committee.

R. E. Munn
Editor-in-Chief
SCOPE Publications

Executive Secretary: V. Plocq-Fichelet

Secretariat: 51 boulevard de Montmorency
75016 Paris, France

Contents

PART 2 CONTRIBUTED CHAPTERS

Foreword

Pesticides continue to play major roles both in maintaining a high level of agricultural productivity and in public health programmes. However, these chemicals are designed to be biologically active, and given the widespread and increasing use worldwide, there is a great potential for affecting non-target organisms, including humans.

The International Programme on Chemical Safety (IPCS) has for many years given the evaluation of risks to human health and the environment from pesticide exposures an extremely high priority. The data available to IPCS regarding the adverse effects of pesticides on the total environment is often sparse; and, where available, they are often collected by methods not necessarily accepted worldwide nor supported by present day scientific knowledge.

In this monograph, the Scientific Group on Methodologies for the Safety Evaluation of Chemicals (SGOMSEC) has tackled an extremely complex problem, that is, the evaluation of methods to assess the adverse effects of pesticides on non-target organisms. This scientific evaluation and its recommendations for future studies will hopefully encourage scientists worldwide to address an extremely important area of public health and ecotoxicology using appropriate methodologies. I am confident that these activities will generate the much needed data for more complete scientific evaluations by IPCS and national authorities. In addition, these data will hopefully support the development of rational integrated pest management strategies in both developed and developing countries, maintaining the level of public health protection and agricultural production already achieved while at the same time decreasing the level of pesticide use.

Michel J. Mercier
Manager, International
Programme on Chemical Safety

Preface

This report is the result of the seventh project of SGOMSEC, the Scientific Group on Methodologies for the Safety Evaluation of Chemicals, which operates under the general sponsorship of the IPCS and SCOPE. The objective of SGOMSEC is to examine and review critically methods for the evaluation of the adverse predictive effects of industrial and environmental chemicals on human health and on non-human forms of life. This leads to recommendations for future research, and should also be useful to scientists advising policy makers.

SGOMSEC No. 7 addresses the problems which pesticides may pose to non-target organisms, humans, animals, plants, microorganisms, and to ecosystems. Pesticides consist of a large group of chemicals designed specifically to control pest organisms and to be deliberately released in the environment. Quantities used yearly are estimated now at 3 million tons, and are increasing steadily in industrialized as well as in developing countries. It is estimated that over 99 per cent of the amounts applied do not reach their targets, thereby producing actual and potential negative effects on human health, livestock, and ecosystems.

This book includes a number of contributed papers plus a joint report expressing the consensus reached after a workshop held on 3–7 October 1988 in Céské Budějovice, Czechoslovakia.

The topics covered include the assessment and control of exposure of human and non-human organisms to pesticides, acute toxicity in humans (mostly neurotoxicity and dermal toxicity), chronic toxicity in humans (mostly on reproduction and development), and damage to ecosystems.

Recommendations are made not only on research needs but also on ways and means of mitigating the problems due to chemical control of pests, in particular through the development of integrated pest management, applications of biotechnology, and improved communication with, and training of, users. The application of these recommendations to developing countries is emphasized.

Thanks are due to the authors of the contributed papers and to those who prepared the joint report: R. Albert, S. Baker, J. Doull, G. Butler, N. Nelson, D. Peakall, D. Pimentel, and, in particular, R. G. Tardiff, who also edited the volume.

Special thanks are expressed to Vladimir Landa and his colleagues who organized the workshop in Céské Budějovice.

The help of agencies which contributed funding for this activity—IPCS, SCOPE, the US EPA and the US National Institute of Environmental Health

Sciences, and the Commission of the European Communities—is gratefully acknowledged.

This workshop was the last to be organized and attended by the founder of SGOMSEC, Professor Norton Nelson. Homage is given here to his scientific merits and human qualities.

Philippe Bourdeau   Bernard D. Goldstein
Coordinator, Health and   *Vice-Chairman, Scientific*
Ecotoxicology Cluster   *Group on Methodologies for*
SCOPE   *the Safety Evaluation of*
Chairman, Scientific Group   *Chemicals*
on Methodologies for the
Evaluation of Chemicals

Acknowledgements

The editors would like to acknowledge the assistance received from:

C. David Fowle
J. Galvin
S. Johnson
T. Kneip
N. Nelson
P. Roney
C. Stapleton
B. Tardiff
L. Wakefield

Scientific Group on Methodologies for the Safety Evaluation of Chemicals

*George Becking
Interregional Research Unit, International Program on Chemical Safety, World Health Organization, MD-A206, PO Box 12233, Research Triangle Park, NC 27709, USA (Secretary)

N. P. Bockov
Director, Institute of Medical Genetics, Kasirskoesosse 6A, Moscow 115478, USSR

*Philippe Bourdeau
Directorate General for Science Research and Development, Commission of the European Communities, rue de la Loi 200, B-1049 Brussels, Belgium (Chairman)

Gordon C. Butler
4694 West 13 Avenue, Vancouver, BC V6R 2V7, Canada

*Bernard Goldstein
Professor and Chairman, Department of Environmental and Community Medicine, UMDNJ-Robert Wood Johnson Medical School, 675 Hoes Lane, Piscataway, NJ 08854, USA (Vice-Chairman)

Gareth Green
Professor and Chairman, Department of Environmental Health Sciences, The Johns Hopkins University, School of Hygiene and Public Health, 615 North Wolfe Street, Baltimore, MD 21205, USA

*Miki Goto
Professor, Department of Chemistry and Director, Institute of Ecotoxicology, Gakushuin University, 1-5-1 Mejiro, Toshima-ku, Tokyo 171, Japan

J. R. Hickman
Bureau of Chemical Hazards, Environmental Health Center, Department Health and Welfare, Tunney's Pasture, Ottawa, Ontario K1A 0L2, Canada

---

*Member of the Executive Committee

xxii SCIENTIFIC GROUP ON METHODOLOGIES

Alf G. Johnels
Royal Swedish Academy of Sciences, The Swedish Museum of Natural History, S-104 05 Stockholm 50, Sweden

Theodore Kneip
New York University Medical Center, Institute of Environmental Medicine, 550 First Avenue, New York, NY 10016, USA

Vladimir Landa
Czechoslovak Academy of Sciences, Institute of Entomology, Branisovska 31, 370 05 Cĕské Budĕjovice, Czechoslovakia

*C. R. Krishna Murti†
Cancer Institute (wia), Canal Bank Road, Gandhi Nagar, Adyar, Madras 600 020, India

Aly Massoud
Professor and Chairman, Departments of Community, Environmental and Occupational Medicine, Ein Shams University, Abbassia Cairo, Egypt

*Michel Mercier
Manager, International Program on Chemical Safety, World Health Organization, 1211 Geneva 27, Switzerland

*Norton Nelson†
New York University Medical Center, Institute of Environmental Medicine, 550 First Avenue, New York, NY 10016, USA

Thomas Odhiambo
Director, International Centre for Insect Physiology and Ecology, PO Box 30772, Nairobi, Kenya

*Blanca Raquel Ordonez
Lopez Cotilla 739, Col. del Valle 03100 DF, Mexico

Dennis V. Parke
Head, Department of Biochemistry, University of Surrey, Guildford, Surrey GU2 5XH, UK

David B. Peakall
Head, Toxicology Section, National Wildlife Research Centre, Canadian Wildlife Service, Ottawa, Ontario K1A 0E7, Canada

Jerzy Piotrowski
Lodz Medical Academy, Institute of Environmental Research, Narutowicza 120A, 90-145 Lodz, Poland

---

*Member of the Executive Committee
†Deceased

*Emmanuel Somers
Director General, Drugs Directorate, Health Protection Branch, Health and Welfare Canada, Tunney's Pasture, Ottawa, Ontario K1A 0L2, Canada

*Robert G. Tardiff
Director, RiskFocus® Division, Versar Incorporated, 6850 Versar Center, Springfield, VA 22151, USA (Editor)

René Truhaut
Laboratoire de Toxicologie et d'Hygiène Industrielle, Faculté des Sciences, Pharmacéutiques et Biologiques de Paris, Université René Descartes, 4 avenue de l'Observatoire, 75006 Paris, France

---

**Member of the Executive Committee

Participants of the Workshop

Roy E. Albert
Institute of Environmental Health, University of Cincinnati, Kettering Laboratory (ML-56), 3223 Eden Avenue, Cincinnati, OH 45267-0056, USA

Jeffrey Allender
1905 Brenda Drive, North Augusta, SC 29841 USA

Scott Baker
RiskFocus®/VERSAR Inc., 6850 Versar Center, Springfield, VA 22151, USA (Vice-Chairman)

George Becking
Interregional Research Unit—MD A206, International Programme on Chemical Safety, World Health Organization, PO Box 12233, Research Triangle Park, NC 27709, USA

Philippe Bourdeau
Directorate General for Science Research and Development, Commission of the European Communities, rue de la Loi 200, B-1049 Brussels, Belgium

Thomas Brown
Clemson University, Department of Entomology, 114 Long Hall, Clemson, SC 29634-0365, USA

Gordon C. Butler
4694 West 13 Avenue, Vancouver, BC V6R 2V7, Canada

David Calamari
University of Milan, Institute of Agricultural Entomology, Via Celoria 2, 20133 Milano, Italy

Christopher DeRosa
US Environmental Protection Agency, 26 West Martin Luther King Drive, ECAO, Cincinnati, OH 45268, USA

John Doull
Department of Pharmacology, University of Kansas Medical Center, 39 Rainbow Boulevard, Kansas City, KS 66103, USA (Co-Chairman)

J. Finkelman
Pan American Health Organization, World Health Organization, Apartado Postal 249, Toluca, Mexico

Bernard Goldstein
*Department of Environmental and Community Medicine, UMDNJ-Robert
Wood Johnson Medical School, 675 Hoes Lane, Piscataway, NJ 09954, USA*

Charles Hagedorn
*Department of Plant Pathology and Agronomy, Virginia Polytechnic Institute
and State University, Prince Hall, Room 401, Blacksburg, VA 24061, USA*

Alf G. Johnels
*Royal Swedish Academy of Sciences, The Swedish Museum of Natural History,
S-104 05 Stockholm 50, Sweden*

Robert Kroes
*National Institute of Public Health and Environmental Hygiene, Antonie van
Leeuwenhoeklaan 9, Postbus 1, 3720 BA Bilthoven, The Netherlands*

George Lacey
*Department of Plant Pathology and Agronomy, Virginia Polytechnic Institute
and State University, Prince Hall, Room 416, Blacksburg, VA 24061, USA*

Vladimir Landa
*Institute of Entomology, Czechoslovak Academy of Sciences, Branisovska 31,
370 05 Cĕské Budĕjovice, Czechoslovakia* (Co-Chairman)

Dr. Lichatchev
Petrov Institute of Oncology, Ministry of Health, Leningrad, USSR

Aly Massound
*Department of Community, Environmental and Occupational Medicine,
Ein Shams University, Abbassia Cairo, Egypt*

Myron Mehlman
*Environmental Health Sciences Laboratory, Mobil Corporation, PO Box 1029,
Princeton, NJ 08540, USA*

John A. Moore
*Office of Pesticides and Toxic Substances, US Environmental Protection
Agency, 401 M Street SW-TS 788, Washington, DC 20460, USA*

Victor Morley
*London Research Center, Agriculture Canada, 1400 Western Road, London,
Ontario NG6 2V4, Canada*

Norton Nelson†
*New York University Medical Center, Institute of Environmental Medicine,
550 First Avenue, New York, NY 10016, USA* (Chairman)

---

†Deceased

Blanca Raquel Ordonez
161 Guerrero and Department 102, Col. del Carmen Cogacan,
Mexico 04100 DF, Mexico

David Peakall
National Wildlife Research Centre, Toxicology Research Division,
Canadian Wildlife Service, Ottawa, Ontario K1A 0H3, Canada

David Pimentel
Cornell University, College of Agriculture and Life Sciences,
6126 Comstock Hall, Garden Avenue, Ithaca, NY 14853, USA

Jerzy Piotrowski
Lodz Medical Academy, Institute of Environmental Research,
Narutowisza 120A, 90-145 Lodz, Poland

J. Russell Roberts
Senior Science Advisor, Revenue Canada, 123 Slater Street, Ottawa, Ontario
K1A 012, Canada

Margaret Rostker
US Environmental Protection Agency, Office of Pesticides and Toxic
Substances, Room 635, East Tower, TS 788, 401 M Street SW, Washington,
DC 20460, USA

Stephen Saunders
RJR Nabisco, Corporate Center of Toxicology, Bowman Gray Technical Center,
Winston-Salem, NC 27102, USA

Bernard Schwetz
National Institute of Environmental Health Services, PO Box 12233,
Research Triangle Park, NC 27709, USA

Tomas Soldan
Institute of Entomology, Czechoslovak Academy of Sciences, Branisovska 31,
370 05 Cěské Budějovice, Czechoslovakia

Robert G. Tardiff
RiskFocus® /VERSAR Inc., 6850 Versar Center, Springfield, VA 22151, USA

Jiri Veleminsky
Institute of Experimental Botany, Czechoslovak Academy of Sciences,
Vltavska 17, 150 00 Praha 5, Czechoslovakia

Part 1

JOINT REPORT

1 Introduction, General Conclusions, and Recommendations*

1.1 INTRODUCTION

For purposes of this discussion, a pesticide is any compound or formulation used to control pests which contains active ingredients and other substances (e.g., solvents, emulsifiers, buffers) to aid its delivery to target organisms and hence minimize pests. The major types of pesticides are herbicides, fungicides, rodenticides, molluscicides, soil bacteriostats, disinfectants, and living organisms with pesticidal activity. In practice, mixtures of pesticides rather than single agents are often applied; this practice can lead to synergism or potentiation resulting from interaction between pesticides or among the ingredients of a formulation.

Through the careful use of pesticides, humans have benefited considerably by having an increased abundance of assorted foods. In some places, pesticides have assisted in assuring a continued supply of nutriment to the local population. An estimated 5 million tons of pesticides have been applied to world agriculture. Yet, pests around the globe still destroy about 35 per cent of all potential crops before harvest, indicating that the use of pesticides has been only marginally successful at improving agricultural productivity.

People cannot survive with only their plants and livestock. Natural biota in the ecosystem number 5–10 million species in the world and 500 000 in the United States alone. Most of these natural species are essential for a quality environment and the survival of humankind. Natural biota perform a diversity of essential tasks including: decomposition of wastes, recycling nutrients, maintenance of biological diversity, stabilization of soil and water resources, continuation of energy flow in natural ecosystems, pollination of crops and natural vegetation, and stabilization of climatic conditions.

---

*This section was prepared by R. Albert, S. Baker, J. Doull, G. Butler, N. Nelson, D. Peakall, D. Pimentel, and R. G. Tardiff.

Methods to Assess Adverse Effects of Pesticides on Non-target Organisms
Edited by R. G. Tardiff
©1992 SCOPE Published by John Wiley & Sons Ltd

Despite their value to agriculture, pesticides have also in some circumstances posed direct and indirect threats to the health of humans and to the environment around the world. Workers, because of ignorance or neglect, have been injured—even killed—by pesticides as a result of improper mixing, loading, and application techniques. At times, those consuming pesticide-tainted foods have been over-exposed, even to the point of illness. In other circumstances, pesticides—agents generated to destroy unwanted organisms—have destroyed beneficial organisms in the delicate web of nature, leading in some instances to changes in the human environment that reduce, rather than promote, human well-being. These beneficial species are the non-target organisms (NTO) which are the subject of this report.

The occurrence of such unwanted side-events is of sufficient magnitude to warrant attention from scientists and public officials alike to improve the safety in the manufacture, use, and disposal of pesticidal substances. This volume is dedicated to that objective. In Chapter 2, the ways by which humans come into contact with pesticides are addressed, as are the scientific procedures by which human exposures can be documented to determine later whether injury to people and their environment has been, or is likely to be, manifest. Chapter 3 is devoted to an analysis of the intricacies associated with documenting injuries to humans exposed either only one time or repeatedly for the major part of a lifetime. Chapter 4 pays comparable attention to diverse approaches by which to measure injurious changes at various locations of ecosystems, upon which people depend inextricably for growth and development of a global civilization. Chapter 5 provides an overview of integrated pest management, a complex practice that makes more efficient use of pesticides and reduces the likelihood of over-exposure of humans and other non-target organisms.

Presented below is the consensus view of a global representation as to the major conclusions and recommendations associated with the impacts of pesticides on non-target organisms.

1.2 GENERAL CONCLUSIONS

1.2.1 PESTICIDE USE

1. Approximately 1000 pesticide formulations are in use throughout the world today for virtually all forms of agricultural commodity. The annual worldwide agricultural use of pesticides has been estimated to be of the order of 5×10^6 tons with a value of about $16.3 billion (US).

2. Despite the use of pesticides, about 35 per cent of crops have been estimated to be lost. Nearly 50 per cent of food in the world may be lost annually despite all pest control procedures. It has been estimated that less than 0.1 per cent of the pesticides applied to crops reach the target pests; thus, more than 99 per cent of applied pesticides have the potential to impact NTOs and to become widely dispersed in the environment.

3. Delineating toxic effects of the use of any pesticide is complicated by the existence of some 5-10 million species in the environment, most of which are potential unintended targets of the toxicity of pesticides.

4. Approximately 5 million ton of pesticides (perhaps 70 per cent herbicides and only 5 per cent insecticides) are applied annually in the world, of which about 70 per cent is used for agriculture, and the remainder by public health agencies and government agencies for vector control and by home owners. Agriculture and forestry, which occupy approximately 70 per cent of the land area in some countries, are the primary source of pesticides in ecosystems.

1.2.2 INJURIES TO HUMAN AND NON-HUMAN NTOs

1. In developing countries, acute pesticide poisoning is a major public health problem, because it is so frequent (i.e., more than one million cases annually in the 1980s). Classically, acute toxicity has been restricted to morbidity and mortality in those individuals exposed directly; recently, that definition has been enlarged to include injury to developing fetuses.

2. Although not yet well documented, pesticide-induced chronic toxicity is emerging as a public health concern of major proportions. The toxic manifestations that capture the greatest attention include cancer, reproductive impairment, and irreversible neurotoxicity.

3. Acute and chronic injury to non-target organisms other than humans has been pronounced over the past few decades. The most affected organisms have included fish and birds; and the most prevalent mechanisms of such damage have been depression of reproduction of beneficial organisms and stimulation of reproduction of natural enemies.

4. The extent of ecosystem damage is illustrated by the observations that invertebrate NTOs are often killed by pesticides used against insects and acarine target pests; foliar applications of broad spectrum insecticides produce nearly total depletion of arthropod populations in crops such as cotton; microorganisms are most susceptible to fungicides and bactericides aimed at target plant pathogens in the field.

5. The measurement of adverse consequences in ecosystems is extremely difficult because of the biological complexity of the biosphere. Consequently, considerable resources need to be directed to efficient and reliable methods to identify early effects that may propagate injury throughout the ecological web.

1.2.3 CONTROLLING EXPOSURES TO PESTICIDES

1. Damage caused to NTOs from the use of virtually all forms of pesticides is large and needs to be reduced appreciably in developing and developed countries. The costs of such unwanted injuries are enormous.

2. Reductions in exposures to pesticides used for agriculture and in the home are possible through education about the proper use of pesticides, the use of

application techniques that reduce the environmental dissemination of aerosols, liquids, and powders, and the appropriate use of protective equipment.

3. Limitations on the overall use of pesticides is not only desirable but also achievable through the diverse approaches offered by integrated pest management.

4. The use of techniques developed for recombinant DNA in the biological control of plant pathogens is currently a promising area of research in both academic and industrial institutions. The application of molecular genetics to selected biocontrol systems can potentially provide an understanding of the genes involved in biological control phenomena; an establishment of a genetic basis for biological control is a prerequisite to further molecular studies that centre on the enhancement of biological control phenomena.

1.2.4   ASSESSING EXPOSURES TO PESTICIDES AND ASSOCIATED UNCERTAINTIES

1. Two major approaches exist by which to determine the means through which NTOs come into contact with pesticides and the doses that the NTOs obtain: (a) computerized modelling of the numerous phases of environmental fate and transport, and (b) monitoring specific NTOs for the presence and concentration of pesticides of interest.

2. Models are available at three levels of sophistication, from the more qualitative to the most rigorous quantitative site-specific models. Level three is the most data-intensive, level one the least. While level one models are useful to obtain a sense of trends, site-specific models are needed to provide accurate and precise estimates of exposure that permit an authoritative evaluation of possible damage to NTO species such as humans.

3. The validation of computer models remains a difficult and challenging prospect, because the complexity of environmental processes that govern mobility of chemicals is still poorly understood. Nevertheless, progress is being made in predicting, with substantial quantitative accuracy, exposures in environmental compartments of limited scope.

4. Monitoring represents the most confident means of describing the degree and magnitude of exposures to humans and other species. However, such an empirical approach is quite costly.

5. In humans, exposures are characterized either at the human interface by monitoring the presence of substances in media such as air, food, water, and contact surfaces in the human environment (this is known as 'media monitoring') or within the organisms of interest by measuring the presence of pesticides in easily obtainable samples of biological materials such as urine, blood, hair, adipose tissue, and breast milk ('biological monitoring'). Despite the need to assure the application of appropriate ethical constraints to the use of biological monitoring, this approach provides the most precise estimate of dose to the individuals of interest.

6. Of the two approaches, modelling and monitoring, the latter generally contains fewer uncertainties in fully characterizing the patterns of exposure to pesticides.

1.2.5   ASSESSING ACUTE TOXICITY FOR HUMANS

1. The adverse health effects of acute exposure are generally well recognized. Although the incidences of mortality and morbidity are more severe in developing countries, the primary effects—insecticide-induced neurotoxicity and dermal toxicity—are universal.

2. Most known associations of pesticides with neurological effects involve insecticides. Neurotoxicologic methods currently under development provide the opportunity to characterize neurotoxicity for other pesticide classes and to enhance our understanding by examining neurologic endpoints, other than those that are cholinergic, such as behaviour.

3. The clinical features of dermal toxicity are moderately well characterized. Techniques exist to determine skin penetration, correlation of urinary metabolites with dermal exposure, and histological changes after exposure. However, techniques to determine cellular proliferation, the presence of biomarkers, and allergic reactions of skin are presently inadequate.

4. The impact of pesticides on the immune system is less clear than that on other organ systems.

5. Biomarker techniques and toxicokinetics can help to enhance the predictive value of risk assessments for acute exposures and effects.

1.2.6   ASSESSING CHRONIC TOXICITY FOR HUMANS

1. Interference with normal reproduction and development from the manufacture, use, disposal, and misuse of pesticides is a rapidly growing area of concern to public health officials and toxicologists. As the database has grown, the level of concern has increased rather than decreased.

2. A significant shortage exists of epidemiologic studies on exposed humans and of animal toxicologic studies using state-of-the-art methods. Actually, for most pesticides and other chemicals in the environment, epidemiologic data confirm neither the absence nor presence of significant risk, because of (a) the high background and variability and adverse reproductive events in humans, (b) the problems posed by confounders, and (c) the limited power of many epidemiology study designs.

1.2.7   ASSESSING DAMAGE TO ECOSYSTEMS

1. Methods to detect and quantify damage caused by pesticides on terrestrial and aquatic ecosystems are complex and costly depending on the species involved and the pesticides that are targets of investigation.

2. Because less than 0.1 per cent of all applied pesticides are estimated to reach target pests, more than 99 per cent contaminate the environment and are available to disrupt various natural ecosystem processes.

3. Pesticides injure particular ecosystems by upsetting natural stability, destroying natural enemies and key species in the ecosystem, and altering normal trophic structure resulting possibly in the resurgence and outbreak of undesirable species.

4. Furthermore, pesticides may influence the normal decomposition of organic wastes produced by humans, livestock, and other biota. The resulting situation may lead to accumulation of organic wastes and pollutants in the environment. One consequence may be a reduction in the productivity of the ecosystem, because of a critical shortage of elements necessary to support life.

5. Common pesticides may reduce the diversity of food chains, including reductions of parasites and predators at the top of the food chain. In certain cases, this alternative may result in excessive numbers of organisms at the low end of the food chain.

6. Energy is an essential requirement for the normal function of all natural ecosystems. In some situations, pesticides, like herbicides, may reduce plant populations and thus the primary food production. Therefore, the total productivity and survival of a natural ecosystem may be influenced adversely.

7. Cross-pollination is essential to the reproduction of many plants. For example, 90 US crops, valued at $20 billion (US) (in 1988 dollars), are dependent upon insect pollination (mostly wild bees and honey bees). In addition, a large number of wild plants depend upon insect pollination. Pesticides may upset this delicate balance.

8. The implications of the above observations for those who choose to use predictive models in the assessment of exposure are that it is unlikely today that models of complex environmental systems will have the precision required to predict ecosystem exposure patterns in widely different ecosystems to chemicals with widely differing properties. However, comparative qualitative models for preliminary assessment of trends and optimization of monitoring programs can be useful.

9. There is a need to refine (a) correlative relationships based on calculated properties of a chemical and (b) empirical data on the properties of both chemicals and ecosystems. Carefully constructed and performed studies on models describing kinetics of processes, rather than models of environmental systems, are undoubtedly the most important step in expanding our predictive capabilities.

10. Situation-specific models of troublesome situations for comparative purposes have a role. Such models can provide tests of the usefulness of the data, and form a basis for the prediction of patterns from one chemical to another.

11. Model validation is dependent on carefully designed field experiments that examine pollutant levels under conditions producing significantly different exposure patterns.

12. Models of environmental systems must depend largely on empirical determinations of the descriptive processes. Hence, the results will be highly system-specific. This outcome makes their use unreliable to predict patterns in highly differing ecosystems. Yet, highly predictive models can be established for a specific ecosystem, if sufficient effort is focused on characterizing the processes.

13. Some progress has been made to introduce (a) insect development inhibitors, many of which are very selective and nonpersistent, (b) genetically engineered microbes and plants with insecticidal activity, and (c) pesticide resistance in plants, natural enemies, and chemical ecology mediators. Evidently, these approaches are also subject to developed resistance in pests; thus, caution must be exercised in their management. In general, there is a great need to improve understanding of the factors most influential in the perturbation of ecological systems by pesticides and in developing less disruptive pesticides.

1.2.8   INTEGRATED PEST MANAGEMENT

1. Winning increasingly broad support are alternatives to conventional agriculture, often referred to as integrated pest management (IPM) which minimize the use of pesticides.

2. IPM prescribes six forms of controls: cultural, biological, behavioural, biotechnological, environmental, and chemical.

1.3   GENERAL RECOMMENDATIONS

1.3.1   CONTROLLING EXPOSURES TO PESTICIDES

1. As a prerequisite, the development of either new pesticides or new uses of existing pesticides should include means for exposure control proportional to the hazard potential of the chemical. This effort should consider physical form, prepackaged quantities for direct use in the field, closed transfer systems, and application procedures that deposit the pesticide primarily on a specific target.

2. The success of procedures for pesticide exposure control depends on a proper understanding and motivation of individuals using these substances. Rudimentary education is needed to impart general principles to prevent exposure; these fundamentals can be presented through visual and textual aids and in the language and social style of the populace. The recent initiative under the aegis of the Food and Agriculture Organization (FAO) is an example of this approach.

3. High priority should be given to developing pesticides with increased selectivity toward pest species and greatly reduced damage to non-target species. Furthermore, pesticide management should increasingly prevent the development of resistance in pests, because this phenomenon impairs selectivity.

4. State-of-the-art technologies to apply pesticide are designed to reduce the potential for human exposure. The best available and most cost-effective technologies should be applied to reduce the occurrence of acute poisoning, and new technologies should be encouraged to continue reduction of exposures.

1.3.2   ASSESSING EXPOSURES TO PESTICIDES AND UNCERTAINTIES

1. An international agency, such as the United Nations Environmental Program (UNEP) or the Organization of Economic and Community Development (OECD), should conduct a workshop aimed at developing environmental sampling guidelines for monitoring studies. Participants should include regulatory officials, modellers, epidemiologists, and chemists.
2. Improved methods are necessary on an international scale to provide developing nations with the capability to screen dietary exposures and identify sources of potential hazard in the diet.
3. Serious attention must be given to the effects of pesticide exposures on subgroups, such as infants and children, who are known to be exposed to relatively higher doses of pesticides through dietary and household exposures.

1.3.3   ASSESSING ACUTE TOXICITY FOR HUMANS

1. To characterize the problem of acute pesticide poisoning, conventional public health practices must be monitored. Recognizing that there are geographic, population, climatic, and agricultural differences around the world that influence patterns of pesticide usage, the best approach to study acute pesticide poisoning is from the 'bottom up', i.e., beginning at the local level with support from state and national levels.
2. Many immunotoxicity procedures have been developed for classes of chemicals other than pesticides. These techniques need to be adapted to examine the response of the immune system to pesticides. Because of evidence of auto-immune responses in humans after exposure to pesticides, reliable animal models are needed to detect and quantify such effects in a manner predictive of human responses. Newer biochemical techniques need to be incorporated into the investigation of pesticidal effects on the immune response.
3. While technologies for measuring the effect of chemicals on immuno-suppression and immunosensitization exist, they have yet to be validated or used to examine the effects on the immune system of acute exposures to pesticides. Measuring functional impairment of the immune system should be part of the evaluation of pesticide toxicity.

4. Tests of acute toxicity in major organs such as the lungs (except for the paraquat effect), blood and blood-forming tissues, the cardiovascular system, kidney, endocrine organs, and musculoskeletal system need to be part of test batteries.

5. Adequate techniques are unavailable to determine in skin cellular proliferation, the presence of biomarkers, and allergic reactions; hence, research is needed into the numerous functions of skin.

1.3.4 ASSESSING CHRONIC TOXICITY FOR HUMANS

1. For the spectrum of pesticides, reproductive and developmental toxicity should be assessed in animals and humans.

2. The current assessment of developmental toxicity focuses primarily on structural rather than functional endpoints. Methods are needed to assess the effect of *in utero* exposure on the functional development of organ systems in addition to the nervous system.

3. Reproductive toxicity screens should be expanded beyond tests in rodents used to evaluate fertility. Specific methods must be enhanced to detect effects on spermatogenesis and oogenesis to help identify site(s) of action of reproductive toxicants and to distinguish primary (i.e., direct effect) from secondary (i.e., due to other toxicity) reproductive toxicants.

4. Animal models are needed to evaluate the effect of pesticides on lactation— both on its quality and as a source of exposure of neonates to chemicals in the milk. Human milk is an extremely important source of nutrition worldwide, and is probably the most critical source of exposure to neonates, a highly vulnerable age-group.

5. Further development and validation of *in vitro* tests for developmental toxicity is strongly recommended. Test systems which provide useful mechanistic data would potentially improve our understanding of those mechanisms by which developmental toxicity is caused in animals and humans.

6. Improved reliability is needed for short-term *in vitro* and *in vivo* qualitative and quantitative tests for promoters of cancer.

7. Reliable short-term *in vivo* qualitative and quantitative genotoxicity tests are needed to detect and quantify oncogenes and anti-oncogenes; for *in vitro* genotoxicity tests, research should focus on quantitation of cancer potency.

8. The current scientific basis should be greatly enhanced to extrapolate carcinogenic responses from laboratory animals to humans and to extrapolate effects at high doses to those at low doses.

9. Additional epidemiological studies are required of pesticide-exposed populations to establish the presence or absence of cancer induction.

10. Biological markers of carcinogen exposure and effect need to be improved, particularly to detect changes that occur early in the latent period.

11. Public health should be promoted by implementing appropriate monitoring and epidemiologic surveillance, initially to identify improved control measures.

12. In developing countries, local pesticide control boards should be established with representation of all interested parties having authority to implement and supervise the policies and regulations established by national regulatory agencies.

1.3.5   ASSESSING DAMAGE TO ECOSYSTEMS

1. The ecological consequences of pesticide use must be evaluated from the level of a single species to that of multiple species and finally to the level of the ecosystem. Many methods are available to test for susceptibility of NTOs, and some tests are already required for pesticide registration. The effects of pesticides on ecosystem structure and function should be measured in the agroecosystem of interest for a pesticide. Decisions on surveillance of the broadest ecosystem should be based on the hazard of each pesticide.

2. Microcosm studies cannot be relied upon solely to determine complex ecosystem responses to pesticides; however, microcosm methods are appropriate, and are recommended for general information on the relative persistence, bioaccumulation, and ecological kinetics of pesticides in model organisms.

3. Studies of soil subsystems are recommended, because direct and indirect complex processes are caused by pesticide treatments and their residues. Changes in the community structures of soil biota are reflected by altered biological and chemical processes, as well as by their rates of change. These changes could be measured in microcosms (e.g., leaching of nutrients and humic substances) and, albeit less easily, in the field by changed ecosystem parameters such as diversity, CO_2 production, and decomposition rate.

4. The development and application of genetically engineered pesticidal organisms require research to evaluate ecological risks, if any, posed by such organisms. Risks should be evaluated on the bases of (a) ecosystem effects, (b) fate and survival of population, (c) intraspecies and interspecies gene transfer, (d) contaminant and mitigation, (e) transport and dispersal, and (f) detection and enumeration.

5. Natural ecosystems must be investigated and protected from pesticide damage, because they play an essential role in maintaining a quality environment for humans, agriculture, and forestry.

6. A distinct need exists for a widely accepted procedure to assess ecological effects of pesticides on NTO species in terrestrial and aquatic ecosystems. From the myriad of possibilities that could comprise ecosystem effects, certain factors should receive priority and are amenable to research using biogeochemical cycling, trophic structures, decomposition rates, and transport into non-target environments.

1.3.6   INTEGRATED PEST MANAGEMENT

1. To alleviate public and scientific concern, prior to the approved release of engineered microorganisms into the environment, the efficacy and safety of

biological control agents should be fully evaluated, and the risks and benefits carefully assessed.

2. To implement biological control programs based on the biotechnology of IPM, the following must be improved: (a) understanding of total ecosystems, (b) mass production and delivery of control agents, (c) selection and enhancement of control agents, and (d) the specificity of control agents to only one disease on one crop in a small geographic area.

2 Methods to Assess Exposure to Pesticides: Data Acquisition and Monitoring Techniques*

The distribution and eventual fate of a chemical released into the environment is governed by a variety of processes, the rates of which are determined by many factors. These processes consist of those that remove the chemical from the environment (e.g., biodegradation or photodegradation) and those that govern the distribution of the chemical (e.g., chemical sorption by soil or sediment). The processes are competitive and may be complex. Their relative importance is dependent upon the physico-chemical properties of substances, the environment in which they are released, and the time lapsed since their release.

Actual exposure subsequently encountered is dependent not only on the application rate and method and on the time since application, but also on the nature of the environment in which a substance is introduced. Depending on the relative influence of each process in a given situation, the behaviour of a pesticide varies drastically from one location to another, and the duration and magnitude of exposure are highly variable. Since considerable information is available on the processes which may attenuate the concentration of a pesticide after its release, pesticide exposure can be examined in terms of the particular environment in which the substance is introduced.

Because pesticides must be registered in many countries, information is generally available on the transformation of the pesticidal agents in mammals and soils, including their degradation and persistence under assorted environmental conditions. A detailed review of the fate and distribution of pesticides is beyond the scope of this report, and exhaustive reviews of the behaviour of pesticides in the environment already exist. Furthermore, the International Union of Pure and Applied Chemistry (IUPAC) has released a critical examination of this testing procedure, and the reader is referred to this material for specific details.

---

*This section was prepared by G. Becking, P. Bourdeau, G. Butler, D. Calamari, V. Morley, and R. Roberts.

Methods to Assess Adverse Effects of Pesticides on Non-target Organisms
Edited by R. G. Tardiff
©1992 SCOPE Published by John Wiley & Sons Ltd
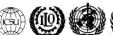

Within different environments, exposure to a pesticide can be determined either directly by quantitative measurement or indirectly by predicting the nature and magnitude of its presence from an understanding of its behaviour under alternative environmental conditions. The usefulness of large collections of data and of current monitoring approaches to characterize exposures has been raised to a high degree of importance. Since an understanding of exposure patterns is a prerequisite to any risk–benefit analysis, this issue needs to be resolved before risk–benefit analysis can be accomplished successfully.

2.1 MODELLING TECHNIQUES TO ESTIMATE PESTICIDE EXPOSURES†

For many years, information on the distribution and fate of chemical substances was acquired largely through retrospective studies involving large-scale monitoring that incorporated an enormous number of chemical analyses. The retrospective approach leaves wide margins for error in the environmental management of chemical substances, for it provides a weak base from which to anticipate problems.

One approach to reduce this difficulty is to forecast the environmental behaviour of a pesticide through the use of computerized models. Over the past decade, some investigators have advanced the idea that one can predict the behaviour of a chemical on the basis of comparisons of measured properties with those of compounds for which greater amounts of environmental data are available. For example, the concept was introduced for the use of hypothetical 'evaluative models' based on properties of stylized environments and pollutants to provide quantitative approaches to exposure estimation.

2.1.1 MODELS AND MODELLING—WHY USE THEM?

Environmental scientists must assess impacts of pesticides in a multiplicity of situations. It is not practical to establish the associated exposure profiles through direct measurement except in rare cases. Thus, environmental scientists and pesticide regulators require tools to estimate exposures to pesticides from one situation to another.

Tools are needed first to optimize the design of monitoring programs, and secondly to test the validity of (a) study designs used in existing monitoring programs and (b) compilations of data to estimate environmental pollutant levels. A valid study design must include the sampling of at least the matrices in which the pesticide is most likely to be found at any given time. In complex systems, which matrix, stratum, or sampling site is most likely to be contaminated is not necessarily obvious. Models provide the analyst with the

---

†This section was prepared by P. Bourdeau, D. Calamari, G. Lacy, R. Roberts, and T. Soldan.

tools to optimize the design of monitoring schemes and hence to increase the chance of detecting a compound, should it be present.

Such tools are predictive models that depict how a pesticide may behave in various environments. These models may vary in complexity from structured conceptual models of a pesticide's behaviour in a specified situation to complex mathematical integrations that attempt to describe various processes of translocation and removal. The descriptions of processes can be simple, empirically determined relationships; or they can be complex, theoretically-based relationships, reflecting a chemical's properties and their influence on its translocation and degradation. The exposure models currently used are composed of (a) simple ones that characterize a single input, transport, and removal process controlling the fate of a chemical, and (b) complex models of numerous, simultaneous environmental influences on the ultimate distribution of a chemical. The usefulness of a model is dependent on its ability to provide correlations between the nature of a chemical and its mobility and persistence in a given matrix.

A hypothetical model of the environment, sometimes called the 'environmental system' is first constructed by conceptualizing several environmental 'compartments' considered to have distinct, uniform characteristics, such as pH, percentage of organic matter, or temperature. The discharge, loading, or emission rates of a chemical are then described by discrete models. Finally, mathematical relationships are developed to describe the intercompartmental transfer and removal processes that influence the dynamics of a chemical.

Today's modelling can be categorized into three levels of increasing complexity:

1. qualitative conceptual comparative distribution models,
2. generic quantitative situation-specific models, and
3. site-specific quantitative models.

The first group of models provides general qualitative descriptions of a chemical in fixed scenarios. They are used as basic screens for ranking pesticides according to their affinity for various ecological compartments, as well as for the evaluation of data available for understanding the distribution, translocation, and transformation processes.

The second group of models has flexible mathematical bases not fixed to specific scenarios. That is, the user can adjust a scenario to develop a comparative base of exposure profiles. Conceivably, they can also be used as a first approach to predict field distribution and planning studies.

The third group, the site-specific models, are the most difficult to develop, for they are directed at providing detailed descriptions of a pesticide's behaviour in a specific complex ecosystem. The number of processes and compartments in such models requires the use of complex approaches such as sensitivity analysis. Development of such models requires that the ecosystem be described in detail and that measures be available to define the transfer and degradation processes operative within various compartments. This modelling is normally achieved through specific empirical measurement of the rates.

The conclusions resulting from the use of such models are being questioned at present, and their usefulness is questioned by some. At least two reasons exist for this scepticism. First, some managers and scientists have extended conclusions beyond the limits of the assumptions and errors inherent in the models. Second, modellers have added complexity to models without fully evaluating either the implications of the limitations of the input data or the assumptions used to construct the models. Both groups of individuals seem to forget that models are evaluative tools that are useful only within the boundaries of their limitations in their output.

The first two types of models are relevant in hazard assessment schemes, while the third is required in the estimation of risks or benefits.

2.1.2   VALIDATION OF ENVIRONMENTAL FATE AND DISTRIBUTION MODELS

The validation of a model and the modelling process must be performed at different levels depending on the type of model and its ultimate use. In levels 1 and 2, qualitative results are sought; hence, the accuracy of trends identified by the models is the focus of attention rather than the numerical values themselves. At level 3, the convergence between the quantitative output of the models and actual field exposure patterns must be examined.

In either case, two types of error must be examined: first, that resulting from the use of incorrect model structure and assumptions; and secondly that resulting from inaccuracies of the input data.

In levels 1 and 2 qualitative models, trend analyses may be generated from correlations of the sorptive and partition properties of the chemicals with their chemical properties. Generally, correlations based on empirically determined characteristics of chemicals are relatively imprecise, particularly when chemicals with widely differing properties are compared. These correlations have been found to be so imprecise as to fail to characterize trends between isomers. This finding may be of particular concern in hazard assessment at level 2, for a chemical's toxicity can be highly dependent on its isomeric structure.

Correlations based on theoretically calculated properties of a molecule (e.g., fragmentation constants) may provide a sound basis for developing qualitative submodels. The use of non-empirical correlations provides improved internal consistency for comparisons, thereby leading to increased accuracy to predict patterns and trends between chemicals of differing structure. In the qualitative models, the most useful trends are generated when sorptive and advective, rather than degradative, processes dominate, because of the paucity of knowledge about relationships among degradative biological processes.

None of the level 3 models are truly validated. Several models can show convergence between field studies and their output; however, arbitrary decisions are generally made about the characteristics of an ecosystem, a chemical's properties, and the models. Hence, the apparent convergence does not constitute validation.

Laboratory studies can be of considerable value in improving the accuracy of correlations between the physical-chemical parameters and partition-sorption, translocation, and kinetic data. The accuracy of the input data and the models should be based on the objective of the modelling. Simulation chambers and small-scale pilot experiments have a role in demonstrating the validity of trends predicted by the levels 1 and 2 models.

An iterative process exists for the validation of models between their refinement and testing in simulation chambers, small-scale experiments, and field trials. Refinement will occur only through an interactive process of testing and adjustment.

2.1.3 USEFULNESS OF MODELS TO PREDICT EXPOSURE PROFILES

The most accurate models address equilibrium soil-sorption and fish bio-concentration relationships. Models of the sorption of pesticides by other components of aquatic systems are, at best, site-specific; and general predictive relationships are limited. The dynamics under non-equilibrium conditions and at high rates of degradation are at best site-specific and empirically determined. Thus, accurate quantitative predictions are unlikely, given the level of sophistication of today's general models. With sufficient study, site-specific models of a given situation can be developed in which empirical descriptions of the processes are utilized. The degree of precision of such models make them useful for projecting trends within the system, but the results generally cannot be extrapolated to dissimilar situations.

A reason for the limitations is the lack of focus on descriptions of models of the processes. Only as these descriptions improve will models provide useful generic qualitative predictions of exposure.

2.1.4 VALUE OF MODELS TO DESIGN MONITORING PROGRAMMES AND TO EVALUATE DATA

The design of an optimal monitoring program requires the ability to predict the distribution and fate of a chemical at various times within the area to be monitored. Conceptual models of expected equilibrium distribution patterns and dynamic models are both of value.

Those models are particularly useful prior to loss or degradation of significant quantities of a chemical, for it is during this period that simple distribution processes are most likely to govern chemical distribution. In such cases, the accuracy of the evaluations is directly related to that of the description of the relationships between a chemical's partitioning in various phases of an ecosystem. The correlations can be relatively precise and simple.

The predictive relationships for pesticide distribution patterns have sufficient accuracy to be generally useful when the descriptions of the ecosystems are accurate. The difficulty is that accurate models are difficult to obtain in large, complex systems such as rivers and ground-water aquifers. For example, the migration rate of a pesticide through a clay matrix is dependent on understanding the degree of fracturing, a parameter that can only be obtained after detailed geological studies. In the case of a river, good hydrological models are required to predict the location of matrices most likely to contain a pesticide at a given time after its introduction. Where such models exist, they can be very useful to optimize the design of sample programs.

2.2   METHODS TO MEASURE EXPOSURE TO PESTICIDES*

The sophistication of current analytical and separation techniques makes the acquisition of exposure data relatively simple. Unfortunately in many cases, this has resulted in data collection being an end in itself rather than a means to an end.

Some people view monitoring as simply the collection and storage of data; actually, it is much more. The United Nations defines monitoring as 'the collection of analytical data according to an agreed plan of sampling in time and space'. Thus, monitoring data are gathered in response to a defined need or objective, established in consultation between data users and analysts. The definition implies that data should be generated in the most appropriate units to ensure comparability and that a sampling program should be constructed prior to analysis by users of the data.

Consequently, data should be as relevant as possible, and the number of analyses performed should be the minimum compatible with the intended purposes. Because these criteria have not yet been employed, much of the data gathered in the past regrettably cannot be used by modellers, regulators, or others.

2.2.1   USES OF MONITORING DATA

The three principal users of monitoring data are:

1. Regulators wanting measurements of chemicals in various media either to determine regulatory compliance or to predict concentrations and environmental behaviour,

---

*This section was prepared by G. Becking, P. Bourdeau, G. Butler, D. Calamari, V. Morley, and R. Roberts.

2. Environmental scientists seeking knowledge of concentrations in environmental compartments either to validate environmental transport models or to describe environmental processes, and

3. Risk analysts characterizing risks to NTOs from the use of pesticides.

2.2.2 PURPOSES OF MONITORING DATA

Data obtained from well-designed monitoring programs can be used for numerous purposes in the fields of public health and environmental protection. For example, these objectives include determinations of trends in environmental concentrations, persistence of bioaccumulation of residues, environmental transport and fate, and estimation of doses to NTOs. Furthermore, monitoring data should be an integral part of validating predictive models.

These data must be collected at appropriate time intervals and in correct environmental compartments to answer authoritatively questions raised by users of this information; otherwise, the measurements of pesticide levels at one point in time in various environmental compartments may be of little value to characterize the dose regimen or to validate the models. Monitoring pesticide concentrations in various environmental compartments (i.e., food, air, biota, water) is required to obtain baseline values and trends over time, thus providing information from which to identify emerging problems.

Most pesticide monitoring programmes analyse only the parent active ingredient, thus failing to take into account any environmental transformation products or other potentially toxic compounds used in pesticide formulations. Either group of substances may be not only persistent but also of toxicological importance. Such information would help identify NTOs at risk, thereby characterizing more comprehensively the overall risk posed by pesticide formulations. Such data would also provide information on environmental persistence and transport, thereby having intrinsic value to validate predictive models.

The mobility, persistence, and distribution of pesticides (e.g., herbicides contaminating ground or surface waters) in the environment can be ascertained through adequate monitoring.

The establishment of causal relationship uncovered in environmental epidemiology studies depend on appropriate definitions of dosage. However, to date, environmental epidemiological studies have suffered from a lack of such information. For example, determining exposure from measurements at one point in time causes much uncertainty in the determination of dose.

Accurate assessment of integrated dosage requires monitoring programs designed from inputs obtained from epidemiologists and chemists. Such measurements need to be frequent and extensive, with samples collected from relevant locations. Such information can, in turn, be used to refine the design of epidemiological studies.

2.2.3   FATE AND TRANSFORMATION: HUMAN*

As pesticidal NTOs of considerable public health concern, humans have come under considerable study to ascertain how and to what extent they are exposed to pesticidal substances. Monitoring human exposures has most often taken the form of measuring the presence of the substance of interest in one or more environmental media: air, food, water, or consumer products. Monitoring has taken place not only at home and at play but also at work. Recently, such monitoring has focused on characterizing human doses most closely associated with injurious consequences, namely, the biological or tissue dose. By using all reasonably accessible tissues, a relatively precise definition of body burden can be obtained, and can aid in deciding appropriate occupational and environmental policies.

2.2.3.1   The concept of exposure monitoring

The term 'exposure' refers to the quantity of a foreign chemical entering the organism for a specified duration. Depending on the monitoring methods, other terms may prove useful. 'External exposure' may be expressed as concentrations in inhaled air, intake from food and water, or contamination of the skin surface. 'Internal dose' is the amount that enters the circulation, and may be computed using the respective transfer coefficients for retention in the lungs, uptake in the gastrointestinal tract, or absorption through the skin.

With a continuous flux of a foreign chemical into the organism, the term 'dose rate' represents a satisfactory measure of exposure, irrespective of the route by which the contact occurred; the term is also applicable when two or more routes of entry occur. In real-life situations, however, the information is often insufficient for such computations, and fractional data from each route are used. The 'internal dose' or 'dose rate' may be measured as concentration(s) of the chemical and its metabolites in tissues and body fluids, including blood and urine. In principle, the procedure, called 'biological monitoring', represents the simplest way by which dose rates received by various routes can be integrated, depicting total exposure. A link between the data obtained from biological monitoring and those of external environmental monitoring is often secured by studying respective correlations obtained under field conditions. Such investigations are possible, however, with only one route of entry. For multiple exposure routes, individual transfer coefficients are needed.

Other important factors to interpret biological monitoring data in relation to external exposure are duration of exposure and time interval after termination of exposure. Chemicals in general and pesticides in particular differ dramatically in their toxicokinetic properties, which are manifest as the presence or absence

---

*This section was prepared by B. Goldstein, J. Moore, J. Parizek, J. Pietrowski, M. Rostker, and S. Saunders

of accumulation in the body during repeated and prolonged exposure, and as slow versus rapid disappearance following cessation of exposure. Biological monitoring may be based on the measurement of either the unchanged substance or selected metabolites in a particular biological medium. For instance, DDT exposure may be measured as 'total DDT' in blood or fat tissue (biopsy or autopsy)—e.g., during occupational high exposure—or as the ultimate metabolite, DDA, in urine. In practice, any such determination may be useful, with the method chosen based on availability.

Contemporary trends in biological monitoring of organic chemicals focus on the products of microsomal metabolism. As a result of activation in the system of cytochrome P_{450}-dependent oxygenating enzymes, several organic chemicals yield 'active metabolites' such as epoxides or oxidation products of N-hydroxy-derivatives of aromatic compounds. These active metabolites may bind covalently with macromolecules, such as nucleic acids or proteins, resulting in relatively stable 'adducts' that may be measured selectively.

Two separate lines emerge in these trends, of which one centres on adducts with DNA (measured in the white blood cells) and the other on adducts with haemoglobin (measured in the red blood cells). This type of monitoring requires sophisticated methodologies such as ^{32}P-post-labelling linked with thin layer chromatography or mass spectrometry of the hydrolysis products of the adducts. Therefore, the development of such methods is largely confined to a few advanced and well-equipped laboratories. For pesticides, the best known example of such monitoring has been the fumigant ethylene oxide, which yields DNA adducts.

One important property of macromolecular adducts is their relative stability. For instance, adducts to haemoglobin persist in a red blood cell throughout its life-span (approximately 4 months); therefore, the readings are likely to increase greatly with the duration of exposure. This situation offers a convenient way of integrating individual doses received over time, yielding the average daily exposure level.

2.2.3.2 Patterns of exposure

In practical terms, the collection of information relevant to human exposure to pesticides can be assigned to two broad categories: environmental (or external) measurements such as air, water, and diet; and biological (or internal) measurements. Biological measurements can be conveniently divided into actual measures of the pesticide (or metabolites) or physiological variables. The latter are surrogate measures that must have an established causal relationship with a chemical of interest to be relevant to exposure.

In many situations, pesticide exposure results from multiple sources. In an agricultural setting, for example, workers may receive dermal and inhalation doses from pesticide spray application. In the home, exposure can occur through ingestion of unwashed garden produce that contains pesticide residues and from inhalation of indoor pest control sprays. Dietary exposure to pesticides occurs for almost all members of the population.

Depending upon the use pattern, one or two exposure routes may be of dominant importance and account for a majority of exposure. Nevertheless, secondary or relatively minor routes may also be influential in the summation of total exposure.

Designs for exposure studies must consider statistically correct sampling schemes, and include sufficient numbers of samples to account for loss or attrition, control or baseline measures, and potentially small but significant variations in exposure patterns. To study cholinesterase inhibition, it is frequently important to have baseline or control samples for comparison with those from potentially exposed individuals. Multiple samples are useful to establish ranges of biological variability and to reduce uncertainties surrounding the biological significance of measurements. Many blood variables exhibit cyclic and diurnal patterns; multiple samples taken through time help to distinguish among pesticide exposure-induced changes and normal variability.

Ultimately, total exposure is the relevant measure for assessment. Integration of all routes of exposure, along with characterization of the frequency and duration of exposure, leads to a complete exposure assessment. Knowledge of the endpoint or effects of exposure is important to structure study designs that are statistically strong and relevant to the nature of the exposure. At present, many methodologies are still primarily focused upon single-route exposures. To some extent, an approximation of total exposure is calculated via summation of exposure routes. While this technique is a good start toward total assessment, better understanding of the ways to integrate different routes of exposure is needed. Growing use of carefully designed monitoring and assessment studies which utilize repeated sampling regimes, and which are sensitive to small variations in patterns, is one way to promote improved dosimetry.

2.2.3.3 Specimen selection

A variety of human tissues and excreta can be sampled for determination of exposure to pesticides.

Chemical characteristics

The chemical characteristics of a xenobiotic such as a pesticide are of primary importance to determine how the compound and its metabolites are distributed in and excreted by the body. A major characteristic is lipophilicity (hydrophobicity), which to a large extent governs distribution in adipose tissue. Lipophilic compounds tend to be stored in fatty tissues, and are not excreted into the urine unless metabolized to a relatively water soluble form (e.g., glucuronides). Excretion of fat soluble compounds may occur through the bile duct, but in most instances such compounds are reabsorbed through the enterohepatic circulation. Accordingly, highly lipophilic compounds that are also poorly metabolized, such as DDT, may persist in the body for many years, and may be measurable only through sampling of adipose tissue; however, water soluble compounds or metabolites may be immediately detectable in urine.

Other important chemical characteristics include the presence of specific chemical moieties capable of being acted upon by the human metabolic machinery. In some cases, metabolism can produce a specific detectable product in blood or urine; in others, it can act too rapidly and completely degrade a xenobiotic, so that it cannot be readily detected in biological media. Varying rates of metabolism resulting from differing genetic or environmental backgrounds can produce wide variations in the relationship between measured metabolites and external dose, thereby complicating exposure assessment.

The choice of environmental or personal monitoring approaches often depends on technical feasibility. Protecting the worker by measuring a chemical in exposure media is particularly problematic for pesticide applicators and agricultural workers, because exposures usually occur outdoors. Thus, the standard approach in an enclosed workplace of using air measurements is relatively impractical. Furthermore, worker exposure to pesticides is often through skin contact, which is difficult to measure under any circumstance. These problems, as well as the technical problems related to human monitoring, are detailed elsewhere in this document.

Ethical aspects of human monitoring sampling approaches

Some sampling approaches are far more feasible than others in terms of technical difficulty. However, a major overall principle in selecting a human monitoring approach is the absolute need to do no harm to the person undergoing the procedure. This principle restricts the sampling media to excreta and to those tissues that can be sampled with little or no risk to the subject. In the case of blood, venipuncture is considered to be a small risk, as long as proper sterile techniques are followed and the amount of blood withdrawn is appropriate for the age, size, and health status of the individual. If analytical procedures permit, use of capillary blood obtained by finger puncture should carry less risk. Willingness to undergo human monitoring often depends on perceived risk, discomfort, or inconvenience of the procedure. Implicit in this discussion is that any sampling of an individual must be to that individual's direct benefit. Fully informed consent must always be obtained.

Multi-media and multi-pesticide considerations

Pesticide exposures do not always occur through one medium. A single field pesticide application may result in a body burden through (a) inhalation during spray application, (b) passage through the skin resulting from direct skin contact or contact with treated soil, (c) ingestion in food or water consumed by field workers, and (d) ingestion of contaminated soil particularly by children. Exposure to multiple pesticides occurs when workers use mixtures of pesticides on different crops, and when the consumer ingests food purchased at the supermarket or uses pesticides while gardening as a hobby. These different, and sometimes unexpected, routes of single or multiple exposures must be considered when selecting specimens for study. Furthermore, human monitoring is necessarily the required approach for significant multiple exposures.

Composition of pesticide products

Specimen selection should also consider the various inerts, solvents, and other ingredients in pesticide formulations, since they are almost always a composite of several chemicals. Pesticide formulations may contain the following:

1. One or several chemicals that possess the desired pesticidal property, i.e., chemical 'A' for destruction of broad-leafed plants and herbicide 'B' for grassy plants;
2. Chemicals that enhance the pesticidal properties, such as surfactants or stabilizers;
3. 'Trace contaminants' contained in the base chemicals used in the synthesis of the pesticide or formed during the synthetic process, and
4. Solvents or carriers that facilitate the application of the pesticide; these materials often constitute 90–99 per cent of the total volume of pesticide.

Solvents may possess toxic properties that are of human or ecotoxicity concern. Perchloroethylene is an example of the former, toluene one of the latter. Trace contaminants may include nitrosamines and chlorinated dibenzo-*p*-dioxins.

Regional differences

A number of cultural aspects determine specimen selection. In certain parts of the world, obtaining a blood specimen is particularly difficult because of local beliefs about the importance of blood. In less-developed countries, there might be regions in which it is not technically feasible to obtain, handle, or store certain types of specimens. There are also areas of the world in which legal and administrative burdens are sufficiently imposing as to hinder certain types of human monitoring.

2.3.3.4 Specific media

The following media are addressed briefly to indicate their respective merits for biological monitoring: urine, hair, blood, adipose tissue, and breast milk.

Urine

Urine is a useful medium for human monitoring of water soluble pesticides or metabolites. An example is chlordimeform, which can be monitored through measurement of its urinary metabolite, chloro-*o*-toluidine. Several countries require such monitoring for workers using chlordimeform. The profile of urinary metabolites of a single pesticide can sometimes be helpful in distinguishing the pattern or time of exposure.

The advantages of using human urine to determine exposure include its ready availability, the non-invasiveness of sampling, and, in some countries, reduced legal or cultural impediments. A major disadvantage is the need for refrigerated storage, to prevent bacterial contamination. The extent and timing of urine collections will often depend on the exposure pattern and toxicokinetics of a pesticide.

The use of human urine as a means of measuring exposure to pesticides should be encouraged increasingly. Enhanced understanding of the toxicokinetics of environmental chemicals in recent years permits increased confidence in extrapolation of measurement in various body compartments to the initial dose. This knowledge has been accompanied by rapid advances in analytical chemistry to detect ever smaller amounts of parent compounds and their metabolites.

Hair

Hair is a useful matrix to detect the presence of metals and metaloids such as mercury and arsenic, each of which has been an active ingredient of some pesticides. Hair can be obtained easily and non-invasively. Furthermore, one can take advantage of its relatively slow growth to differentiate from chronic exposure by analysing different hair segments.

Nevertheless, a number of problems exist with the use of hair for the determination of exposure. Foremost is the need to distinguish between substances that have been incorporated into the hair matrix during its formation and those that have been added to the hair as part of grooming preparations or through the deposition of dust. Great care must be taken to clean and remove added substances, a process that can be technically difficult.

Blood

Monitoring humans exposed to pesticides is frequently performed through blood sampling. Both direct measurement of the pesticide or its metabolites, and indirect approaches through the measurement of a biological effect of a pesticide (e.g., acetylcholinesterase (AChE) activity) are used.

Blood is a tissue containing cellular and plasma components that can be assayed separately or together. It contains components that will attract both hydrophilic and hydrophobic substances. Thus, not only will water soluble compounds travel readily in the plasma, but highly lipophilic substances can be accommodated in such hydrophobic matrices as the red blood cell membrane, serum albumin, and lipoproteins.

Recent interest in biomarkers has led to the study of potential macromolecular adducts of environmental chemicals using human white blood cells as a source of DNA and albumin or red cell haemoglobin as a source of protein. Haemoglobin is of particular interest, because it is present in very large quantities in routine blood samples, is readily purified, and has a normal lifetime in the blood of approximately 120 days, thereby allowing it to be used to integrate exposure over 4 months and, by density-red-cell-age-separation techniques, theoretically permitting detection and dating of a brief exposure.

By contrast, the term 'biological monitoring' refers to the measurement of an effect in the indicator medium, especially in the case of organophosphate pesticides. So far, the only effect utilized has been the inhibition of the AChE in the red blood cells. This measurement is a special example where the effect of real concern (inhibition of the AChE at nerve synapses) is reflected also in the inhibition of the enzyme contained in the blood, which serves as the indicator medium.

When interpreting the results of such an 'effect monitoring', one has to distinguish it clearly from data on 'chemical monitoring'. Both phenomena differ in their toxicokinetics; therefore, a simple relation can be found only in the steady state of the AChE activity. The inhibition of AChE activity occurs to varying degrees in response to equal doses of varous OP pesticides. Therefore, this method is used, for practical purposes, as a self standing (i.e., independent) measure of exposure.

Adipose tissue

Analysis of body fat samples is a valuable approach to characterize the body burden of lipophilic compounds with relatively long half-lives in the body, such as chlorinated hydrocarbon pesticides. While occasionally used for diagnostic purposes or as part of a research protocol, fat biopsy is too invasive a procedure to be acceptable for routine monitoring of work populations exposed to pesticides.

Adipose tissue banks have been found to be particularly useful for trend analysis, such as following the body burden of DDT, DDE, and PCBs over time when regulatory controls were imposed. These banks, for the most part, depend on obtaining a fat sample during an operative procedure or autopsy. Archiving tissues is also valuable for future use as new analytical techniques become available. The sampling strategy must be responsive to the specific aims of the fat bank; i.e., for trend analysis, one needs a sampling approach that considers age, sex, health status, and occupation, and one that does not change from year to year. As with any tissue bank, archival integrity is as crucial as the storage process. To be used successfully, adipose tissue banks need to combine archival expertise with the ability to develop and test relevant hypotheses.

Breast Milk

Various lipophilic substances have been shown to be eliminated from the body in breast milk, thereby posing a potential health risk to the nursing infant. Breast milk concentrates body stores of lipophilic substances, acting to displace these stores from the mother to the infant who, with much less total body fat, may well have a higher fat concentration of the unwanted substance. In essence, monitoring of breast milk permits estimation of pesticide exposure to both mother and infant. Water soluble pesticides might also appear in breast milk, but the mobilization and concentration phenomena for lipophilic substances would not be anticipated.

Nursing mothers may be exposed to pesticides in the food they eat or through occupational exposures that occur before or during pregnancy and lactation. In many of the lesser developed countries and in migratory farm workers in developed countries, mothers with babies may actively participate in agricultural efforts including pesticide use; thus, the infant in the field may be at risk both from direct exposure and, if the pesticide is lipid soluble, from breast milk as well. Presently, techniques to obtain breast milk are relatively straightforward, although care must be taken in storage of samples. The usual approach is to relate the concentration of the chemical to milk fat content rather than to total volume. Unfortunately, analytical techniques to measure fat soluble substances, including pesticides, in mother's milk are now technically difficult and costly. A high priority should be given to development of monitoring techniques useful for the detection of pesticides in the breast milk of nursing mothers engaged in agriculture.

The value of assessing breast milk in exposure monitoring for pesticides should be considered in the context of the overall benefit of breast feeding for infant development.

2.2.3.5 Occupational exposure

Occupational exposure to agricultural chemicals is generally recognized as having the potential for high doses to the individual, because of the magnitude and frequency of contact. Thus, the number of acute illnesses among agricultural workers reported to national health agencies is a significant public health matter.

The basic approach to estimate occupational exposure is passive dosimetry, biological monitoring, or a combination of the two approaches. Passive techniques are generally used to satisfy regulatory requirements rather than as a means of personal exposure monitoring. As such, these techniques are useful to establish a likely dose under a defined set of field conditions; however, they are not commonly used to monitor exposures of workers on a continuing basis.

Biological monitoring approaches have been discussed fully in previous sections. These techniques may be applied to evaluate occupational exposures as a means of establishing doses of a compound; however, the manner or route of exposure cannot be established by this method alone. The newer immunoassay methodologies hold promise for use as personal monitoring devices. One approach utilizes a small card that, using Enzyme-Linked ImmunoSorbent Assay (ELISA) techniques, can measure pesticide concentrations in virtually any medium. The general approach includes having an individual carry a card containing appropriate antisera and reagents; after exposure to the pesticide, the card changes colour; the colour may then be compared to that on a chart to estimate the concentration of pesticide in the sample. Such cards have already been developed for parathion and paraquat, two chemicals which account for a significant number of acute poisonings in the field. This approach could be used to quickly monitor residues on skin or in urine, and hence to estimate doses to individuals in the field. This approach may prove especially useful in developing nations where access to analytical equipment may be limited.

Occupational exposures to pesticides can be reduced through protective clothing, engineering controls, and modification/refinement of application techniques. Absorption through the skin, in particular the hands, is the major route of exposure for most pesticides. Depending on the specific pesticide and occupational activity, estimates of exposure through the skin of an unprotected hand range from 25 to 98 per cent of total dermal exposure. The use of protective gloves would greatly reduce occupational pesticide exposure; however, care must be taken to select a glove that is impermeable to the pesticide. For pesticides that are volatile or form aerosols, the use of respirators may be necessary to reduce exposure. However, these devices are limited by the requirement for periodic maintenance and a lack of compliance among workers because of discomfort and heat.

In tropical climates, full protective gear may be impractical because of the potential for heat stress in the worker. In such instances, a reduction in exposure can be achieved only through engineering controls and improved application techniques. The use of pre-weighed packages reduces exposure by eliminating the need to handle large volumes of pesticide while weighing out or measuring the amounts necessary for application. In addition, the potential for spills is reduced. The use of emulsifiable concentrates rather than wettable powders reduces inhalation exposure, as does pumping rather than pouring the pesticide from the mixing tank into an application apparatus.

The use of closed-cab ground application systems, rather than airplane or airblast, can also reduce exposure to the applicator and reduce drift onto non-target areas. When airplane applications are used, mechanical rather than human flaggers should be employed to direct the spraying.

Since plants carry a negative electrical charge, the use of an electrostatic device to create an airblast mist that carries a positive electrical charge can cause an electrical attraction between the pesticide mist and plants. This attraction minimizes drift, improves application efficiency and coverage, and ultimately reduces the volume of pesticide required to achieve an effect.

Reducing worker exposures through engineering controls and improved application techniques also leads to a reduction in the overall environmental impact of the pesticide application specifically, less drift, fewer spills, and a reduced potential for accidental exposure of other unprotected individuals. Improved techniques for personal monitoring, such as the currently evolving immunoassay methodologies, are desirable to ensure the efficacy and safety of engineering controls and application techniques.

2.2.3.6 Non-occupational exposure

In some instances, pesticides used in and around the house can result in meaningful exposure. The practice of treating houses for the control of structural pests has resulted in persistent elevated exposure to the cyclodiene pesticides aldrin/dieldrin and to chlordane/heptachlor.

Periodic application of insecticides for control of vermin is a potential source of exposure to persistent chlorinated hydrocarbon and other products such as chlorpyrifos.

Small children may receive the more significant levels of exposure as a consequence of repeated contact with room perimeters, carpets, and soil. In addition, hand to mouth manipulations are common at this age, as is the tendency to taste, chew, and ingest objects. Children of all ages also have the potential for more frequent exposure to pesticides in the home yard, particularly treated lawns or treated soil.

The casual use of pesticides by home owners on the lawn, in the flower garden, or in the vegetable plot, must be considered in determining sources of pesticide exposure. Failure to heed instructions for use of protective clothing, preparation of correct concentrations, and proper disposal can result in levels of exposure equivalent to those present in large-scale agricultural applications. Such lax practices may also result in increased exposure residues on foods harvested from the home garden.

2.2.3.7 Dietary exposure

An ideal system to estimate dietary exposures to pesticides should consist of two main components: sufficient data on food consumption that accurately reflect the diverse eating habits and patterns present in a population and its subgroups; and accurate data on the concentration of pesticide residues present in food at the time it is eaten.

Food consumption data used to derive dietary exposure estimates should reflect the diverse eating habits of a population. In some cases, such diversity can be accounted for by using safety factors or exaggerated estimates of residues in food. In such cases, the use of a single population average for food consumption in combination with exaggerated residue estimates will provide adequate protection for all individuals. The result of using this approach is to greatly overestimate dietary exposures.

In other cases, however, it is desirable to obtain the most accurate estimate of exposure possible because of concern for potential toxicity in a particular population subgroup. For example, infants and children are known to consume more food per kilogram of body weight than do adults. Using a population average for food consumption will always under-estimate consumption in children and generally over-estimate consumption in adults. In addition, infants and young children tend to receive a greater portion of their total diet from a small number of foods than do adults. This restriction of the diet to a few foods, mainly milk products and certain vegetables and fruits, can also magnify pesticide exposures in infants and children, since, if these foods have been treated with a pesticide, a greater portion of the infant diet will contain pesticide residues than that of an adult. Since children are known to be uniquely sensitive to some forms of toxicity (e.g., lead neuropathy), it is important to have accurate consumption data for this group to assess the impact of pesticide residues in their diet. Similarly, for reproductive toxicants, accurate data on food consumption must be obtained for women of child-bearing age.

The toxicity produced by a pesticide can be caused by either a single exposure or multiple exposures over time. Aldicarb is a carbamate insecticide that can produce toxicity after a single exposure, as has been demonstrated by incidents involving the misuse of this chemical on watermelons and cucumbers. To protect against this type of occurrence, it is necessary to have data on the amount of a particular food consumed at one time. In addition, within any population subgroup, a distribution of consumption will exist for any particular food. Some approaches to regulating pesticide residues in food use the 90th percentile of consumption to protect the individuals who eat more food than the average for the population. For chemicals that produce toxicity after multiple exposures, data on average food consumption over time would be more relevant.

Pesticide residues occur in food as a result of commercial agricultural practices and, in some cases, as a result of home gardening. Commercial agricultural practices are generally regulated by national governments, and are influenced by international groups such as the WHO/FAO Joint Meeting on Pesticide Residues (JMPR). These groups generally recommend Acceptable Daily Intakes (ADIs) and Maximum Residue Limits (MRLs), which are the upper limits of pesticide residue expected on raw agricultural commodities consistent with good agricultural practice.* In general, these MRLs are mainly for enforcement purposes, that is, to assure that pesticides are not used in excessive amounts. However, since the MRL (a tolerance) is an upper limit, it is not a useful value for calculating actual dietary exposures.

---

*In the US, this value is legally defined as a 'tolerance' and is established by the Environmental Protection Agency (EPA).

An accurate estimate of exposure should reflect the effects of washing, peeling, processing, and cooking on pesticide residues. In general, these steps will produce a large decrease in the amount of pesticide present in food at the time of consumption, compared to the amount of residue present in the field. In certain other cases, a pesticide may actually concentrate during processing, or it may be converted to toxic metabolites. The ethylene *bis*-dithio-carbamate (EBDC) class of fungicides is known to form the toxicant ethylene thiourea (ETU) during the processing of food treated with these fungicides. Similarly, the growth regulatory daminozide will form unsymmetrical dimethyl hydrazine (UDMH) upon processing (e.g., conversion of apples into apple sauce). In these cases, sampling of field residues alone would not provide an accurate estimate of exposure at the time of consumption. Rather, measurements of field residues combined with studies on the effect of processing and cooking are necessary to accurately predict final residue concentrations at the time of consumption. The residue estimate should also reflect the extent of use of the pesticide. An MRL may be established for a chemical on tomatoes; however, every tomato grown and marketed will not be treated with that chemical.

In addition to residues on fresh and processed produce, pesticide residues may occur in meat, milk, and eggs as a result of feeding items treated with pesticides to domestic cattle and poultry. In certain cases, pesticide residues can occur in meat and milk at significant concentrations. In one instance, dairy cattle were inadvertently fed grain that had been treated with the insecticide heptachlor, resulting in the appearance of heptachlor in milk. In another instance, pineapples treated with heptachlor produced no appreciable residues in the edible fruit; however, when byproducts from a pineapple cannery were fed to cattle, heptachlor residues were detected in milk. In many countries, wastes from food processing are routinely used as cattle feed, resulting in a significant potential for producing secondary residues in domestic food animals. This issue is especially important where residues occur in milk, since milk products form a significant part of the diet for infants and children, who will also receive an exaggerated dose because of their higher rate of food consumption relative to body weight.

In many countries, food has been sampled at the consumer level and analysed for pesticide residues as a means of estimating dietary pesticide exposures. Such techniques include 'market basket surveys', which monitor residues in food purchased from stores and markets, and 'dual diet studies' in which a portion of prepared food is analysed prior to consumption. These approaches provide the most accurate data on pesticide residues at the time of consumption, but are limited by the cost of obtaining and analysing large numbers of samples necessary to achieve statistical validity.

For most individuals, pesticide residues in the diet occur as a result of agricultural practices. However, some individuals may receive significant dietary exposures from other sources. The organochlorine pesticides, which are quite persistent in the environment, will concentrate in fish because of bioaccumulation. Commercial and sport fishermen, who regularly consume such fish from lakes or rivers that have been contaminated with these pesticides, may receive a significant dose of the chemical. Hunters who consume wildfowl may receive similar exposures. In one instance, wild geese were discovered to contain significant residues of the organochlorine endrin as a result of eating grain from fields treated with this pesticide. Some birds died from this exposure; surviving birds that were later eaten caused human illness.

The overall impact of such episodes is difficult to assess. Because few individuals within a population obtain their food from these 'wild' sources, statistical population surveys of food consumption will not provide reliable estimates of consumption. However, fish and wild game can be a source of significant hazard to the individual, and should not be overlooked in an assessment of the impact of environmental contamination.

Home gardening, although not a major source of food in most households, may also present a significant hazard to an individual. Generally, the same laws and regulations apply equally to home and commercial agricultural practices. However, some home gardeners, because of a lack of knowledge or through carelessness, have occasionally introduced significant pesticide residues into a food, resulting in illness.

Finally, drinking water is a source of dietary pesticide exposure that has become of concern in many nations. In agricultural areas of high pesticide use, sampling of ground- and surface-water supplies has generally revealed the presence of pesticides. The problem may become especially serious in areas with sandy soil, which is easily penetrated by pesticides, and/or areas with relatively high water tables. For example, in Suffolk County (New York), aldicarb was found in about 25 wells sampled at concentrations of up to 515 p.p.b. In California, a state with pesticide manufacturing facilities and a large number of agricultural operations, more than 50 pesticides were detected in the ground water of 23 counties. One pesticide, DBCP, was found in over 2000 wells (25 per cent of the total number sampled), with the highest concentration of 1.24 p.p.b. near a DBCP manufacturing facility.

Efforts are currently under way in many nations to monitor ground- and surface-water for pesticides and other chemicals. The monitoring of water for pesticides must consider the largely seasonal application of pesticides. For example, agricultural runoff may produce relatively higher concentrations of herbicides early in the growing season, since pesticides are frequently applied to bare ground, which has a greater potential for runoff. The utility of such monitoring efforts is clear to assess hazards to a population resulting from dietary pesticide exposure. For some subgroups with high water consumption, such as infants fed formula prepared with water, such data are vital to an accurate assessment of dietary exposure.

2.2.4 ECOSYSTEM MONITORING

Of the numerous issues confronted in the monitoring of something as diverse, variable, and complex as an ecosystem, the most difficult is sampling. Adequate principles and guidelines exist for sampling human environments for epidemiological studies; nothing comparable exists for non-humans.

Because of the concern for incidental dietary intake by humans of pesticides, considerable attention has been given to developing accepted procedures for sampling foodstuffs for chemical analysis. Guidelines, indicating substantial agreement over procedures to sample foods, exist in international commerce. The Codex Committee on Pesticide Residues has been prominent in this quest for international agreement and standardization. No such agreement has been reached with regard to ecosystem sampling. The OECD program on wildlife sampling and monitoring partially dealt with the matter, but no guidelines or procedures emerged from this study. Environmental sampling has also been the subject of an IUPAC study.

The paucity of guidelines on ecosystem monitoring, the natural complexity and variability of ecosystems, and the diversity of monitoring methodology makes comparisons of result among investigators virtually impossible. Many existing environmental sampling procedures are carryovers from the randomized, unbiased sampling procedures employed in agriculture to measure endpoints such as crop yields; standard textbooks are devoted largely to such sampling techniques. Environmental sampling requirements are similar to those of epidemiology, namely, reliance on biased non-random sampling, which applies to both spacial distribution and time. For instance, the impact of aerial spraying of a forest on NTOs is likely to be maximal at treetop height and just after spraying; similar considerations apply to the use of pesticides to control biting flies in a fast-flowing river. The failure of some laboratory model systems to extrapolate results to the field may be largely attributed to the failure to include sampling criteria.

The basic need for guidelines for environmental sampling would best be met by a workshop organized by an international agency such as UNEP or OECD. The membership of such a workshop should include a broad array of expertise with particular representation among those specialists who make the greatest use of monitoring data.

2.3 RECOMMENDATIONS

The following detailed recommendations supplement those presented in Chapter 1 of this Joint Report.

1. The complexity of the models should be limited to what is rquired, given the objectives of the study.

2. Research should be oriented mainly toward the development and validation of predictive descriptions of the key processes that influence behaviour, including sorption, photolysis, and biodegradation, rather than on models *per se*, as well as on the validation and improvement of the quality of the databases.

3. Research to test the convergence between predictions and field results should be focused on the identification of those refinements that are essential for improved forecasting.

4. Methodologies that correctly integrate exposure from all routes into a total dose need to be developed and validated. A generally accepted and validated procedure does not exist. Implementation of this recommendation is expected to lead to a better recognition of the relative importance of individual exposure routes in specific pesticide uses.

5. The majority of basic exposure data has been developed in the temperate climate zones of the world. In many instances, the major applications (and toxic effects) of pesticides occur in the semitropical and tropical zones. Since some physiological and biological properties and rates are dependent upon temperature, humidity, and other environmental characteristics, a substantial need exists to adjust for, and verify, the basic data developed in one climate zone before use in other zones.

6. Simple, reliable, and economic measures to indicate level(s) of exposure in the field are needed to affirm the effectiveness of exposure control techniques in practical situations.

7. Advances are needed in the methodology to assess human exposure to pesticides through biological monitoring. A better understanding of the basic biological mechanisms governing the interaction between pesticides and human tissues would allow the extent of exposure to be inferred confidently from the biological endpoint or understood from toxicokinetic data relating to parent compound or metabolite levels in biological fluids. Improved analytical techniques to determine lower concentrations of a compound, its metabolite, or its macromolecular adduct should be sought.

3 Methods to Assess Toxic Effects of Pesticides in Humans

Pesticides, like most other chemicals, have the potential to produce both acute and chronic injury to health. Generally, acute toxic effects are those caused shortly after a single dose or a few doses;* however, some compounds have been known to cause delayed manifestations of injury after a single large dose. Illustrations of delayed toxicity are neuropathy caused by organophosphate esters, lung damage by paraquat, and sensitization by pyrethroids.

Within this framework, acute and chronic effects can be separated in general terms as presented in Table 3.1. These groups form the basis for the discussion in the following sections on the acute and chronic effects of pesticides on human health.

3.1 ACUTE TOXICITY†

Assessing exposure and dose–response relationships for acute toxicity is generally more easily accomplished than that for chronic toxicity. Because acute exposure is restricted, by definition, to a short time interval, estimates of exposure can

Table 3.1. Acute and chronic toxic effects of pesticides

Acute toxicity	Chronic toxicity	Target organ toxicity
Mortality and morbidity	Carcinogenicity	Lungs
Neurotoxicity	Mutagenicity	Cardiovascular system
Immunotoxicity	Development toxicity	Endocrine system
Dermal toxicity		Haematopoietic system
Reproductive toxicity		Musculo/skeletal system
		Liver
		Kidneys

*Acute exposure is defined as a single dose or multiple doses within a short time (e.g., 24 hours); acute effects are those that generally occur shortly after acute exposure.
†This section was prepared by S. Baker, J. Doull, J. Finkelman, and A. Massoud.

Methods to Assess Adverse Effects of Pesticides on Non-target Organisms
Edited by R. G. Tardiff
©1992 SCOPE Published by John Wiley & Sons Ltd

often be made more confidently in occupational, non-occupational, and laboratory settings. For example, dermal exposure in the workplace is 20 to 1700 times greater than inhalation exposure (Feldman and Maibach, 1974). Since exposure of the lungs to pesticides almost always results in effects at remote sites rather than in the lungs, this organ is not considered to be a major target for acute pesticide toxicity. Dermal exposure, either with or without skin lesions, resulting in systemic effects is of particular concern for public health.

The dose–response characteristics for acute effects, unlike those for most chronic effects, are also definable in terms of severity, potency, and existence of thresholds. Consequently, risk assessment or hazard evaluation procedures used to establish margins of safety for acute effects are relatively straightforward and accepted as standard practices by different national and international advisory bodies. In the succeeding sections of this chapter, current methods for determining acute effects noted in Table 3.1 are identified and critiqued for their predictive applicability in assessing risk of acute exposure to pesticides. On the whole, the available methods are highly predictive, although some contain shortcomings that lessen their predictive utility for risk assessment.

3.1.1   MORBIDITY AND MORTALITY: MAGNITUDE OF THE PROBLEM

Acute pesticide poisoning, particularly in developing countries, is frequent, and thus has an elevated importance in public health. Most intoxications occur in workers. WHO estimates that the worldwide incidence of acute pesticide intoxications has doubled in the last decade, from 500 000 cases per year in the 1970s to over 1 000 000 annually in the early 1980s. The case fatality ratio has been estimated to be between 1.5 and 2 per cent. In some countries, the incidence of pesticide poisoning has exceeded the demographic growth and the rates of agricultural production.

Preliminary data from recent studies conducted in the Central American countries by the Pan American Health Organization (PAHO) suggest that the morbidity of acute pesticide poisoning is greater than expected. In 1987 in Costa Rica's Hospital of Gaupiles, 733 of 5000 (i.e., 14.7 per cent) emergency room patients were treated for acute poisoning; numerous fatalities were recorded. An epidemiologic surveillance program was established in five communities of the same Costa Rican area, having a total population of 1505 (including 528 farmers). These communities are located in a banana-producing area of about 490 hectares where, in one year, 286 tons of fungicide and 107 tons of insecticide (mostly organophosphates—OP—such as aldicarb) were applied. All of the insecticides applied are considered 'extremely hazardous' based on the WHO classification of the toxicity of pesticides. In 1987, 63 individuals of these five communities were clinically diagnosed as having been acutely intoxicated, to varying degrees of severity, by pesticides. While there were no fatalities, 58 poisonings were due to occupational exposure, 4 to accidental non-occupational exposure, and 1 to a suicide attempt (rates of poisoning per 1000 are as follows: occupational, 109.8; non-occupational, 2.65).

Pesticides associated with these cases were OP (48 cases), paraquat (4 cases), mixtures (6 cases), and not identified (4 cases). In Honduras in 1986, field tests on 1100 farmers have shown that about 32 per cent of those examined had a decrease in AChE activity of 25 per cent or more.

3.1.1.1 Factors contributing to morbidity and mortality

The magnitude of the public health problem depends on a number of contributing factors. Among them are the type of crop, pesticide regulations, agricultural practices and technology, awareness of the degree of danger, training to minimize exposure, and availability of medical treatment facilities.

Some crops require more pesticide than do others. For example, growth of cotton in Latin America, Egypt, Sudan, and other developing countries consumes about 60 per cent of total insecticides used in these regions. Resistance of pests also contributes to the selection of the pesticide used.

The selection of a particular pesticide is also critical. Quite often, this decision is made by individuals with no professional or technical training, which may lead to improper use of pesticides. Cost of a chemical and its effectiveness (number and quantity of applications) are also important elements contributing to the selection of pesticides. In general, the more toxic a pesticide, the lower its cost.

The most common pesticides used in Latin America and the Middle East are:

Carbamates: aldicarb, carbofuran, carbaryl
Herbicides: 2,4-D, 2,4,5-T
Organochlorines: dieldrin, lindane, DDT, heptachlor, aldrin, endrin, toxaphene
Organophosphates: parathion, fenthion, diazinon, fenitrothion, malathion, methylparathion
Pyrethroids: desmethrin, δ-methrin
Pyridyls: paraquat, diquat

Most developing countries have inadequate pesticide regulations and the inability to enforce the existing ones. Pesticides are openly marketed, and minor verifications are applied. Restricted pesticides are frequently used for purposes other than those intended or approved.

At times, good agricultural practice requires less pesticide usage than is the common practice. Large areas containing single crops such as cotton or bananas are usually treated by professional pesticide applicators. This situation does not imply that all precautions are taken. Quite often, aerial spraying will not spare neighbouring residential areas, Smaller farms do not use professional pesticide applicators. In these cases, the farmer applies the chemicals, which are usually mixtures selected by the individual.

Lack of vital knowledge of toxicity and of procedures for the safe use of pesticides plays a critical role in obtaining direct exposure. Furthermore, labelling practices in developing countries are often inadequate.

Since most of the exposure events occur in distant rural areas, medical facilities to diagnose and treat the patients are likely to be quite distant. In the absence of locally trained personnel, there is greater likelihood that increased mortality results from acute over-exposure.

Typical cases of acute pesticide poisoning occur in males between 14 and 50 years of age, who are usually applying OPs with a backpack sprayer. If they live in an area of Latin America where pesticides are used intensively, their chance of acute intoxication (from clinically detectable to severe intoxication) on a yearly basis is about 10 per cent. This percentage may be as high as 30 per cent, if one includes subclinical levels of intoxication such as AChE depression.

3.1.1.2 Methods for investigation and surveillance of morbidity and mortality

From a practical perspective, the first goal is to reduce to the minimum possible the number of fatal cases caused by pesticides; the second goal is to significantly reduce the risks that may lead to acute intoxication. Bearing these goals in mind, the strategy recommended is to establish proper surveillance programs that take into account the role and needs of all involved parties.

At national and state levels, it is essential firstly to decide which pesticides will be licensed, restricted, or banned, making certain that proper resources are made available to supervise compliance with these decisions; secondly to communicate and enforce sound labour practices regarding the safe use of pesticides; and thirdly to establish reference laboratories to support field testing activities of pesticides.

At the local level, a surveillance program requires additional efforts. In an effective surveillance program, the *first* step is collection of the following data:

1. Crops per agricultural cycle,
2. Possible pests to be controlled,
3. Recommended pesticides to be applied in the sector of concern,
4. Indentification of sources of distribution of pesticides,
5. Identification of applicators, including the non professional,
6. Identification of other individuals or populations who may be exposed, and
7. Identification of health facilities in the sector of concern.

The *second* step should include the following activities:

1. Training of pesticide applicators (professional and non professional) in safety and in the proper handling of pesticides, including periodic review of equipment used for the application;

2. Training of health personnel in early diagnosis and proper treatment of acute poisoning; this training should also include proper field testing of AChE activity or other appropriate biomonitoring, as well as assuring the availability of antidotes;
3. Establishment of a registry and of follow-up procedures to ensure that each reported case of acute intoxication is fully investigated; each case should be considered as part of a cluster that may indicate the need for additional studies, and
4. Establishment of a pesticide control group with legal representation, with authority to supervise and regulate the use of pesticides at local or state levels, and responsive to public and private concerns.

3.1.2 EPIDEMIOLOGICAL STUDIES

Major difficulties exist in performing epidemiological studies on pesticide exposures, including the assessment of doses, the variability and unpredictability of agricultural exposures, and, in some instances, the migratory lifestyle of some of the agricultural workers. For epidemiological surveillance to be effective, measurements of exposure and characterization of risk must be improved. Design of epidemiological studies depends on the nature of the questions to be addressed and the availability of time and resources. Once the exposed population groups are defined, population registries might be established for follow-up and for cohort studies. These registries might contain information on periodic medical examinations of individuals obtaining high doses. Epidemiological follow-up of individuals exposed or diagnosed as having acute poisoning may stimulate further studies of acute delayed toxicity.

3.1.3 TESTS FOR ACUTE TOXICITY

The traditional means of measuring acute toxicity have been the observation of mortality per unit of single dose in groups of experimental animals; the details for such tests have been reviewed extensively by others, and are not addressed herein. Specialized tests for neurotoxicity and immunotoxicity have been developed recently, and will be discussed in some detail below.

3.1.3.1 Tests for pesticide neurotoxicity

Pesticides may produce either acute or chronic neurotoxicity in non-target species. A single exposure can produce immediate symptoms of neurologic poisoning, as well as delayed manifestations of injury. Chronic, low-level exposures usually produce symptoms of chronic poisoning and, in some cases, even acute poisoning, because the body burdens of the pesticide are so large.

Most cases of acute poisoning from pesticides in human result from exposure to insecticides rather than herbicides, fungicides, and other pesticide classes. The reason is that the neurotoxicity of insecticides (such as the organochlorine compounds, OPs, carbamates, and pyrethroids) results from the primary mechanism of action being at either or both the peripheral and central nervous systems, leading directly to motor, sensory, autonomic, cognitive, or behavioural disturbances. By contrast, neurotoxicity from other classes of pesticides is usually a secondary, non-target effect.

Neurotoxicity testing is aimed at detecting and quantifying changes in both structure and function of the central and peripheral nervous systems that are produced by exposure to a test chemical such as a pesticide. Although there are many animal testing methods for detecting neurotoxicity, few methods have been sufficiently standardized and validated to serve as protocols for regulatory purposes. Most current neurotoxicity test methods use indices of neurochemistry, neurophysiology, neuropathology, behaviour, and specific psychological effects (such as perception, motivation, habituation, learning, and memory) to detect toxicity. To adequately assess neurotoxicity as an adverse non-target effect of pesticides, simple non-invasive methods are needed to identify all types of neuronal dysfunction and to quantify effects such as impaired vigilance, reduced concentration, memory deficit, linguistic disturbances, depression, and irritability.

Depression of AChE activity in serum, whole blood, or erythrocytes has been used extensively to detect exposure to cholinergic pesticides (i.e, carbamates and OPs) and to quantify the magnitude of exposures. Interpretation of these findings requires some clinical judgement, since the effects depend on the class of pesticide (e.g., carbamates produce a briefer depression than do OPs), the specific agent (some OPs depress serum esterase but not erythrocyte esterase); the route and duration of exposure (repeated and prolonged exposure at relatively low doses may depress esterase without producing cholinergic symptoms); the effect of treatment (oxime reactivators such as 2-PAM will modify the esterase effect); and the formulation (concomitant exposure to mixtures of some pesticides may produce either potentiation or inhibition of the effect). Nevertheless, measurement of AChE inhibition is a useful and well-validated method for assessing exposure; it can be used in the field for relatively low cost.

Delayed neurologic sequelae (e.g., paraesthesia, tremors, and equilibrium disturbances) have been reported with organochlorine pesticide exposure; delayed neuromuscular paralysis which can be detected by non-invasive nerve conduction studies has been produced by exposures to OPs such as phosvel, leptophos, and mipafox. *In vivo* tests, such as the leghorn chicken test, and *in vitro* enzyme studies can be used to detect the neuromuscular effects of OPs, and are useful to predict similar effects in humans. However, other neuronal dysfunctions may also occur as a delayed response to acute or chronic exposure to cholinergic insecticides.

Acute exposure to the organochlorine insecticides such as DDT, cyclodienes, and chlordecone may produce acute convulsive seizures with residual neuronal cell loss and brain ischemia and anoxia. These effects can result in a variety of behavioural changes (irritability, loss of recent memory, depression, anxiety, EEG modifications, and learning impairment in humans; difficulty in performing complex tests in animals), which may persist for many years. Chronic exposure to these agents can produce similar effects, but the persistence and severity of these changes appear to be related to the incidence of convulsive seizures in both acute and chronic exposure situations.

3.1.3.2 Tests for immunotoxicity

Aside from producing hypersensitivity, relatively little indication exists that pesticides produce anything other than minimal dysfunction of the immune response in humans. Current technologies make it possible to detect immuno-modulation or disease that results from modulation of the immune system.

Pesticides were among the first environmental chemicals to be tested for immunotoxic effects. Because the immune systems is so complex, a single test is inadequate to evaluate immune alterations caused by pesticides. Rather, a battery of tests is required to examine specific endpoints. The occurrence of immunotoxicity is influenced by pre-existing toxicity; conversely, the immune response might predispose individuals to diseases such as cancer. This situation suggests the need for a dose–response characterization of the relation between pesticides and immune function.

Preliminary screening tests for immunotoxicity before undertaking detailed testing is scientifically reasonable firstly because specific immune function tests are costly and time-consuming, and secondly because relatively little is known about the ability of the majority of pesticides to alter specific immune functions, thus creating a need for broader-scale screening for effects on the immune system.

Advantages have been identified for several screening tests. These tests can be conducted as a part of subchronic or chronic dosing regimens, few experimental animals are required, and a measure of immune response can be obtained by weighing critical organs and performing simple pathological examinations on them. From regulatory and risk assessment perspectives, however, relatively few endpoints included in subchronic toxicity studies are direct indicators of immunotoxicity.

Evidence of immunomodulation is extensive. Specific points along the sequence of events characterizing immune response are susceptible to pesticidal influence. These loci include antigen contact and macrophage processing; antigen recognition by T- or B-cells; clonal proliferation of immunocompetent cells; production, storage, and release of lymphokines; cell–cell communication; and tissue damage. Sensitivity may vary among different cell populations, leading to the possibility of a biphasic immune response (immunostimulation at low dose; immunosuppression at high dose). Such a phenomenon makes tests for immunotoxocity mechanisms highly desirable for understanding the immune response potential of pesticides.

From risk assessment and regulatory perspectives, relatively few immunologic endpoints are considered useful. For a preliminary screen, however, the following are useful: differentiated leucocyte count, total serum protein, organ weights and cellularity, histopathology, and haematology as a measure of pesticide-induced anaemia. Additional tests, such as serum immunoglobulin levels, and possible premature mortality of dosed animals from immunosuppressive effects would yield more definitive screening results.

If the screening procedures show an immunologic alteration, then more comprehensive data to support risk assessment would be required. These tests include host resistance, both specific and non-specific cell-mediated immune response, and time-course for recovery from immunologic effects.

Several clinical endpoints are useful for screening tests. Haematology, spleen cell, and bone marrow evaluations can provide clues to an altered immune response via lymphocyte transformation, mixed lymphocyte response, or *in vitro* antibody formation. *In vitro* macrophage functions can also be evaluated in pesticide-dosed animals. While *in vitro* phagocytosis and immunoglobulin profiles (identified with ELISA) are also useful, these techniques are less sensitive for evaluating immune response after antigenic challenge, because they are not as responsive as the immune system sensitized by pesticide pretreatment. Finally, host-resistance models, including the use of tumour cells, bacteria, viruses, blood parasites, or *E. coli* endotoxin, may indicate a thymus-dependent immunity and thus may also be useful as a screening tool.

Specialized tests for immunotoxicity

Batteries of targeted tests are available for comprehensive investigation of immunological effects. These include tests for humeral and cellular immunities, macrophage responses, and biochemical mechanisms. In each intance, the following features must be carefully crafted or considered for proper application of a test:

1. Experimental design,
2. Antigen selection,
3. Treatment dose, route of delivery, and duration of exposure,
4. Immunization dose and route,
5. Number of dose levels (several are desirable for a period of at least two weeks before antigenic challenge),
6. Whether to use suboptimal antigenic levels to induce both immuno-stimulation and immunosuppression,
7. The time of sampling (time-dependent studies can result in effects on different immunologic endpoints during the complete sequence of events in the immune response,
8. Organ pathology and other forms of target organ toxicity,

   9. Gastrointestinal damage (leading to possible endotoxin absorption and mmunotoxicity),
  10. Food consumption,
  11. Endocrine function (e.g., circulating corticosteroids), and
  12. Effects on the developing immune system.

Techniques involving the use of human cells and *in vitro* metabolism are somewhat unreliable, because of inconsistency due to individual variation and potential confounding effects.

Tests for autoimmunity and hypersensitivity

Autoimmunity has been reported in workers with chronic pesticide exposure. The development of autoantibodies against liver and kidney occurs after organochlorine or OP insecticide exposure and usually follows pathologic changes in tissue.

Similarly, hypersensitivity in humans has been reported. However, in contrast to autoimmunity, for which no reliable animal model has been identified for testing, there is an experimental basis for examining hypersensitivity in animals. Cutaneous or pulmonary hypersensitivity in animals caused either by pesticides or industrial solvents has been observed. Standardized protocols for detecting hypersensitivity in the guinea pig are available from USFDA and OECD.

3.1.4 SKIN ABSORPTION OF PESTICIDES AND ACUTE POISONING

The skin is one of the main routes of systemic exposure to pesticides. Feldman and Maibach (1974) showed that spraying or dusting of pesticides causes doses 20–1700 times greater than that reaching the respiratory tract. The lipophilic component of the skin diffuses non-polar molecules, while the intracellular proteinaceous material of the skin permits diffusion of polar molecules, a process that is enhanced by the moisture content of the outer layers of the skin.

Many factors play a role in the percutaneous absorption of pesticides: among them are the nature of a chemical substance (e.g., chemical structure, concentration, total dose, application frequency, and duration of contact), and the characteristics of exposed individuals (e.g., individual variation, temperature, humidity, surface area potentially exposed, site of application, and skin condition including pH and cleanliness). Dermal absorption of pesticides can be greatly enhanced by solvents or other ingredients in a formulation.

3.1.4.1 Clinical forms of acute exposure of skin to pesticides

In the clinical setting, cases of acute exposure may show different symptoms. Contact dermatitis (Baginsky, 1978) is the most common of these symptoms, manifested either as non-allergic irritation or allergic contact dermatitis. This latter effect is a form of delayed hypersensitivity resulting from the low molecular weight of a chemical, usually a hapten conjugated with protein in blood (Morison *et al.*, 1981). Localized or generalized urticaria, pigmentation (discoloration, increase or decrease of melanization), and occupational acne (halogen acne and chloracne) are also known to occur (Yonemoto *et al.*, 1983; Echobichon *et al.*, 1977). Cutaneous parasthesia (i.e., delayed transient itching sensation mostly on facial skin) has been reported in case of acute exposure to synthetic pyrethroid (Knox *et al.*, 1984).

3.1.4.2 Methods to assess acute skin exposure

Methods to assess acute exposure include the following.
1. Clinical assessment of symptoms and signs, removal of the worker from the place of exposure for a recovery period, and follow-up after return to work. If a worker shows the same affliction upon return to work, this observation represents strong evidence for causation by this chemical environment. Recurrence of the symptoms and signs will support the diagnosis of chemical exposure. This observation should trigger searches for additional exposures to the same compound and to compounds having the same effects. If other workers have the same symptoms, the evidence for causation is strengthened.
2. Absorbent patch testing will assess only exposure, not absorption.
3. Urinary metabolites such as those detected during exposure to OPs (e.g., alkyl phosphate for parathion exposure or 4,8-h-dimethyl-thiophosphate for azinphos-methyl). This method indicates absorption of the pesticide from many routes of entry including the skin. Franklin (1984) showed that, if a strong correlation exists between the results of this test and those of the patch test, it provides a mechanism for estimating dermal dosage.
4. Histology samples and chemical analyses of biopsy samples can be used as a method to assess the lesion type and any specific findings related to pesticide exposure.
5. Adverse effects of pesticides can be determined using the Draize test in the laboratory.

3.1.5   OTHER TARGET ORGANS OF ACUTE TOXICITY

The previous discussion documents toxicological and epidemiological evidence of acute effects related to acute exposures to pesticides. For other organs and systems (e.g., pulmonary*, haematopoietic and haematological, cardiovascular, renal, endocrine, and musculoskeletal) evidence of toxicity or its absence is often lacking. While the absence of data may indicate that these organs or systems

---

*With the exception of the paraquat effect on the lungs.

are unaffected as a result of a single dose of diverse chemical entities, it is possible that the available methods may be insufficiently sensitive or specific to detect subtle changes in these organs. Thus, before concluding that acute toxic effects are absent in these systems, research should be undertaken to remove uncertainties that surround the issue.

A promising approach to demonstrate subtle effects in these organs and tissues is the use of biomarkers. These techniques have the advantage of providing non-invasive, inexpensive, field-adaptable exposure assessments that could be particularly useful for risk assessment and epidemiological applications. Such procedures also should be useful to identify susceptible populations such as the young, the elderly, or those with pre-existing conditions or predisposition to disease.

Toxicokinetics (the dynamics of absorption, biotransformation, and excretion) represents another promising approach to detect the adverse effects of both acute and chronic exposures. Toxicokinetic information is likely to have particular applicability to single-dose exposures where factors, such as an enzymatic pathway of detoxification, are rate limiting (i.e., saturation kinetics). For example, failure of the kidney to demonstrate an adverse response to acute pesticide exposure may reflect the absence of saturation kinetics which enhances its capacity and efficiency of elimination. By contrast, other primary pathways of exposure may be saturated, leading to the manifestation of secondary toxic responses that would not occur usually, were it not for saturation of the primary target organ or pathway. For example, saturation by one compound of either the sulfhydryl deactivation process or the P_{450} microsomal detoxification mechanism may lead to adverse effects by a second parent compound. Better understanding of these processes would help resolve some of the more difficult scientific issues important for regulation (such as the establishment of a maximum tolerated dose (MTD) for a compound with multiple, dose-dependent metabolic pathways) or for the appropriate design of animals studies. Ideally, an understanding of the mechanisms of toxic action of pesticides and of their specific relation to the consequent adverse effects remains the most effective tool for making interspecies comparisons, conducting low-dose extrapolations, and increasing the predictive value of the risk assessment process.

3.1.6 CONCLUSIONS AND RECOMMENDATIONS

1. Dermal toxicology research should be encouraged to address percutaneous absorption, cellular proliferation, biochemical markers, and allergic and non-allergic reaction of skin to pesticides.

2. The ultimate goal of these approaches to increase the utilization of the recently developed scientific methods to assess the adverse effects of pesticide exposure is to reduce exposure and minimize the adverse human health effects of pesticide exposure. Nevertheless, prevention remains the best antidote for pesticide

poisoning, and innovative engineering (ultra-low volume aerosol techniques, use of granular formulations, and non-respirable pesticide spray generation) is a major determinant in reducing pesticide exposure.

3. Use of sophisticated techniques as biochemical markers (e.g., prostaglandins, leukotrines, phosphodiesterase, cyclic nucleotide, and calcium-dependent endonuclease) should be explored as measures of the impact of pesticide exposure on immune responses.

4. Data gaps exist in our understanding of neurotoxic, immunotoxic, and delayed morbidity and mortality contribution to acute pesticide exposure. Techniques must be developed to measure percutaneous absorption, cellular proliferation, and allergic reaction of skin; to detect and quantify immune responses (including the use of biochemical processes); to identify and quantify behavioural effects of acute exposures; and to search out possible pulmonary, cardiovascular, renal endocrine, haematological, and endocrine effects.

3.2 CHRONIC TOXICITY*

This section deals with the chronic deleterious effects of pesticide exposure. These effects may involve the delayed manifestations of short-term, high-dose exposure or be the outcome of continuous low-level exposure. For some compounds, both acute and chronic exposure involve the same target organ being affected predominantly and similar pathological lesions; however, the toxic potency is often quite different. For instance, short-term, high-level exposure to a carcinogen is generally far less effective at inducing tumours than continuous, low-level exposure for the same total lifetime doses.

This section focuses on four specialized areas in chronic toxicity: reproductive and developmental toxicity, genotoxicity, cancer, and target organ toxicity. Several factors are common to each area:

1. Route of exposure; effects may occur either at the site of initial contact with body tissues (as with some direct-acting carcinogens) or at some distant organ; the latter depends upon the extent of absorption at the initial site of contact and of metabolism.
2. Exposure to multiple chemicals, which collectively may produce interactions resulting in either additive, synergistic, or antagonist effects
3. Individual susceptability to toxic properties; this susceptability may play a role in the rates of absorption and metabolism, and differences in tissue responsiveness
4. Biotransformation and toxicokinetics, which influence the magnitude of effects per unit of dose and the degree of confidence in extrapolating between species.

---

*This section was prepared by R. Albert, R. Kroes, A. Lichacev, M. Mehlman, B. Ordonez, and B. Schwetz.

Knowledge of biotransformation and toxicokinetics of a chemical is vital, since it provides unique insight into mechanism(s) of action of a chemical and its metabolism in target organs. Toxicokinetics also provide a necessary understanding of the relationship between dose and toxicity. Accumulation in the body of pesticides and other chemicals greatly influences the ability of a substance to cause chronic injury; therefore, the extent of accumulation should be determined early in toxicity testing. The degree of tissue accumulation and the steady-state levels of lipophilic pesticides not biotransformed to hydrophobic metabolites define in part the duration of dosing in chronic toxicity tests.

Physiologically-based pharmacokinetic modelling is useful for risk assessments because it describes in quantitative terms the emporal behaviour of a chemical in various body compartments. Analysis of target sites for a parent compound and its metabolite(s) provides information with which to facilitate extrapolation among species, relying on empirically-derived correlations in various species.

3.2.1 REPRODUCTIVE AND DEVELOPMENTAL TOXICITY

The most frequently observed manifestations of reproductive toxicity caused by chemicals are abortions in females and infertility in males. The apparent frequency of these manifestations is due largely to the greater ease of detecting these adverse effects compared to other forms of toxicity. Manifestations of injury to embryonal and fetal development include malformations, decreased birth weight, mortality of the fetus or neonate, and functional changes observed in neonates. The nature of an adverse effect on reproduction and development depends on the chemical, amount and duration of exposure, age, stage of pregnancy, and pre-existing health status. Acute exposure is sufficient to cause significant risk for developmental toxicity because of the narrow 'time windows' of susceptibility. In contrast, repeated and prolonged dosing is more critical for risk of reproductive injury.

To date, most changes in human reproduction or development in humans have been detected initially via anecdotal information or case reports. For example, astute clinicians were largely responsible for the early detection of several noteworthy human teratogens—thalidomide, alcoholic beverages, diethylstilbestrol, and methyl mercury. The effect of dibromochlorpropane (DBCP) on male fertility was first recognized in humans by chemical workers sharing observations about their inability to have children. Many chemicals which are now recognized as human developmental toxicants were first identified as such in animal studies, and were subsequently confirmed in humans by case reports.

Surveillance records and birth defects registries hold promise for future identification of reproductive and developmental toxicants, but to be useful the databases must be much larger than they are today, and researchers must ask the correct questions to produce meaningful answers. Epidemiologic studies have been helpful to confirm chemicals as human developmental toxicants, but have had limited usefulness in their initial identification (Schardein et al., 1986).

3.2.1.1   Animal tests for reproductive toxicity

Adverse effects of chemicals on reproductive organs and function are detected by a variety of test methods. The most direct measurement is made from fertility trials that are part of reproduction studies. Single or multiple generation reproduction studies, having typically one or two sets of litters per generation, are most often conducted in mice and rats.

A protocol for reproductive assessment by continuous breeding of rats or mice, recently developed and validated by the National Toxicology Program in the United States, is another definitive test for reproductive toxicity. According to this protocol, mating pairs of rodents are housed together continuously for 100 days; observations include mean number of litters per mating pair, litter size, body weight, gross appearance, and time between litters. If an effect is noted in any evaluated endpoint, animals are cross-mated to determine whether the effect is transmitted by the male, the female, or both. In this continuous breeding study, rats and mice normally deliver between four and five litters during the period of cohabitation. The last set of litters is saved, raised to sexual maturity, and mated to determine fertility of the F_1 offspring.

A large decrease in sperm count can be tolerated by rodents without altering fertility, whereas human fertility is known to be affected by smaller changes in sperm count. Thus, the absence of an effect in rodent fertility does not preclude the possibility of an adverse effect of importance in humans, even though environmental levels of chemicals are typically much lower than the dose levels used in toxicity studies. The sensitivity of rodent reproduction studies is increased through the use of additional measurements on sperm and testis. Changes in testis weight, sperm motility, and sperm count have been found to be correlated positively with changes in fertility of rodents (Morrissey et al., 1988). Significant changes in these parameters, even in the absence of an adverse effect on rodent fertility, should be considered predictive of a potential effect on human fertility. Compared to the database for males, our knowledge of the effects of chemicals on reproductive mechanisms in female humans or animals is quite limited. Improved knowledge of normal performance is needed along with enhanced methods to detect adverse effects on reproductive organs and performance in females.

Studies other than those described above also provide useful reproductive toxicity data. Subchronic toxicity studies routinely include histopathologic examination of reproductive organs and measurement of testis weight. Dominant lethal studies, while designed to detect chromosomal damage in males which results in death of the conceptus of untreated females, also provide useful information on male fertility.

In addition to measurements of effects of chemicals on reproductive organs, function, and performance, another adverse effect of considerable consequence to reproduction is the induction of germ cell mutations. While mutations in somatic cells might lead to cancer, those in germ cells may lead to heritable changes of great pathological significance to the offspring. Studies such as the heritable translocation test, the specific locus test, and the dominant lethal test are the most definitive for germ cell mutations. A number of potent mutagens identified by short-term mutagenicity screens have also been shown to cause germ cell mutations.

3.2.1.2 Animal tests for developmental toxicity

The traditional measures of developmental toxicity in animals and humans include malformations, decreased body weight at birth, death of the embryo, fetus or neonate, and alterations of function. Many chemicals shown initially to be developmental toxicants or teratogens (i.e. inducing major structural malformations) in laboratory animals have later been demonstrated to cause the same effects in humans; many agents known to be developmental toxicants in humans act similarly in laboratory animals (with the exception of coumarin derivatives). Thus, chemicals which adversely affect the developing embryo or fetus of animals should be considered potentially toxic to developing humans.

The traditional screening test for developmental toxicity is designed similar to the protocol for the segment II study of the US Food and Drug Administration, a protocol which has changed only minimally over the past 25 years. Studies are conducted in rats, mice, rabbits or hamsters; exposure is generally during embryonal and early fetal development. In all species, fetuses are removed just prior to birth for examinations for external, visceral, and skeletal defects. These studies measure primarily effects on fetal structure, weight, and survival.

Supplemental studies, such as behavioural teratology studies, must be conducted to measure functional changes. In this type of protocol, animals are exposed during organogenesis; the offspring are permitted to be delivered, and are examined for developmental landmarks (tooth eruption, eye opening, vaginal opening, hair growth) and for specific behavioural attributes at various stages during their maturation (auditory and visual function, motor activity, learning skills). Protocols for other functional endpoints are not as well developed as for behavioural teratology.

Short-term *in vitro* tests for developmental toxicity are not used as routinely as genetic toxicity screens to predict carcinogenicity. Systems using cultured whole embryos or limb buds, insects, hydra, *xenopus* larvae, or cultured cells or organs have been evaluated; many of these systems, however, receive more use in mechanistic research than as screens or pre-screens for developmental toxicity. A short-term *in vitro* test first described by Chernoff and Kavlock (1982) and variations of this test are useful to anticipate the needs for reproductive and developmental toxicology tests (Hardin *et al.*, 1987).

3.2.1.3 Extrapolation from animals to humans

While developmental toxicants in humans produce similar responses in laboratory animals (with the exception noted above), animal studies are relatively ineffective at predicting the same type of response in humans (Schardein *et al.*, 1986). For example, from the chemical induction of cleft palate in mice, one cannot infer that the same compound will produce cleft palate in humans. A significant effect in any of the four major manifestations of developmental toxicity is considered sufficient to predict some potential adverse effect in humans. The dose level at which developmental toxicity occurs relative to the dose level at which maternal toxicity occurs is a critical determinant of the type of toxic response seen in another species; there is greater risk to humans from chemicals capable of causing developmental toxicity in the absence of maternal toxicity than from chemicals which are embryotoxic solely as a consequence of maternal toxicity. There are at least two reasons for this:

1. Except for accidents, exposure of humans is deliberately limited to avoid toxicity in adults; thus, for the latter type of chemicals, one would expect no developmental toxicity if exposure succeeds in avoiding maternal toxicity.
2. Chemicals that cause developmental toxicity in the absence of maternal toxicity provide no warning signs to the adult; therefore, the damage to the embryo is discovered only after it has occurred; the association between cause and effect is less likely to be discovered in a population where an adverse effect is occurring.

Many mechanisms exist by which chemicals can cause birth defects, but the critical insult which accounts for the adverse effect on the embryo is known for only a few chemicals. Mutagens are considered to account for very little developmental injury observed in humans (Schardein, 1985).

In contrast to carcinogenesis, developmental toxicity is considered for several reasons to be a process for which there is a threshold. Mutations are not necessary to cause developmental toxicity; most abnormalities are the result of interference with several critical events. Also, the plasticity of the developing embryo makes it very unlikely that a single event in a single cell would result in a recognizable birth defect. As a consequence, extrapolation from animal studies to humans has traditionally been based on some margin-of-safety (MOS) applied to the no-observed-adverse-effect level (NOAEL) in the most sensitive species of laboratory animal tested. A margin-of-safety of 100 or more is usually used, the actual value being selected on the strength of the scientific evidence and the nature of the human exposure to a given chemical.

Compared with that for developmental toxicology, less information is available regarding the agreement between animals and humans for reproductive toxicity. However, limited data are available which support the proposition that animal studies are predictive of at least the types of adverse reproductive effects seen in humans (Amann, 1982; Working, 1988).

The role of route of exposure on the causation of adverse reproductive or developmental toxicity has not been fully investigated; unquestionably these two forms of toxicity are the result of systemic dosing and not of a site-specific effect at a portal of entry into the body (such as may be the case for lung cancer or for dermatitis). Consequently, route of exposure is critical only to the extent that it determines the amount of an agent (parent or metabolite) absorbed into the blood.

Exposures to multiple developmental toxicants is as much a cause for concern as exposures to multiple toxicants with different target organs. The combined toxicity of most mixtures is described by additivity models. When interactive toxicity occurs, either potentiation or antagonism may result, and each is important for public health. Fortunately, each is the exception rather than the rule.

3.2.2 GENOTOXICITY

Historically, *in vivo* laboratory models were developed to detect alterations of transmitted genetic effects. Recently these tests have been directed at, and used as tools to predict, possible carcinogenicity in laboratory animals. By contrast, *in vitro*, short-term tests were further developed, and used as possible supplements or replacements for the identification of possible carcinogens. The introduction of a rapid bacterial test by Professor Bruce Ames has been the impetus for the investigation of possible genetic interactions that might be predictive of carcinogenicity. In a decade, important developments led to plant, microbial, or mammalian cells being used in numerous *in vitro* tests. Other short-term tests such as those aimed at detecting promoting properties (e.g., cell-to-cell communication and cell conductivity) are not discussed here, because this section is deliberately limited to methods to detect genotoxic activity *in vitro* and *in vivo*.

A drawback of *in vitro* tests is their inability to metabolize chemicals whose activity is dependent on initial biotransformation to active electrophilic metabolites that react directly with genes. This limitation was overcome partly by introducing subcellular fractions of liver homogenates to mimic effectively *in vivo* metabolism. Many chemicals require metabolic transformation to produce toxicity in an organism. Indeed, the development of reactive metabolites is believed to be the first step in chemical carcinogenesis, which is believed to be an irreversible alteration of the genome leading eventually to the formation of daughter cells that carry somatic mutations which may later become cancerous.

3.2.2.1 *In vitro* assays for genetic damage

Numerous plants and organisms have been suggested to detect genetic damage. Bacteria, yeast cells, or mammalian cells in culture have been used far more than have plants or plant cells. The *Salmonella* systems are the most frequently used as models for prokaryotes; mammalian or yeast cells are most widely representative of eukaryotes, which are closer phylogenetically to humans. Mouse lymphoma cells (L5178Y), hepatocytes *in vitro*, cultured Syrian hamster embryo (SHE) cells, and Balb/c 3T3 cells are used frequently. Since the cells are either devoid of, or deficient in, metabolic transformation, a liver homogenate must be added to provide that dimension. For most chemicals needing metabolic activation, the inclusion of metabolizing enzyme systems in these assays has been necessary to detect genetic damage. While the inclusion of a metabolic activation system has proven successful, such a system does not completely replace transformation *in vivo*.

In the *in vitro* assays a variety of endpoints can be examined, such as reverse and forward mutations, frameshifts and deletions, chromosome breaks and transpositions, sister chromatid exchanges, unscheduled DNA synthesis, and neoplastic transformations.

Since uncertainty exists concerning the mechanism(s) involved in the induction of neoplastic disease, certainty is low about which genetic toxicity test(s) may be most predictive for carcinogenesis. Therefore, a spectrum of *in vitro* tests that measure different endpoints of genetic toxicity have been proposed for use. Preferably, such a battery should include measurement of at least gene mutations, chromosomal mutations or damage, and DNA damage.

In the past decade, top priority has been given to validation of short-term tests and to the development of laboratory tools whose results could be reproduced around the world. The value of short-term tests for genetic damage as a prescreen for carcinogenicity is now well recognized. When first used, these tests appeared to demonstrate a high degree of concordance between genotoxicity and carcinogenicity. Later evaluations based on collaborative studies indicated far lower concordance. For non-genotoxic carcinogens, short-term tests for genotoxicity will, by definition, be negative. Presently, only chemicals likely to cause cancer by attacking DNA are capable of being identified with some precision using carefully selected short-term tests. On the basis of structure–activity analysis to identify sites on a chemical reactive with genetic material, a correlation (perhaps as high as 60 per cent) is said to exist between the results of the Ames-Salmonella assay and genotoxicity.

3.2.2.2   *In vivo* assays of genetic damage

In vivo assays are useful measures of genotoxicity for several reasons:

1. Metabolic transformation *in vitro* may not mimic transformation *in vivo* completely;
2. *In vitro* systems have serious toxicokinetic limitations which may be overcome *in vivo* systems;

3. *In vitro* genotoxicity provides only qualitative information with respect to possible carcinogenic properties, whereas *in vivo* genotoxicity may yield quantitative information;

4. Evidence of genotoxicity *in vitro* is not necessarily equated with evidence of genotoxicity *in vivo*, since a number of mutagens are not carcinogenic in long-term carcinogenicity tests.

As a consequence, when properly validated, *in vivo* mutagenicity assays may hypothetically replace some lifetime carcinogenicity tests.

In vivo tests for genotoxicity have been developed using insects and mammals, primarily rodents. Tests with insects, primarily with *Drosophila*, are relatively inexpensive and rapid. Large numbers of test subjects can be used; because of their relatively short lifespan and generation time, results of chronic exposure may be obtained within relatively brief periods of time. A disadvantage of the insect as a test model for humans is the often considerable difference in enzymatic mechanisms that activate and deactivate chemicals. Mice and rats are the mammalian species of choice. When only data from mice or rats are available, extrapolation of results to humans is necessary, despite the existence of numerous uncertainties, some of which are related to differences in toxicokinetics and biotransformation.

Several endpoints can be identified in the systems mentioned above. Whereas in *Drosophila* sex-linked recessive lethal mutation is the prime target of investigation, chromosomal aberrations and other discrete endpoints can also be studied. In animals, different cytogenetic effects can be studied, such as chromosome aberrations (including appearances of micronuclei), sister chromatid exchanges, and germ cell mutations. In addition, unscheduled DNA synthesis and adduct formation can be studied. DNA adduct formation seems to be a most promising assay for the detection of both genotoxic properties and unknown exposure to genotoxic chemicals in humans.

All genotoxic compounds including some pesticides bind covalently with cellular macromolecules, and form corresponding adducts with nucleic acids or proteins. Depending on the structure of adducts, various methods of monitoring are applicable.

1. Radiochemistry. Based on the monitoring of adducts by detection of radioactivity, this approach is applicable only in experimental systems which apply a pesticide containing a radioactive label in the electrophilic moiety of the molecule.

2. Spectrofluorometry. This method is sensitive, and can be used only if adducts fluoresce in the UV or visible spectrum.

3. Immunochemistry. This technique is very sensitive and applicable to the detection of adducts formed by reactions between an agent and its corresponding monoclonal and polyclonal antibodies. Modifications of this method depend on the structure of adducts formed.

4. ^{32}P-Postlabelling. This technique is currently the most sensitive method to detect DNA adducts. With this method, DNA is hydrolysed to nucleotides, its phosphorus is substituted by ^{32}P, and the presence of adducts in the hydrolysate is monitored by radiochromatography.

Immunochemical and postlabelling methods are the most relevant to detect adducts formed *in vivo* by pesticides. Immunochemistry also permits detection of adducts with either nucleic acids or proteins, whereas postlabelling detects adducts with DNA only. Adducts can be identified precisely only by comparing them with corresponding reference compounds; because the number of reference compounds available for postlabelling is limited, the number of adducts that can be identified is also limited.

For each type of method, the identification of adducts of interest is the greatest challenge, since only a fraction of them are believed to be biologically significant and even fewer adducts are highly specific and relevant to cancer induction.

3.2.2.3   Carcinogenic risk assessment using results of short-term tests

The overall correlation of short-term tests with carcinogenic potential of various compounds is estimated to be approximately 60 per cent, and application of a battery of short-term tests did not improve the correlation. However, the chemicals that cause cancer by reacting with DNA can be identified with some precision in short-term mutagenicity studies. Because non-genotoxic carcinogens exist, and because level of knowledge about the mechanisms of carcinogenesis is relatively incomplete, short-term genotoxicity testing for carcinogens cannot be a substitute for long-term testing.

Since many human carcinogens initiate cancer by means other than reaction with DNA (e.g., non-genotoxic agents which may induce cancer by processes such as stimulation of growth of dormant initiated cells, an action generically referred to as 'promotion'), short-term mutagenicity tests (e.g., point mutations, chromosome aberrations, germ cell mutations, SCE, and DNA adduct formation) are incapable of identifying them. To uncover such carcinogens, short-term tests for tumour promotors (e.g., cell-to-cell communication, cell conductivity) would be highly relevant.

3.2.3   CHEMICAL CARCINOGENESIS

Cancer is the second leading caue of death in industrialized countries. Epidemiological evidence (as demonstrated by different cancer patterns in various parts of the world and by the changing cancer patterns in migrants) exists indicating that environmental factors (including lifestyle) play a major role in cancer.

Pesticides are used widely. Some small populations receive rather high doses during the manufacture and application of pesticides; by contrast, large populations receive relatively low doses via residues in food, and by contamination of tap water from farm runoff and leaching from hazardous waste sites. Several pesticides produce tumours in animals, and so concern is widespread that the use of some pesticides may cause cancer in humans.

Epidemiological studies provide little evidence about the carcinogenicity of pesticides in humans, because suitable study populations are difficult to find. Except for arsenic, the dearth of direct evidence demonstrating that pesticides do or do not cause cancer in humans reflects in part a lack of adequate studies and the difficulties of epidemiological studies in establishing causal relationships. Therefore, claims that pesticides are or are not carcinogenic in humans are to be viewed with caution.

Cancer is a complex process, and its causes are poorly understood (Pitot, 1986). Years of observations have confirmed that cancer generally arises from single cells whose genetic structure and function have been irreversibly altered, with the resultant loss of control of normal growth. The nature of this genetic damage is poorly understood, although considerable progress has been made in recent years to clarify the role of oncogenes and antioncogenes in neoplastic transformation.

Cancers differ so markedly in their characteristics of differentiation, growth rate, and local and distant (metastatic) invasiveness, that one can only conclude that the normal growth control mechanisms must be exceedingly complicated. Knowledge of these changes is in a relatively primitive state. Cancer is also a progressive disease, such that tumours usually tend to evolve with time toward higher grades of malignancy at times after cessation of exposure.

The multistage nature of cancer has been described as follows:

1. initiation of neoplastic cells, which may progress to malignancies,
2. promotion of initiated cells into benign (non-invasive), grossly evident lesions, and
3. progression of benign lesions into malignancy.

This concept has led to the classification of carcinogenesis process into initiation, promotion, and progression. Some substances are complete carcinogens, having the properties of all three.

Carcinogens differ in the nature of their molecular interactions. So-called genotoxic carcinogens are either electrophilic *per se* (i.e., direct-acting) or are metabolized to an electrophilic form which permits them to interact with nucleophiles in cells, especially DNA. The sites of interaction of electrophiles with DNA are determined by complex chemical factors, which, in turn, determine the type and likelihood of mutations. DNA repair processes are important modifiers of the amount and duration of damage.

The complexity of carcinogenesis is indicated by the number of dissimilar classes of carcinogens: for example, polycyclic aromatic hydrocarbons, aromatic amines, nitroso compounds, direct-acting alkylating and cross-linking agents, metals, fibres, and hormones.

Although electrophilic or genotoxic carcinogens are the dominant class of known human carcinogens, a substantial number of agents are non-genotoxic, and yet have been shown to produce tumour in animals. Promoting agents generally fall into this class. Although there has been a general reluctance to regard genotoxic carcinogens as having a threshold response, there is a growing tendency to regard at least some non-genotoxic carcinogens as having a reversible mode of action and as more likely to have a threshold for cancer induction. The linear non-threshold dose–response relationship is generally adopted for genotoxic carcinogens.

3.2.3.1 Tests to identify chemical carcinogens and prospective carcinogens

The following approaches are used to determine whether a chemical causes cancer or can be judged as likely to cause cancer in a specified species. The approaches include structure–activity analysis, mutagenicity tests, lifetime exposures of laboratory animals, and human epidemiological investigations. Taken together, the findings of these analyses provide the basis for judging the scientific strength of conclusions regarding carcinogenicity and for applying the findings to the quantitative estimation of the magnitude of cancer response.

Structure–activity relationships

This approach attempts to link chemical structure with carcinogenic activity (Ennever and Rosenkrantz, 1989). In some cases, the relationship can be simple, as with direct acting alkylating agents. For instance, the powerful carcinogen *bis*-chloromethyl ether (BCME) was identified as a probable carcinogen before it had been studied in animals or exposed chemical workers on the basis of its being a bi-functional alkylating agent with cross-linking properties. In general, the correlation of chemical structure with mutagenic activity is much more highly developed than with carcinogens; however, a strong correlation exists between carcinogenesis and mutagenesis with genotoxic carcinogens. The structure–activity approach is inexpensive and rapid; however, it is insufficiently developed at present to be reliably used on a routine basis.

Mutagenicity assays

A detailed discussion of these relatively inexpensive, rapid, and widely used assays is found above. Genotoxic agents are very likely to be carcinogenic; however, the results give no reliable estimate of carcinogenic potency. Negative results of genotoxicity assays do not rule out conclusively the possibility that a substance may cause cancer (Tenant *et al.*, 1987).

Whole animal lifetime studies

Tumour induction in laboratory animals is the most relevant biological response to evaluate the carcinogenicity for humans (Sontag *et al.*, 1976). Previously, a standardized study was commonly performed under the following conditions: two doses (the current preference is three or four); both sexes; two species of rodent (e.g., F-344 rats and $B_6C_3F_1$ mice); dosing for 2 years in rats and 18 months in mice; and administration by gastric intubation, incorporation into feed or drinking water, or inhalation. The route of exposure was selected to closely simulate human exposure. These tests are quite costly (each about $500 000 (US)), and require almost five year to complete; consequently, only a limited number of agents can be tested.

Some responses in animals are difficult to relate to humans. Such questionable responses, for example, include the increased incidence of tumours at sites absent in humans, a shortening of the time before tumours occur with relatively high frequency, and the induction of mostly benign tumours unlikely to progress to malignancies. Nevertheless, for all their limitations, long-term animal studies are the mainstay of chemical carcinogen testing.

Epidemiology

This discipline is the most accurate indicator of human carcinogenicity, particularly when positive results are obtained consistently in multiple studies under various exposure conditions and with suitable control over confounding factors (Kalder and Day, 1985). However, epidemiology is relatively insensitive; even under ideal circumstances, it is incapable of detecting less than a 20 per cent increase in cancer. Stringent requirements exist for the execution of rigorous population studies: primarily, an adequate number of exposed subjects with appopriate controls are required, and both groups must be followed long enough to permit the expression and detection of carcinogenicity. Both positive and negative epidemiological studies are useful in quantitative risk assessment, since the negative studies set upper limits on a response. Because the number of agents studied adequately in humans is very limited, the lack of human evidence should not generally be taken as an indication of an absence of carcinogenicity.

Miscellaneous studies

A number of other tests have also been used occasionally to detect carcinogenicity; some are promising though still in the developmental stage. Initiation–promotion studies on mouse skin and in rat liver are used on a selective basis to determine whether an agent has promoting action. Since cancer promotion is organ-specific, other initiation–promotion models used in a limited way include mouse forestomach, bladder, intestine, and mammary gland. Even if the results of these tests were unequivocal, the interpretation of the findings remains complex and controversial. For example, dioxin* produces an excess tumour response in a standard long-term animal feeding study; it also shows strong promoting activity in the rat liver promotion assay. Does this mean that dioxin is only a promotor or could it be a whole carcinogen with strong promoting activity?

Other tests for promoting activity being developed include mammalian cell transformation assays and assays of cell-to-cell communication.

3.2.3.2 Risk assessment methodology

If a substance such as a pesticide is found to cause cancer, the estimation of cancer risks in humans can be undertaken using a framework promulgated by the US National Academy of Sciences (1983) and incorporating four steps that facilitate the analysis: hazard identification, dose–response assessment, exposure assessment, and risk characterization.

Hazard identification deals with the question of how likely the agent is to be a human carcinogen. A weight-of-evidence approach is used to evaluate the quality and quantity of evidence for carcinogenicity. Evidence from studies in rodents and humans are weighted most; but results of structure–activity relationships, short-term genotoxicity assays, and metabolic interactions with DNA are also relied upon. Similar weight-of-evidence schemes are employed by IARC and the US EPA (1986). There is a growing tendency to use alternative regulatory strategies for various grades of evidence.

Estimation of risks below the observed levels of response in animals or humans requires some mathematical model to extrapolate dose–response curves below the observation range. The dominant one in carcinogen risk assessment is the conservative linear non-threshold dose–response model, which implies that there is no risk-free dose above zero. However, the shape of the dose–response relationship is not verifiable by direct observation, and its plausibility depends on an understanding of the relevant aspects of the underlying carcinogenic mechanisms. The use of low-dose extrapolation is particularly uncertain for promotors that show evidence of reversible action. Mathematical models which depend on time patterns of tumour occurrence exist, and are being used to a limited extend in dose–response assessment.

Exposure assessment is one of the major sources of uncertainty in risk assessment with respect to ambient concentrations of pesticides to which individuals are exposed. Toxicokinetics are employed to define target tissue dose, although they are often hampered by a lack of understanding of which metabolite is the aetiologic agent.

Risk characterization combines the integrated dose† with the cancer potency value to obtain estimates of cancer risk as either excess numbers of cancers in an exposed population or excess lifetime risk to an exposed individual. The

---

*Dioxin is the abbreviated name for 2,3,7,8-tetrachlorodibenzo-*p*-dioxin or TCDD.
†For example, the lifetime-average-daily-dose or LADD.

The weight-of-evidence conclusion about carcinogenicity should be included with the risk estimates.

The risk estimates can be used for risk management solutions that may entail the value-laden determinations of acceptability of risks or the weighting of incommensurables such as risks versus benefits or lives versus financial profits.

3.2.4 TARGET ORGAN TOXICITY: LIVER

As a result of chronic exposure to chemicals, the liver may be injured in a variety of ways, such as degeneration, cell proliferation, necrosis, and induction or inhibition of various enzyme activities. The accumulation of lipids in a degenerated liver may have largely undesirable toxic effects in the organ. The herbicide metribuzin is known to cause hepatotoxicity through the process of depletion of glutathione from the liver.

Continued prolonged exposure to pesticides or herbicides at sufficiently high doses can result in accumulation of fat in the liver. This accumulation of lipids may also provide a storage site for these compounds. The accumulation of pesticides and lipid in the liver may result in the alteration of liver function, cell proliferation, necrosis, or some secondary effects which may be manifest as a variety of pathological consequences. In many cases, the damage in the liver results from biotransformation of the parent compounds to toxic metabolites, some of which can be potent mutagens or carcinogens.

Pesticides often undergo metabolic transformation in the liver; for example, DDT is converted to DDE or to DAA by different pathways, and the combined toxicity of the metabolites is considerably less than that of the parent compound (DDT). The observed hepatic tumour formation by chlorinated pesticides is generally caused by effects of metabolites rather than of the parent compound.

Two classes of methods are available to detect chronic toxicity from these substances in the liver: structural and functional. The structural methods involve histological examination of tissues by microscopic techniques specifically developed to measure the structural or compositional changes associated with exposure to these substances. The sensitivity of these procedures is usually limited by the availability of microscopy equipment and trained histopathologists.

In the liver, alkyl pesticides are known to induce a large number of enzymes, such as alkaline phosphatase, that can serve as indicators of biological responses when observing the toxicity of these substances. Key enzyme systems include cytochrome P_{450} monooxygenases, phosphoesterases, glutathione-S-transferases, and O-alkyl and O-aryl conjugation.

3.2.5 CONCLUSIONS AND RECOMMENDATIONS

1. Since genotoxicity tests show significant differences in response to various carcinogens, their utility for carcinogen prescreening is restricted to the qualitative detection of genotoxic activity. To varying degrees, such tests predict

possible carcinogenicity, but certainly do not define carcinogenicity. A relatively small proportion of genotoxic substances is not carcinogenic in animal assays, possibly because such substances, or their metabolites, are not absorbed or are effectively detoxified *in vivo*. Therefore, appropriate and validated short-term *in vivo* tests for genotoxicity are greatly needed.

2. Assuming that *in vivo* tests are more predictive for the outcome of long-term carcinogenicity tests than are short-term tests for genotoxicity, positive findings in the former tests may make the identification of carcinogens in long-term carcinogenicity tests unnecessary in the future.

3. Likewise, the development of short-term *in vitro* and *in vivo* assays for non-genotoxic carcinogens seems very appropriate. Cell transformation using various mammalian, including human, cell cultures as targets seems to be most relevant for predicting possible carcinogenic risk of certain pesticides because the endpoint (i.e., cell transformation) may result from both genetic and epigenetic events; that is, both DNA-reacting and non-reacting carcinogens may be detected. However, proper validation remains to be performed.

4. Although the results of genotoxicity tests are associated qualitatively with carcinogenicity, quantitative association is rather poor.

3.3   REFERENCES

Amann, R. P. (1982) Use of animal models for detecting specific alterations in reproduction. *Fund and Appl. Toxicol.* **2**, 13–26.

Baginsky, E. (1982) *Occupational Disease in California*, Division of Labour: Statistics and Research, California Department of Industrial Relations, San Francisco.

Chernoff, N. and Kavlock, R. J. (1982) An *in vivo* teratology screen utilizing pregnant mice. *J. Toxicol. Environ. Hlth.* **10**, 541–550.

Durham, W. F., Wolfe, H. R. and Elliot, J. W. (1972) Absorption and excretion of parathion by spray men. *Arch. Environ. Health* **24**, 381–7.

Echobichon, D. J., Hansell, J. and Safe, S. (1977) Halogen substituents at 4 and 4′ positions of biphenyl influence on hepatic function in rat. *Toxicol. Appl. Pharmacol.* **42**, 359–66.

Ennever, F. K. and Rosenkrantz, H. S. (1989) Application of the carcinogenicity prediction and battery selection method to recent national toxicology program short-term test data. *Environ. Molec. Mutagen.* **13**, 332–338.

Feldman, R. J. and Maibach, H. I. (1974) Percutaneous penetration of some pesticides and herbicides in man. *Toxicol. Appl. Pharmacol.* **28**, 126–132.

Franklin, C. A. (1984) Estimation of dermal exposure to pesticides and its use in risk assessment. *Can. J. Physiol. Pharmacol.* **62**, 1037–39.

Hardin, B. D., Becker, R. A., Kavlock, R. J., Seidenberg, J. M. and Chernoff, N. (1987) Overview and summary: workshop on the Chernoff/Kavlock preliminary developmental toxicity test. *Teratog. Carcinog. Mutagen.* **7**, 119–127.

Kalder, J. and Day, N. (1985) The use of epidemiological data for the assessment of human cancer risk. In: Hoel, D. G., Merrill, R. and Perera, F. P. (eds), *Risk Quantitation and Regulatory Policy*, Banbury Report 19, Cold Spring Harbor Laboratory.

Knox, J. M., Tucker, S. B. and Flannigan, S. A. (1984) Paraesthesia from cutaneous exposure to a synthetic pyrethroid insecticide. *Arch. Dermatol.* **120**, 744–746.

Morison, W. L., Parrish, J. A. and Woehler, M. E. (1981) The influence of ultraviolet radiation on allergic contact dermatitis in the guinea pig: 1 UVB radiation. *Br. J. Dermatol.* **104**, 161–4.

Morrissey, R. E., Schwetz, B. A., Lamb, J. C. IV, Ross, M. D., Teague, J. L. and Morris, R. W. (1988) Evaluation of rodent sperm, vaginal cytology, and reproductive organ weight data from National Toxicology Program 13-week studies. *Fund. and Appl. Toxicol.* **11**, 343–358.

National Academy of Sciences (1983) *Risk Assessment in the Federal Government*, National Academy Press, Washington, DC.

Pitot, H. (1986) *Fundamentals of Oncology*, Marcel Dekker Inc., New York.

Schardein, J. L. (1985) *Chemically Induced Birth Defects*, Marcel Dekker, New York.

Schardein, J. L., Schwetz, B. A. and Kenel, M. F. (1986) Species sensitivities and prediction of teratogenic potential. *Environ. Hlth. Perspect.* **61**, 55–67.

Sontag, J. M., Page, M. P. and Saffiotti, U. (1976) Guidelines for carcinogen bioassays in small rodents. Carcinogenesis Program, National Cancer Institute, DHEW Publication 16 (NIH) 76–801, 65pp.

Tennant, R. W., Margolin, B. H., Shelby, M. D., Zeiger, E., Haseman, J. K., Spalding, J., Caspary, W., Resnick, M., Stasiewicz, S., Anderson, B. and Minor, R. (1987) Prediction of chemical carcinogenicity in rodents from *in vitro* genetic toxicity assays. *Science* **236**, 933–941.

US Environmental Protection Agency (1986) Guidelines for carcinogen risk assessment. *CFR* **51**, 33992–34003.

Working, P. K. (1988) Male reproductive toxicology: comparison of the human to animal models. *Environ. Hlth Perspect.* **77**, 37–44.

Yonemoto, K., Gellin, G. A. and Epstein, W. L. (1983) Reduction in eumelanin by activation of glutathione reductase and gamma glutamyl transpeptidase after exposure to a depigmenting chemical. *Biochem. Pharmacol.* **32**, 1379–82.

4 Methods to Assess Toxic Effects on Ecosystems*

4.1 INTRODUCTION

Pesticide use has resulted in acute and chronic ecological damage either by direct injury to NTOs such as birds and fish or by indirect effects such as elimination of natural enemies; particularly long-lasting effects have included the depression or stimulation of reproduction in organisms. Methods exist to detect, prior to commercial application, the potential of a pesticide to damage NTOs such as wildlife species.

When designing methods to assess the ecological consequences of pesticides, several issues must be considered. Assessing the toxic effects of pesticides on ecosystems is difficult, because so many species and processes are interacting. When significant changes in important ecological parameters become apparent only after a long time period, they are frequently undetectable in short-term experiments. Natural variation in ecological parameters requires very sensitive measurements and sampling at high frequency. Furthermore, observations made in one location may not apply to other sites because of variation among ecosystems. Finally, highly managed ecosystems may be more or less sensitive to a pesticide than a more natural community in the same site.

Ecological consequences of pesticides can be studied at several levels:

1. Accidental pesticide contamination of the environment may provide clues about how populations might be affected at the lower recommended use levels.
2. Testing of sensitive species can indicate whether new biological or chemical pesticides will likely have side effects.
3. Relying on experimentally created plots, field studies can be designed to measure the effects of pesticides on ecological parameters such as species

---

*This section was prepared by T. Brown, C. Hagedorn, A. Johnels, G. Lacy, V. Landa, D. Peakall, D. Pimentel, T. Soldan, and J. Veleminsky.

Methods to Assess Adverse Effects of Pesticides on Non-target Organisms
Edited by R. G. Tardiff
©1992 SCOPE Published by John Wiley & Sons Ltd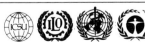

diversity, energy flow, decomposition, trophic structure on indicator or monitored species.

4. Laboratory experiments can be performed with individuals, populations, or model ecosystems constructed from combinations of species chosen to represent the numerous components of natural ecosystems.

Field experiments have detected pesticidal effects on interspecies relationships such as predation. Pest resurgence has been observed following applications of select pesticides that reduce natural enemy populations and subsequently increase pest populations. Such consequences may be anticipated from laboratory investigations that measure susceptibility of a pest of its known natural enemies. Methods that measure susceptibility and use various direct-dosing and self-dosing techniques have been developed, and are recommended against many public health and agricultural pests. Host resistance to pesticides decreases selectivity and effectiveness. Biochemical techniques are under development to rapidly detect and diagnose resistance in the field.

At the ecosystem level, the challenge is to determine whether pesticide use causes changes in viability. Field methods that exist for such ecological studies have been adapted to identify effects of pesticides, and have been applied most often to the soil biota portion of the ecosystem. Soil biota have been observed to be affected in a complex manner; that is, some species increase in numbers, while others are reduced by injury. Thus, long-term observation is required for such studies. Similar effects take place above ground and in a plant host. These findings imply that extensive sampling of the total ecosystem is necessary to obtain a thorough and balanced understanding of the nature and extent of pesticide alterations likely to be manifest.

To understand the effects of pesticides on ecosystems, it is necessary to examine a spectrum of effects from lethality to subtle changes on reproduction, behaviour, and vital organ physiology.

Responses may vary between closely related species or even 'biotypes' of a species, so that careful identification of test specimens is critical to learning much in depth about the genetic characteristics of the species of interest. This objective can be accomplished rapidly with newly developed molecular genetic techniques (e.g., restriction fragment length polymorphisms), so that at least the population genetics of organisms in experimental ecosystems can be taken into account.

Pesticides affect ecosystems by disrupting natural equilibrium; their effects can be observed by measuring the stability of populations, nutrient cycling, species diversity, interspecies food chains, primary production in and energy flow through trophic levels, and pollination. Some pesticides exert their effects on particular components of an ecosystem; for instance, some herbicides affect primary production in plants, and persistent organochlorine insecticides (such as DDT) bioaccumulate in higher trophic levels such as predators. Broad-spectrum OP and carbamate insecticides with high acute toxicity to many species may acutely alter energy flow as well as other ecological parameters.

Prediction and assessment of ecological impacts caused by pesticides alert humans to the dangers of some alterations to the environment. Ecosystems are integrated and stable systems; they include humans, all other species on this planet, and basic biotic and abiotic processes. Components of ecosystems cannot be changed or destroyed without directly or indirectly impacting the human condition. It is to humans' benefit to consider all uses and risks of pesticides to ensure preservation of critical systems in the environment.

4.2 TROUBLESOME PESTICIDES

With about 1000 pesticide formulations in use throughout the world today, the listing of all hazards to ecosystems would be enormous, particularly with most individual pesticides having different effects on various species. Clearly delineating these effects is complicated by the fact that there are 5–10 million species in the environment.

The United Nations offers a list of pesticides considered most hazardous to humans. While valuable, this list is limited, since it is restricted to acutely lethal doses in humans (based on studies in the rat and other laboratory species).

In general, insecticides generally are the most toxic pesticides to the environment, followed by fungicides and herbicides. Exceptions exist for certain herbicides which are highly toxic, and are far more hazardous to the environment than are insecticides. The most hazardous pesticides include those that can be distinguished on the basis of either water or fat solubility. Water soluble compounds are easily transported out of the target area into ground water and streams; fat soluble chemicals are readily absorbed in insects, fish, and other animals, often resulting in extended persistence in food chains.

Some of the most troublesome pesticides to the ecology are:

1. insecticides: DDT, dieldrin, diazinon, parathion, and aldicarb;
2. herbicides: 2-4-D, atrazine, paraquat, and glyphosate, and
3. fungicides: benomyl, captan, mercury, copper, and pentachlorophenol.

4.2.1 MAGNITUDE OF PESTICIDE APPLICATIONS

Approximately 5 million ton of pesticides are applied annually in the world, of which about 70 per cent is used for agriculture, and the remainder by public health agencies and government agencies for vector control and by home owners. Thus, agriculture and forestry are the primary source of pesticides in ecosystems. In many countries, agriculture and forestry occupy approximately 50 per cent of the land area. When croplands are treated, some impacts of pesticides occur on non-target terrestrial and aquatic ecosystems, as well as on adjoining agroecosystems.

Forests are important wildlife habitats. Two broad classes of pesticides are used in forests: insecticides to control insect pests, and herbicides used to suppress the growth of shrubs during the regeneration process. Over the last thirty-five years, two large-scale pest control programmes have been used in forests of eastern Canada and of the north-eastern United States in attempts to control spruce budworm; from 1980 to 1983 in Czechoslovakia, similar programmes were initiated to control the larch bud moth. In the latter programme, a mixture of pyriphosmethyl and permethrin eliminated many invertebrate species, but recovery was relatively rapid (Tonner *et al.*, 1983). In eastern Canadian forests, DDT caused fish mortality (Kerswill and Edwards, 1967) as a result of bioaccumulation through the food chain.

Extensive mortality of canopy-dwelling song birds has been observed with applications of phosphamidon and to a lesser extent, with fenitrothion; ground-nesting birds and small mammals were unaffected (Pearce *et al.*, 1976). Generally, the safety margin of OPs for canopy-dwelling birds is small. Indirect effects of decreasing the biomass of insect food would be expected to affect insectivores, but that has rarely been demonstrated.

The use of herbicides to control broad-leaf plant growth during regeneration alters habitat and food-availability, but is unlikely to have any direct effect except on plants.

Most of the wide variety of other natural ecosystems—ranging from alpine meadows to deserts—are rarely treated with pesticides. Exceptions are programmes to control specific pests. The largest of these are those to control quella and locusts. Quella are controlled largely by the use of OPs; some direct mortality of non-target bird species and some secondary mortality have been reported. Locust control has been carried out using dieldrin-containing bait and by spraying with OPs (i.e, diazinon and fenitrothion). Studies of effects on NTOs have rarely been made. Some direct mortality would be expected, but the residence time under desert conditions is likely to be short.

Around human habitation, pesticides are used heavily; but these areas are so altered that pesticides are unlikely to exert much additional effect. Exceptions are semi-natural areas such as parks and golf-courses. The use of insecticides on the latter can be heavy, and has resulted in mortality of birds and mammals. The use of DDT around human habitation for control of malaria is unlikely to have much impact on non-target organisms, although it adds to the overall burden of this persistent material.

4.2.2 APPLICATION TECHNOLOGIES

The manner in which pesticides are applied is influential in determining the nature and magnitude of injury that may occur in ecological species. Likewise, this process also greatly impacts the effectiveness of pesticides.

According to some estimates, less than 0.1 per cent of all pesticides applied reach the target pests. If so, then a large fraction of applied pesticides may be available to contaminate water, soil, and atmosphere and may disrupt non-target species.

One reason for the small amounts of pesticides that actually reach target pests is the requirement that plant surfaces be thoroughly covered with pesticides to control small arthropods (e.g., aphids and mites) and plant pathogens (fungi and bacteria). To achieve this thorough coverage of plant surfaces requires that sprayed particles be extremely small, a situation that favours dissemination by gentle winds for distances of several thousand meters.

Achieving coverage of crop plant surfaces with pesticides is part of the problem, as is placing the pesticides into the target area. Under ideal conditions using aircraft, for instance, less than 50 per cent of the pesticide applied by aircraft reaches the target crops. With ultra-low-volume sprays (ULV) by aircraft, drift is even more extensive, placing less pesticide in the target area. Under ideal weather conditions, less than 25 per cent of the ULV-applied pesticide reaches the target. Likewise, most drifts often contaminate untreated terrestrial and aquatic ecosystems. Large quantities of pesticides are applied to orchards, vineyards, and similar crops by employing air blast sprayers. Only about 65 per cent of the pesticide applied by use of this equipment reaches the target area, whereas 35 per cent goes elsewhere.

Ground application equipment under normal weather conditions often place 70–80 per cent of the sprayed pesticide into the target area. If, at the same time, a 'plastic blanket' were used to protect the crop and spray boom, perhaps 90 per cent or more of the pesticide could be placed in the target area.

The physical form of pesticide formulations (i.e., wick, dust, granule, and chemigration technologies) greatly influences the extent to which a pesticide will be placed on the target site and be distributed elsewhere. One of the best means of placing pesticides on the target pests is illustrated with herbicides using the 'wick' technology. A wick that has been wetted with the herbicide is drawn over the vegetation in a field. No drift occurs, and the herbicide is placed directly on the weeds without drift problems.

Dusts are highly susceptible to drift because of their extremely low weight. Seldom does 50 per cent of the applied dust remain in the target area when using ground equipment, even under ideal wind conditions.

Granules have become a popular means of applying dry insecticide materials to the surface of croplands and pasture lands. However, granules pose major problems to non-target pests, particularly birds. Birds mistake the granules for gravel, and may consume them with disastrous results.

Some pesticides can also be effectively applied in irrigation water; this practice is referred to as 'chemigration'. Although this is an effective, easy method of applying pesticides to agricultural crops, it is also a means of spreading pesticides in the environment and of poisoning non-target species. In particular, it can contaminate the drinking water of birds, mammals, invertebrates, and humans. Ground and surface waters are also readily contaminated by chemigration.

Clearly, the need exists to improve pesticide application technology to assure that more pesticide reaches the target points and to reduce hazards to human and ecosystem NTOs. Finding the means to place more pesticide on target pests should not be difficult.

4.2.3   SPECIES AT RISK

Invertebrate NTOs are often killed by pesticides used against insects and acarine target pests. The susceptibility of NTOs, such as crustaceans, is due to the similarity of their physiological sites of action among target insects and certain non-target invertebrates; for example, AChE enzymes, octopamine receptors, and moulting processes are all similar insecticide targets in both pest and invertebrate NTOs. Terbufos, chlorpyrifos, and carbofuran are important insecticides for controlling corn rootworm larvae in soil; however, both terbufos and carbofuran are highly toxic to earthworms. Foliar applications of broad spectrum insecticides produce nearly total depletion of arthropod populations in crops such as cotton. While selectivity for herbivorous pests can be gained through systemic insecticides, some of these insecticides, such as aldicarb and oxamyl, are extremely toxic; thus, secondary poisoning can result in predators of treated pests.

Some selectivity of insecticides can be achieved. For example, the insect development-inhibitor methoprene controls mosquito larvae at doses not toxic to most NTO aquatic invertebrate species. Substrains of *Bacillus thuringiensis* are selective for certain insects in a given taxonomic order: *B.t. israeleasis* for mosquito larvae and *B.t. kurstaki* for lepidopterous larvae. Some herbicides and fungicides also affect NTO invertebrates, although they are the exceptions. Bipyridilium herbicides have a non-selective cytotoxic action, as do dinitrophenol pesticides which uncouple oxidative phosphorylation.

For pesticide registration, data are required about toxicity to representative invertebrates such as *Daphnia magna*, earthworms, and decapod crutaceans. Test protocols are specified by various national and international organizations such as the US EPA, OECD, and FAO.

Microorganisms are most susceptible to fungicides and bactericides aimed at target plant pathogens in the field. Some herbicides are effective against both fungi and bacteria by producing the same molecular lesions in each. In general, microorganisms lack the physiological and molecular targets (e.g., AChE and photosynthetic pathways) that render them susceptible to insecticides and herbicides. Insecticides and herbicides can deplete the insect and plant hosts of microorganisms.

Microorganisms are very important in the environmental detoxification and decomposition of pesticides. Soil ecosystems can change because of the enhanced capacity of select soils to degrade pesticides, as observed in the loss of effectiveness developed in certain soils after 10 to 20 years of continuous pesticide use. Some fungicides are known to interfere with the detoxification of

OP insecticides in the soil, adding significantly to the energy flow of ecosystems which may affect species composition at lower trophic levels.

4.2.4 EFFECT AT INDIVIDUAL AND POPULATION LEVELS

Ecosystems, whether plant or animal, can suffer from accrued damage to individuals. As an illustration, the complexities of such interactions among plants is described.

4.2.4.1 Plants

Plants are exposed to pesticides, whether as target organisms or as NTOs such as pathogenic fungi. The routes of contact include the uptake from soil and water and deposition via atmospheric drift.

Toxic and mutagenic effects and changes in the metabolism of plants (including formation of metabolites and residues capable of producing adverse effects) can be observed in NTO plants, even with quantitative and qualitative differences resulting from variations in plant sensitivity, and with the numerous metabolic pathways of pesticide degradation. Differential sensitivity of plant species to toxic and genotoxic effects of pesticides has been shown to cause overall changes in species proportion among weeds in croplands and in natural plant communities, because of the reduced abundance of susceptible species and concurrent increases in naturally tolerant species. However, neither the eradication of a susceptible species nor the occurrence of a new plant species has been established in the experimental plots even after long-term (36 years) spraying with formulations such as the herbicide 2,4-D.

The emergence among susceptible plant species of forms resistant to herbicides has become increasingly important. Pesticides can play a dual role as agents favouring the selection of pre-existing resistant mutants and as potential inducers of genetic changes. Genotoxic pesticides are potentially able to increase the pool of mutations in various qualitative and quantitative traits that could cause genetic instabilities of natural plant populations and in crop varieties.

Elements related to possible ecological damage include the formation of stable mutagenic and toxic metabolites and the accumulation of residues in plants that can be harmful to both human and animal populations via exposure through the food chain. This problem needs to be addressed despite the fact that in plants bound residues formed and incorporated into lignin, hemicellulose, and other carbohydrate components of the cell wall are usually less hazardous to the biosphere.

Pesticides have produced changes in both plant metabolism and nutritional patterns which may have further detrimental effects on the ecology. Several mechanisms are known to lead to this consequence.

1. Some herbicides, when applied at recommended dosages, have increased the attacks of insect pests and plant pathogens on crops. For example, when corn-growing areas were treated with 2,4-D at the recommended dosage of 1 kg/ha, the numbers of corn leaf aphids increased three-fold; corn borers were 26 per cent more abundant, and were 33 per cent larger than those insects present on untreated corn. Larger corn borers produce one third more eggs, and thus contribute to the build-up of corn borers on corn.

2. The insecticides monocrotophos and phosphamidon increased concentrations of nitrogen and phosphorus in rice plants, and these changes were thought to contribute to a resurgence in the numbers of the rice blue leafhopper.

3. Herbicides may increase damage due to plant pathogens. For instance, when corn was treated with a recommended dosage of 2,4-D (1 kg/ha), black corn smut grew five-fold larger than on untreated corn. Also, corn that was resistant to southern corn leaf blight lost its resistance to the blight when treated with 2,4-D.

4. Most nutrients, especially C, K, N, P, and S, are taken up by plants that, in turn, may be eaten by animals. These nutrients are eventually returned to the soil or atmosphere via decomposition of dead organisms. The amounts and forms of nutrients in soils and plants may be changed by pesticides, thereby altering the dynamics of these animals in the ecosystem.

5. Pesticides can alter the chemical make-up of plants. The changes that occur appear to be specific for both the plants and pesticides involved. For example, certain organochlorine insecticides have increased the amounts of some macro- and micro-elements (Al, B, Ca, Cu, Fe, K, Mg, Mn, N, P, Sr, and Zn) of corn and beans. DDT, aldrin, endrin, and lindane have stimulated synthesis of the essential amino acids arginine, histidine, leucine, lysine, proline, and tyrosine in corn, but have decreased the content of tryptophan. The herbicide simazine increased water and nitrate uptake in barley, rye, and oat seedlings, resulting in increased plant weight and total protein content.

Increasing insect pest and plant pathogen attacks on crops by using some herbicides may, in turn, lead to an increase in spraying of additional pesticides, like insecticides and fungicides. Thus, the environmental problem arising from the use of herbicides may involve more than just the herbicide itself.

Methods are available to detect both non-genotoxicity and genotoxicity of pesticides in plants, including their effects on plant reproduction. The toxic effects of pesticides have been measured in plants growing in separated experimental plots using endpoints such as frequency of species and individuals in each species, survival of plants, fresh and dry weight of plants at the harvest, and seed setting. Cytogenetic analyses of mitotic cells in roots and shoots, meiotic cells in pollen mother cells, and postmeiotic cells in pollen represent the most frequently used methods to detect genetic changes caused in natural plant populations and communities or in plants growing in the field. Special plant assay systems are also available to monitor genotoxicity *in situ*.

About 150–160 pesticides have been tested on plant genotoxicity assay systems. About 90 per cent of the test agents produced some kinds of changes in the chromosome structure, about 60 per cent caused disturbances in the meiosis and seedset reduction, and about 70 per cent caused gene mutations. Compared with other assay systems (e.g., microbial cells, mammalian cell cultures, insects, and whole animals), plant assays appear to be the most efficient to detect pesticide-related genotoxicity. Seasonal variation in cytogenetic endpoints have been correlated with the application of herbicide mixtures.

4.2.4.2 Animals

The more obvious effects of pesticides (i.e., reproductive failure caused by DDT and mortality caused by OPs and carbamates) have, so far, been the basis of concern and regulatory action.

The major adverse effects of organochlorine (OC) pesticides have been manifested through effects on reproduction. DDT has caused eggshell thinning in several high trophic level avian species and sufficient impact on reproduction to result in population declines (Risebrough, 1986). Likewise, the effects on fish occurred largely during the reproductive cycle (i.e., at the time that the yolk sac was absorbed) (Burdick et al., 1967).

By contrast, the major effect of OPs and carbamates has been direct mortality. The mechanism of action of these insecticides is the inhibition of AChE activity which causes the disruption of nerve function. Acute inhibition of 80 per cent and chronic inhibition of 50 per cent has been associated with mortality (Ludke et al., 1975; Hill and Fleming, 1982). Other esterases are also inhibited, and the inhibition of brain neurotoxic esterase (NTE) has been related to delayed neuropathy (Johnson, 1975). Lotti and Johnson (1978) compared the toxicity of inhibition of AChE and NTE for a range of OPs. The ratio of inhibition of the two enzymes varies over several orders of magnitude, but the degree of inhibition of AChE correlates well with the LD_{50} and that of NTE with delayed neurotoxic damage. For those pesticides causing neurotoxic effects, inhibition of NTE can be one to two orders of magnitude more sensitive than that of AChE.

The relationship between dosage of the pesticide and degree of inhibition of AChE has been used to assess the impact of insecticide spray programme on forest songbirds (Mineau and Peakall, 1987). The data show a severe collection bias in favour of birds with inhibition of the enzyme of less than 30 per cent. This manifestation is probably due to behavioural effects on birds having AChE inhibition greater than this value.

Since behaviour is the result of integration of many inputs, it has long been considered as a potentially sensitive indicator of pesticide toxicity (Warner et al., 1966). For OPs, behavioural alterations are demonstrated only at AChE inhibition of 40–50 per cent (Grue et al., 1982; Rudolph et al., 1984). The conclusion that behavioural effects are not particularly sensitive has been confirmed by a review of the effects of toxic chemicals on birds (Peakall, 1985). While it can be stated that behavioural changes will reduce an organism's ability to survive in the wild, little direct evidence exists to confirm this hypothesis. In some cases, predation experiments have been conducted in the laboratory (Brown *et al.* 1985); there remains a major extrapolation to field conditions. Furthermore, in this experiment a significant increase in predation was not seen until the concentration equivalent to half the LD_{50} was used.

4.2.5 MEASURES OF EFFECTS ON STRUCTURE AND FUNCTION OF ECOSYSTEMS

Terrestrial and aquatic ecosystems are generally self-sufficient basic living units of nature that include a complex of species dependent on one another, and interacting with the physical-chemical environment. Pesticides may alter the structure (species richness, density, and biological diversity) and functional activities of an ecosystem. Pesticides may alter the self-sufficient nature of natural ecosystems that include plants (producers), herbivores, parasites and predators, and decomposers*.

Some pesticides are capable of destroying some species totally or of significantly reducing the populations of others. When the diversity of the ecosystem is reduced sufficiently, then food chains may be shortened or altered in diverse ways. When food chains are changed, the stability of ecosystems may be reduced, leading a susceptible ecosystem to extinction by a variety of mechanisms such as invasion by other complexes of species.

A critical component of all ecosystems is energy flow. Plants collect energy from the sun for growth, metabolism, and reproduction. Energy fixed by the plants eventually becomes available to herbivores and other species that make up the ecosystem. The more energy the plants collect, the more productive, diverse, and complex is the ecosystem. In aquatic ecosystems, eutrophication—a form of energy cycling—may enhance or limit diversity. If a pesticide influences the growth of the plant populations, then the food/energy supply for the ecosystem is reduced, lowering its productivity and stability.

Another essential component of an ecosystem is the decomposition of organic matter. The basic elements (e.g., C, Ca, H, K, Mg, Mn, N, O, P) are vital to the proper functioning of all life, including ecosystems. Thus, the decomposers are essential to keep the vital nutrients in circulation for use and reuse by an ecosystem.

Some essential nutrients are in the atmosphere. Plants and other organisms may obtain some essential elements (C, H, O, N) from the atmosphere for use throughout an ecosystem. Other nutrients may be obtained directly from soil or water, and are cycled through the biota. Pesticides may be capable of reducing

---

*Decomposers are organisms (microbes, earthworms, insects, etc.) responsible for the decomposition of organic compounds other than their nutrients.

the variability of one or more organisms involved in the recycling process in an ecosystem. If this occurs to a large extent in an ecosystem, it may function at such a reduced rate as to threaten the entire web in the ecosystem.

Methods to quantify ecological effects of pesticides on terrestrial and aquatic ecosystems are generally complex and costly, the magnitude and complexity being dependent on the nature of the pesticides and on the characteristics of the particular terrestrial and aquatic ecosystem in which pesticide is used.

Presently, ecosystem parameters are not among those data developed prior to registration of pesticides in most countries. The effects on two ecosystem components seem most urgently to require assessment prior to pesticide registration: these are the effects on the trophic structure (plants, herbivores, parasites, and predators), and on decomposer organisms, because of the unique vulnerability demonstrated by these components for ecosystem integrity and survival.

Any new pesticide, whether biological or chemical, should first be assessed for ecosystem effects in the particular agroecosystem of proposed primary use (e.g., an apple orchard or a cotton field). This approach requires the measurement of population dynamics for a representative number of resident species in addition to the target pests and their natural enemies. The number of species to be sampled should be in proportion to the complexity of the agroecosystem of interest. Effects on decomposers can be determined by cellulosic sampling by litterbag methods, for a minimum of three growing seasons.

4.3 RECOMMENDATIONS

Non-chemical pest controls, such as biological, cultural, and environmental controls and host plant resistance, should be improved and used in order to reduce pesticide use.

4.4 REFERENCES

Brown, J. A., Johansen, R. H., Colgan, P. W. and Mathers, R. A. (1985) Changes in the predator-avoidance behaviour of juvenile guppies (*Poecilia reticulata*) exposed to pentachlorophenol. *Can. J. Zool.* **63**, 2001–2005.

Burdick, G. E., Harris, E. J., Dean, H. J., Walker, T. M., Shea, J. and Colby, D. (1964) The accumulation of DDT in Lake Trout and the effect on reproduction. *Trans. Amer. Fish Soc.* **93**, 127–136.

Grue, C. E., Powell, G. V. N. and McChesney, M. J. (1982) Care of nestlings by wild female Starlings exposed to an organosphosphate pesticide. *J. Appl. Ecol.* **19**, 327–355.

Hill, E. F. and Fleming, W. J. (1982) Anticholinesterase poisoning of birds: field monitoring and diagnostic of acute poisoning. *Environ. Toxicol. Chem.* **1**, 27–38.

Johnson, M. K. (1975) The delayed neuropathy caused by some organophosphate esters: mechanism and challenge. *Crit. Rev. Toxicol.* **37**, 113–115.

Kerswill, C. J. and Edwards, H. E. (1967) Fish losses after forest spraying with insecticides in New Brunswick, 1952–1962, as shown by caged specimens and other observations. *J. Fish Res. Bd. Canada* **24**, 709–729.

Lotti, M. and Johnson, M. K. (1978) Neurotoxicity of organophosphate pesticides: predictions can be based on *in vitro* studies with hen and human enzymes. *Arch Toxicol* **41**, 215–221.

Ludke, J. L., Hill, E. F. and Dieter, M. P. (1975) Cholinesterase (ChE) response and related mortality among birds fed ChE inhibitors. *Arch. Environ. Contamin. Toxicol.* **3**, 1–21.

Mineau, P. and Peakall, D. B. (1987) Review: an evaluation of avian impact assessment techniques following broadscale forest insecticide sprays. *Environ. Toxicol. Chem.* **6**, 781–792.

Peakall, D. B. (1985) Behavioral responses of birds to pesticides and other contaminants. *Residue Rev.* **96**, 45–77.

Pearce, P. A., Peakall, D. B. and Erskine, A. J. (1976) Impact on forest birds of the 1975 spruce budworm operation in New Brunswick. *CWS Progress Note #61.*

Risebrough, R. W. (1986) Pesticides and bird population. *Current Ornithology* **3**: 397–427.

Rudolph, S. G., Zinkl, J. G., Anderson, D. W. and Shea, P. J. (1984) Prey-capturing ability of American Kestrels fed DDE and acephate and acephate alone. *Arch. Environ. Contamin. Toxicol.* **13**, 367–372.

Tonner, M., Vavra, V., Syrovatka, O. and Soldan, T. (1983) Einfluss der Luftbespritzung genen grauen Larchenwicker (*Zeiraphera diniana*) auf die Entomofauna des Rhithrons in Krkonose (Riesengebirge). *Vest. Cs. Spol. Zool.* **47**, 293–303.

Warner, R. E., Peterson, K. K. and Borgman, L. (1966) Behavioural pathology in fish: a quantitative study of sublethal pesticide toxication. *J. Appl. Ecol.* **3**, (Suppl), 223–247.

5 Management Technologies: Integrated Pest Management

Integrated management strategies have as their goal providing maximum economic yields to the farmer, while improving or maintaining the production site and protecting the environment. Examples of integrated pest management (IPM) procedures to improve economic yields while reducing inputs include: the integration of pesticides with cultural techniques for disease control; and biological, behavioural, and environmental controls of pests such as weeds. Biotechnology promises to have a major impact on IPM through the use of recombinant DNA techniques to genetically engineer microbes for the control of diseases, insects, and weeds, and to generate plants that resist insects, pathogens, and herbicides. Examples of each management procedure follow:

1. Cultural controls: crop variety selection or host-plant resistance, double cropping and/or crop rotation patterns, minimum or reduced tillage, use of organic fertilizers, and prescription pesticide application.
2. Biological controls: natural pathogens or predators of insects and weeds. Several cultural techniques mentioned above (such as variety selection) relate directly to biological control.
3. Behavioural controls: release of sterile insects, pheromone traps, and development of lethal natural products that attract insects. These techniques have only recently received attention in IPM; they relate to pest behaviour modification based on insect communication.
4. Biotechnology: microorganisms with novel features that are currently impacting IPM strategies include viruses and bacteria that were developed for control of insects, weeds, and/or fungal pathogens. These practices are likely to impact substantially on IPM procedures regarding the development of plants having novel characteristics such as herbicide tolerance and insect resistance.
5. Environmental controls: alterations of soil pH, moisture status, use of topography, temperature, and light intensity are among the environmental approaches. However, such manipulations are difficult to perform. While closely related to cultural practices, environmental controls relate to alterations in the physical environment to maintain yields and reduce stress.

Methods to Assess Adverse Effects of Pesticides on Non-target Organisms
Edited by R. G. Tardiff
© 1992 SCOPE Published by John Wiley & Sons Ltd

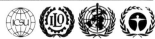

Finally, an excellent opportunity exists to introduce expert systems and computer-aided decision-making processes into IPM strategies. Many different IPM options should be assembled into a stepwise approach that evaluates each practice, and recommends the most appropriate choice. The best options for a specific cropping system will always depend on the probability that desired results will occur; thus, computerized applications are an obvious choice for future IPM planning and implementation.

5.1 CULTURAL CONTROLS

Cultural methods can be modified by using knowledge of the ecology of cultivated plants for control of diseases, insect pests, and weeds. The five major ones are as follows.

Early planting

Sowing crops over the winter provides a plant that is more physiologically active at an earlier period than plants sown in the spring. Accelerated crop-growth in the spring may break the plant-damaging cycle of key pests at cenoses and thus avoid the disease-susceptible stages of the crop. As an example, short season cotton has been incorporated effectively into IPM programs for cotton farming in Texas (USA) to control the boll weevil and pink bollworm. Similarly, fall sowing of sugar beets decreased damage caused by pests and diseases, including beet yellow disease and mildew of beet.

Late planting

This technique may uncouple plant–pest synchronization. For example, if wheat is sown late, it is less likely to be attacked by Hessian flies that emerge in the spring.

Crop rotation

Sequential crop rotation may be used to reduce insect pests, plant pathogens, and weeds. Maintaining crop rotation in alternate years or at other intervals can effectively control pests. For example, planting sugar beets decreases the effects of weeds, diseases, and pests that survive in the soil and on crop debris. Crop rotation provides an inexpensive control for important weed species such as *Avena fauna* and *Elytrigia repens*, as well as for pests such as eelworms and for diseases like black leg.

Soil cultivation

Cultivation can achieve a plentiful harvest by acting as an effective control for late infestations of weed and diseases that would lower the sowing density of emergent plants. However, if the sowing density of seeds per unit area is too low, the risk of damage from other pests increases. For example, if a sugar beet crop is planted at too low a density, then the crop can be attacked more frequently by aphids.

Reproductive control of pests

Technology is available to reduce the reproductive success of pests. The normal reproductive process of pests is affected more by simple, biologically effective agrotechnical operations, and less by chemical means. For example, such techniques have been used experimentally for control of *C. pomonella* and *C. molesta*.

Crop variety selection for resistance to insect and plant pathogens

For example, the technique has been employed against the Hessian fly and cabbage yellows.

5.2 BIOLOGICAL CONTROLS

Biological control is agricultural management using a biological agent to reduce the impact of a specific pest or pathogen. These methods include numerous procedures such as production and introduction of insect or weed parasites, predators, and pathogens into the agreocosystems. Alternative methods include the use of pesticides that do not reduce a natural population of indigenous biological control agents and the development of more vigorous, pesticide-resistant plants, and microbes that foster plant productivity. Much recent research has focused on the use of microbes that either enhance plant development or protect plants from chemicals, pathogens, or pests. Plants and organisms used for biological control may also have the ability to cause environmental injury either through careless development or by self-replication in a susceptible environment.

Research and development projects aimed at biocontrol and utilized in IPM are:

1. Mechanisms of biocontrol, such as parasitism, antibiosis, competition, stimulation of plant defences, or a combination of these factors;
2. Ecology of biocontrol agents, such as suppressive soils, physical and chemical environmental factors, composition of the soil microflora, interspecific competition, saprophytic competence, and plant stimulating or repressive effects, and
3. Formulation of biocontrol agents, such as delivery systems, carrier development, and application technology.

5.3 BEHAVIOURAL CONTROLS

Behavioural controls utilize some chemicals to modify insect pest behaviour, and control pests without the use of toxins, thereby playing an important role in area-wide control systems. At present, behavioural modification methods (e.g., pheromones) have been used to confuse or trap the male population. This technique has been applied successfully for control of *Pestinophora gossypiella* in cotton, *Cydia pomonella* in apple orchards, and *Eupoecillia ambiquella* in vineyards. These methods are not effective with extremely large insect pest populations.

Recently, chemists and entomologists have focused on relationships between plants and insects, with the aim of altering insect–plant communications (i.e., antifeedants, plant attractants, and plant repellents) with chemical behaviour mediators. A series of possibilities includes reducing the success of female insects in finding plant hosts, altering reproductive physiology, or both. Attractants have also been developed to capture female insect pests; for example, in vineyards some weed plants are more attractive to female European grape vine moths. This approach may form the basis for removing female populations that cause damage by generating offspring that directly damage commercial crops.

The visual orientation and colour preference of insects may also be used for effective control. Whitefly populations in greenhouses, cherry fruit flies in cherry orchards, and sarfly in plum orchards—each has been controlled effectively employing colour attractants.

5.4 IMPACT OF BIOTECHNOLOGY ON IPM

Microbial biocontrol agents are equipped to survive and to perform the role that nature has intended. However, providing high levels of disease control in genetically uniform crops exposed to massive quantities of pathogen inoculum is not equivalent to natural evolution. Characteristics of some possible benefit to an organism in the natural state may be of little use or even detrimental when employed in agriculture. The tailoring of biocontrol agents to meet the requirements of current agricultural practices will most likely entail genetic alteration of those microbes. Although lagging somewhat behind the advances made in the genetic manipulation of bacteria, this process has already begun in fungi.

Several researchers have used mutants of biocontrol agents, either to understand mechanisms in the biocontrol process or to enhance the efficacy of a biocontrol agent. The difficulty in making mutant fungi is that mutagenesis is a relatively non-specific process: all too often, silent mutations are made in addition to the desired ones. A mutant strain may perform well when assayed for a given trait *in vitro* (such as antibiotic resistance or antibiotic production), but it may be unable to sustain itself in nature, because other undetected and later expressed mutations may make it less competitive.

5.5 FUTURE PROSPECTS FOR BIOCONTROL

Research on biocontrol has provided a wealth of information, not the least of which is how little we know about this phenomenon. If successful strategies for biological control of plant diseases are to be developed, much research needs to be aimed at the following questions:

1. What mechanisms are responsible for the observed effects of biocontrol agents on plant pathogens?
2. How do biotic and abiotic environments alter the viability and metabolism of biocontrol agents, and the mechanisms involved in the biocontrol process?
3. What genes are responsible for the production of biocontrol mechanisms? Can these genes be isolated, transferred, and expressed in other genomes?
4. Will genetic manipulation of biocontrol agents result in superior biocontrol strains?
5. How can biocontrol agents be mass-produced most efficiently, economically, and safely?
6. What are the most effective formulations for storage, application, and activity of biocontrol agents?
7. What are the optimum timings, frequencies of application, and treatment concentrations for biocontrol agents?
8. How readily can biocontrol agents be integrated in agriculture with other means of disease control and with crop production practices?

With definitive responses to these questions, agriculture will probably be able to make practical and economic the use of fungal and other agents to control plant diseases. The biocontrol agents alone or in combination with other means of disease control may achieve this end.

Research on population ecology and genetics of parasite–host and predator–prey systems has provided new and exciting information for the control of insect pests and weeds. Authoritative responses to the following questions would probably improve substantially the value of biological pest control.

1. How can 'new association' parasites (predators) from related hosts of the pest species be selected to obtain successful biocontrol agents that will provide effective, permanent control of insect pests and weeds without further manipulations?
2. Relative to 'new associations', how important are the ecology and genetics of searching, transmission, reproductive capacity, and virulence?
3. Are there different regions (continents versus islands) where 'new association' biological control agents should be sought?
4. Since viruses, bacteria, fungi, and protozoa can be genetically engineered to improve their pathogenicity for insect and weed control, what

ecological and genetic characteristics will make these microbes effective biocontrol pathogens?

5. How is it possible to genetically engineer microbes as biocontrol agents that provide effective, permanent control of a pest?

IPM clearly represents a highly promising approach that requires patient and careful application to reap high crop yields while minimizing injury to ecosystems.

Part 2

CONTRIBUTED CHAPTERS

6 Pesticides: A General Introduction

H. V. MORLEY

London Research Center, Agriculture Canada, Ontario, Canada

6.1 OBJECTIVE AND SCOPE

The primary objective of this chapter is to identify the problems, evaluate the methodology available, and indicate priority areas for research required to assess potential or actual adverse effects of pesticides upon non-target organisms (NTO). The breadth and scope of the subject necessitates extensive reliance upon reviews and texts as references for the reader.

NTOs will be taken to mean man, other vertebrates, invertebrates, microorganisms, and plants which are unintentionally exposed to pesticides or toxic derivatives. Voluntary exposure resulting from occupational sources such as manufacture, formulation, and application will not be covered here, because, although the people thus affected are NTOs, their exposure cannot be said to be unintentional; the risk is accepted, and full safety precautions can be followed to minimize exposure (Holden, 1986). Ambient exposures near manufacturing sites, landfills, and sewage treatment plants have been discussed (NRCC, 1982c). Occupational health risks and the problems and errors associated with epidemiological studies have been described (Elwood, 1986; Roberts *et al.* 1985a). The risks associated with re-entry of agricultural workers to recently sprayed areas have also been amply reviewed (Kahn, 1979; Gunther, 1980; Gunther *et al.*, 1977). Methods for evaluating human exposures to pesticides are dicussed elsewhere in this volume.

6.2 THE NATURE OF THE PROBLEM

The annual worldwide agricultural use of pesticides has been estimated to be of the order of 5×10^6 tons with a value of about \$16.3 billion (US) (Helsel, 1987). The same source estimates that some 52 per cent of applied

Methods to Assess Adverse Effects of Pesticides on Non-target Organisms
Edited by R. G. Tardiff
©1992 SCOPE Published by John Wiley & Sons Ltd

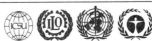

pesticides are herbicides, 26 per cent insecticides, 17 per cent fungicides, and 5 per cent other. Global pesticide use continues to grow, especially in developed countries that account for about 80 per cent of the total use (Helsel, 1987).

Despite the use of pesticides, about 35 per cent of crops are estimated to be lost (Pimentel and Pimentel, 1979). Approximately another 20 per cent of the crops are lost post-harvest. Thus, nearly 50 per cent of food in the world is being lost annually despite all pest control procedures.

It is estimated that less than 0.1 per cent of the pesticides applied to crops reach the target pests (Pimentel and Levitan, 1986). Thus, more than 99 per cent of applied pesticides have the potential to impact NTOs and to become widely dispersed in the environment.

Exposure routes include inhalation, dermal absorption, ingestion, and systemic action through plant surfaces and roots and cell surface of microorganisms. Direct exposures through dietary intake of food or water are of particular concern to all organisms since they cannot be avoided. The young may be at particular risk. Levels of persistent organochlorine compounds in human milk (Jensen, 1983) suggest that suckling vertebrates may be exposed to low levels of pesticides in areas still using organochlorine pesticides. Many third world countries still continue to use DDT and other persistent organochlorine pesticides. Levels in soil and water are of special concern to NTOs confined to these media and thus subjected continually to a pesticide, its contaminants, and its decomposition products.

Acute adverse effects on NTOs are more easily measured and have been reasonably well documented in many cases, albeit mostly through laboratory studies. Regulatory authorities now require such data as part of the registration submission.

The potential for subtle, sublethal effects has been increasingly recognized. These effects are far more difficult to measure, and adequate models for their measurement are lacking. Attempts have been made to use behavioural responses to sublethal levels of pesticides as indicators of potential adverse effects (Beitinger and Freeman, 1983; Peakall, 1985; Haynes, 1988). It is likely that behavioural parameters are sensitive indicators of ecosystem damage, but they are more difficult to investigate than biochemical or physiological parameters. The roles of biochemical indicators and their development and validation as indicators of ecosystem health has been reviewed (NRCC, 1985a). Baseline data from which comparisons can be made are universally lacking. For this reason, it is difficult to determine impacts on communities and populations which are ecologically more significant than effects on a few individuals.

In the 'real world', NTOs are subjected to a wide number of pesticides and byproducts together with a larger number of non-pesticide industrial chemicals. This chemical barrage occurs via a variety of routes, at varying levels of exposure, and over most of the life-span of the organism. These chemicals are present in very small quantities, often at the limit of analytical detection. The impact, if any, on NTOs remains to be established and awaits the development of suitable methodology. This problem has been addressed at length in a recent publication which identifies the limitations, methodologies, practicalities, and utility of dealing with chemicals in mixtures (Vouk *et al.*, 1987).

The pesticides themselves consist of hundreds of compounds differing significantly in structure, chemical and physical properties, modes of action, persistence, and toxicity. Thus, the effect of over 600 insecticides, herbicides, defoliants, acaricides, and fungicides on honeybees has been described (Johansen, 1977; NRCC; 1981). The basic active pesticide ingredients are formulated with surfactants, carriers, solvents, and other adjuvants that can affect persistence and toxicity in an unpredicted manner—a topic that has not been extensively investigated (Graham-Bryce, 1987; Hartley and Graham-Bryce, 1980; Matthews, 1979).

Pesticides themselves have varying levels of impurities depending on the purity of the starting materials, synthetic routes, and quality control by the manufacturer. Some of these impurities, such as the dioxins and nitrosamines, are extremely toxic to animals. Furthermore, after release to the environment, there may be formed a wide variety of products by a range of mechanisms resulting in materials with toxicities different from the parent compound. Thus, simple cause–effect relationships in the 'real world' are virtually impossible to establish, making the findings of much of the control laboratory experimentation at elevated dosage levels of questionable value.

The levels of exposure to NTOs vary considerably over time, ranging from fully registered application rate arising from drift or soil application, to the nanogram or picogram levels usually found by environmental monitoring. These lower concentrations, while usually insignificant to large organisms, are potentially more significant to microorganisms weighing approximately 10^{-12}g.

6.3 PESTICIDES

Many compilations of pesticides exist (CPCR, 1986; Reynolds, 1987; Spencer, 1982; Worthing, 1987). Classification of pesticides may be based on structural similarity (e.g., organochlorines, OPs, carbamates, and pyrethroids) or by function (insecticides, herbicides, and fungicides). Structural similarities are convenient, but many compounds do not fit into the main categories. Functional organization is helpful for the user, but may hide the fact that the compound has several activites (e.g, pentachlorophenol is an insecticide, fungicide, defoliant, and a herbicide).

From the point of view of the potential impact of pesticides on NTOs, the mode of action is the most significant parameter. This approach, however, has the difficulty that in most cases the mode of action is unknown in detail, but nevertheless still identifies the potential area of concern for environmental impact on NTOs. In some cases the mode of action is completely unknown. The lack of detailed knowledge regarding the mode of action of most pesticides highlights

Table 6.1. Illustrations of pesticides and their sites of action

Site of action	Pesticide(s)
Nervous system	Organophosphorus compounds, *N*-methyl or *N,N*-dimethyl carbamates, pyrethroids, most organochlorine compounds, avermectins, nicotine, and chlorodimeform and related compounds
Respiration	Arsenicals, copper compounds and those which can form copper chelates, oxathiin carboxanilides, dinitroaniline herbicides (secondary site of action), dinitrophenols, pentachlorophenol, tri-substituted organotins, hydroxybenzonitriles, rotenone, hydrogen cyanide, phosphine
Photosynthesis	Herbicides: straight chain, substituted and cyclic ureas, triazines, acylanilides, phenylcarbamates, triazinones, phenolic herbicides, nitrodiphenyl ethers
Cell growth and development	Benzimidazoles and related compounds, dicarboxamides, N-phenyl-carbamates, dinitroanilines, phosphoramidates, sulphonylureas, maleic hydrazide, juvenile hormones and analogues and precocenes
Biosynthesis	Acylalanines, hymexazole, cycloheximide, pyridazinones, aminotriazole, thiocarbamates, imidazoles, triazoles, pyrimidines, dichlobenil, diflubenzuron, glyphosate, ethirimol, and tricyclazole
Non-specific	Mercury compounds, sodium fluoride, captan-type fungicides, petroleum and tar oils, long-chain guanidino fungicides, chloracetanilides, chlorinated short-chain aliphatic carboxylates, alkyl *bis*-dithiocarbamates, chlorthalonil

one of the areas of research requiring intenive effort. Table 6.1 summarizes current thoughts on modes of action but does not detail secondary effects or uncertainties (Coats, 1982; Corbett *et al.*, 1984; Hassall, 1982).

Thus, although primarily used in crop protection, many organophosporus compounds are of low toxicity to vertebrates and are used to control animal pests. Some are too phytotoxic for use on crops but may be fed to cattle to control a variety of parasites (e.g., fenchlorphos).

Unfortunately, laboratory determination of LD_{50}s on a limited number of laboratory species does not usually allow extrapolation of potential effects on other species under field conditions (Moriarty, 1983). Thus the exceptional sensitivity to grain contaminated with carbophenothion of grey geese but not other game birds, pigeons, corvids, rabbits, or rats was discovered after the death of overwintering geese in Britain (Dempster, 1987).

One of the great unknowns in measuring the potential impact of pesticides on NTOs and the environment is the almost complete lack of data on the effect, if any, of the so-called non-active ingredient in formulations. This is not altogether surprising, since laboratory studies aimed at establishing simple cause–effect relationships are much easier to perform using solutions of analytical grade material. Such experiments, while useful to provide clues as to real-world possibilities, are often extrapolated beyond the limits imposed by the experimental conditions and those intended by the original workers.

The primary purpose of a formulation is to improve the efficiency of the pesticide, but in so doing, another large unknown is introduced for NTOs. There are literally thousands of possible adjuvants which may be used, many of them complex mixtures whose composition is not known fully. No information is more subject to secrecy than the composition of pesticides' formulations. It is an accepted maxim in the pesticide industry that no active ingredient can perform more efficiently in the field than its formulated ingredients will allow.

Formulated ingredients may include emulsifiers, dispersing agents or stabilizers, spreading or wetting agents, sticking agents, humectants, synergists, activators, inert mineral carriers, and organic solvents. These adjuvants are used to formulate the active ingredient as dusts, granules, aqueous concentrates, wettable powders, emulsifiable concentrates, and less frequently as aerosols, poison baits, and microcapsules (Hassall, 1982). The use of microencapsulated materials caused massive bee kills, because foraging bees took the capsules back to their hive and stored them in brood frames together with pollen. Thus foraging bees were killed transporting and collecting contaminated pollen; young hive bees were killed by the poisoned food (Aitkins *et al.*, 1978; Johansen, 1977).

In other cases granular formulations, but not the emulsifiable concentrate of carbofuran, have been implicated in bird kills. The potential influence of surfactants on soil and aquatic organisms with regard to the biological availability of the active ingredient is obvious, especially those solvents or surfactants that modify cell membranes and protective coat properties. The degree of impact on both game and useful insects by the fungicide triphenyltin hydroxide has been shown to be greatly influenced by the nature of the formulation (Pieters, 1961). The relative phytotoxicity of solvents has been described (Krenek and King, 1987).

The method of application is also important, since, in the majority of cases, efficiency is poor: most of the formulation is not applied to the target organism, but is lost through drift or fall out. The types of machinery and structure of equipment have been described (Matthews, 1979). High, medium, low, and ultra-low volume sprays, and fumigation, each pose a different set of problems for NTOs (Corbett *et al.* 1984; Hassall, 1982; Vander Hooven and Spicer, 1987).

6.4 ECOSYSTEMS

To determine the impact of pesticides on NTOs, one must first know much about the ecosystem in which the NTOs exist. Such information is lacking due to the complexity of the problem and the absence of multidisciplinary research teams.

The intended direct impact of pesticide application is the reduction of target pests below economic thresholds. An indirect effect of this treatment is to kill NTOs since by their nature most pesticides are broad spectrum toxicants designed to kill living organisms. Many indirect effects are not measurable as acute toxicity. Thus, biocontrol agents not directly affected by an application may find that their food supply has been either seriously depleted or contaminated with sublethal levels of pesticides. Herbivores feeding largely on weeds may find that their food supply has virtually disappeared. Additionally, sublethal levels of pesticides may continue to exert subtle effects, reducing the ability of the NTO to reproduce, feed, or avoid its predators.

Ignorance of the population dynamics of NTOs and of the interactions with the microecosystem of which NTOs are components make it extremely difficult to predict from laboratory studies the impact of pesticides. Such studies cannot mimic 'real-world' situations and should simply serve to establish priorities for large-scale and lengthy field studies conducted by multidisciplinary teams. Laboratory studies focus on effects on relatively few individuals, usually using pure materials under artificial conditions. Ecological effects occur in populations or communities, necessitating a knowledge of population dynamics.

Some of the problems encountered in studying the impact of pesticides on NTOs in soil, water, air, and forest ecosystems will be briefly discussed. Many publications now adopt the ecosystem approach and identify deficiencies and research priorities (NRCC, 1975b, 1978a,b, 1979, 1983a; Osborne, 1986).

6.4.1 SOIL

Soil constitutes a medium of such complexity and variability that relatively few scientists have attempted to work in this area. It has been stated that on average a temperature zone meadow in mid-summer will have the following population per 100 m^2: approximately 150 000 individual plants, several hundred guilds of herbivores and carnivores; diverse populations of insects, birds, and mammals totalling approximately 30 000; above and below ground, 1000 billion bacteria, fungi, algae, and protozoa; and around the plants' roots, a billion nematodes, 5 million microarthropods, 2 million oligochaetes, and 30 000 earthworms (Rhoades and Cates, 1976; Swain, 1977). Much of the communication and interaction between this ecological complex will occur by chemical signals which may be interrupted or modified by the influx of outside chemicals in a pesticide formulation. Attention has been focused on soil microorganisms because of the vital role these organisms play in the recycling of wastes, nitrogen, and carbon. The literature on the impact of pesticides on soil microorganisms is voluminous (Butler, 1977; Edwards and Thompson, 1973; Lal and Saxena, 1980; McCann and Cullimore, 1979; Padhy, 1985; Rajagopal et al., 1984; Tu and Miles, 1976). Ignorance of ecological interaction and population dynamics of soil organisms makes it difficult to achieve definitive conclusions, but attempts to develop ecologically-based 'yardsticks' are vital (Domsch et al., 1983).

6.4.2 WATER

The aqueous medium probably has been studied more than any other, due to the relative ease of investigation in the laboratory. This has led to the development of a multiplicity of experimental techniques utilizing static, recirculation, renewal, and flow-through systems. Comparison of results from different workers is virtually impossible, and whether laboratory results can in fact be extrapolated to field conditions is doubtful. These problems are discussed, and the evaluation in the field of the pesticide impact on many pest control projects internationally is given by Muirhead-Thomson (1987).

The behavioural avoidance of fish to sublethal levels of pesticides has been demonstrated (Beitinger and Freeman, 1983) and an evaluation made of the various experimental designs used to examine behavioural responses (Giattina and Garton, 1983).

The impact of pesticides on NTOs in aquatic ecosystems under field conditions has also been the subject of numerous publications and reviews (Hart and Fuller, 1974; Hurlbert, 1975; Hurlbert *et al.*, 1972; Mulla *et al.*, 1979; Mulla and Mian, 1981; NRCC, 1982b, 1983b, 1985b,c, 1986; Smith and Stratton, 1986). The same difficulties discussed under soil apply here, and are just as difficult to resolve.

6.4.3 TERRESTRIAL

It is impossible to study the infinite variety of complex subsets of the terrestrial ecosystem. Application of pesticides for crop (food and forestry) protection and health purposes covers a wide range of climatic, cultural, social, and economic conditions. The transport and transformations of pesticides in the environment have been reviewed recently (Jury *et al.*, 1987). Of necessity, studies have focused on systems where the greatest impact might be expected on NTOs. Forestry has been the subject of many such studies, because of the large areas involved and of the use of aerial application techniques (NRCC, 1975a, 1977, 1982a; Norris, 1981; Symons, 1977). Pesticides are distributed widely, and organisms in vegetation, forest floor, soil, water, and air are exposed to levels of pesticide not necessarily allowed on food crops. The general impact of pesticides on NTOs in a forest ecosystem is well documented, but again inadequacies in knowledge and detailed understanding of the forest ecosystems' population dynamics and their interactions with climatic factors present do not allow predictions of the impact on NTOs, especially at the sublethal level of exposure.

Because of these deficiencies, Symonds (1977) has suggested that use of bacterial insecticides, such as *Bacillus thuringiensis* (BT), would be beneficial for NTOs because of its more specific toxicity. However, the field effects of BT on non-target insect populations has been reviewed, and the conclusion reached that the same incomplete picture emerges (NRCC, 1976). Similar studies on the impact of pesticides on a large variety of agricultural food crops have been carried out with essentially the same conclusions, namely the inability to predict the likely impact of an applied pesticide stems largely from our ignorance of the basic ecology of most species, their interactions, and population dynamics. Arthropod community structure complexity in agricultural crops has been reviewed (Liss *et al.*, 1986).

6.5   RESISTANCE

One of the impacts of pesticides on living organisms has been the widespread development of resistance. Pesticide resistance occurs when some individuals of the target species are no longer killed by the pesticide at the prescribed dosage formerly found to be lethal. Resistance results in higher rates of application to effect control with potentially larger impact on NTOs. Ultimately control breaks down.

Since the first reported case of resistance to a pesticide (Melander, 1914) there has been an exponential increase in reported cases with a doubling in the number of resistant arthropod species from 1970 to 1980 (Georghiou and Mellon, 1983). Over 432 insect species have been found to be resistant to insecticides, to a total of 829 pesticide groups. Fungicide resistance has also developed with some 90 species resistant to 34 fungicides and bactericides (Ogawa *et al.*, 1983). Herbicide resistance is also slowly developing with the triazines and other classes of herbicides (Lebaron and Gressel, 1982).

While some progress has been made in understanding the biochemical basis of resistance, very little is known about the genetic basis for resistance (Plapp and Wang, 1983; Tsukamoto, 1983). Such an understanding is required before biotechnology can be used effectively. Most of the research on pesticide resistance has understandably been directed at the target species due to the impact this phenomenon has had with regard to increased pesticide use, breakdown of crop and animal protection, and the useful life of new materials which may have limited marketability due to cross resistance, e.g., pyrethroids and DDT.

One effect of pesticides on soil microorganisms has been the acceleration of their ability to degrade pesticides. This rapid breakdown of pesticides may have been confused with resistance problems in some cases, since the results are the same: breakdown in control and increased use of the pesticide. Evidence for this has been accumulating since the early 1970s, and has been the subject of many recent publications (Williams *et al.*, 1976; Read, 1986; Camper *et al.*, 1987).

Increasingly, with the emphasis on integrated pest management (IPM) and biological control, there is a need to know more about mechanisms of resistance in NTOs. It appears that less than 3 per cent of the published literature is involved with NTO resistance (Booth *et al.*, 1983). Pesticide resistance in NTOs that are beneficial insects or other types of biocontrol agents is an obvious advantage, if these agents are to be used in conjunction with pesticides in an IPM program

(Hassan, 1987). In the laboratory, attempts to induce resistance to pesticides has usually resulted in failure or, at best, a low level of resistance which regressed rapidly back to the original level within a few generations. In the 1970s, resistance of predatory phytoseiid mites to organophosphorus pesticides was confirmed, and has been utilized in IPM programs. Toxicology and mechanisms of resistance and the application of resistant biocontrol agents in IPM programs has been reviewed by Croft and Strickler (1983).

6.6 INTEGRATED PEST MANAGEMENT

IPM has become a buzz-word with a multiplicity of meanings ranging from intensive monitoring studies of insect pest populations as a prerequisite to pesticides use to a total holistic approach. The latter involves detailed knowledge of the microecosystem of crop-pest-biocontrol-climatic factors. Such holistic approaches are difficult to organize due both the complexity of the systems being examined and to the difficulty in assembling the multidisciplinary teams required to carry out the long-term research essential to answer the problems.

Many definitions have been used for IPM. The term was coined some time in the 1950s, although the concept has evolved over thousands of years (Newsome, 1975). Typical of the many definitions used is the following (Flint and Van den Bosch, 1981):

> IPM is the use of the best possible combination of methods to reduce and maintain pest populations below a level that would cause economic damage. It is based on a principle of optimum rather than maximum pest control. It constitutes a major component in an agricultural production system which will allow sustained agricultural production with minimal deleterious effects on the producer, consumer, the agrosystem, and the environment in general.

Such a definition leaves open the choice of the 'best possible combination of methods', and what would constitute an economic threshold of damage would vary on geographic and market conditions. Most workers agree that pesticides will continue to be used as part of IPM.

One aftermath of the influx of new pesticides available in the 1950s and 1960s was the loss of the IPM approach and the adoption of the philosophy of eradicaton rather than reduction of pest levels to below economic thresholds. More importantly, the concept of the older pest control methods (cultural, biological, host resistance, mechanical, monitoring) were discarded in favour of prophylactic treatment of pesticides with rigid spray schedules that resulted in maximum impact on NTOs, including biocontrol agents, and in the development of resistance.

One of the impacts of the prophylactic use of pesticides is the destruction of the natural abiotic and biotic natural control mechanisms (Brown, 1978; Van den Bosch et al., 1982), many of these controls being insects themselves.

Naturally, these are targets for broad spectrum pesticides and often result in species normally controlled naturally becoming significant pests (MacPhee *et al.*, 1976). Furthermore, destruction of natural biocontrol agents may allow rapid repopulation of target pest populations due to destruction of controlling NTOs by the pesticide treatment. This lack of understanding of the arthropod pest–predator complex often results in outbreaks of non-target pests. Thus use of synthetic pyrethroids against the main pest of apples has resulted in outbreaks of phytophagous mites. This has been ascribed to destruction of natural control agents or sublethal effects on their behaviour (Hull and Starner, 1983; Hull *et al.*, 1985).

Thus the movement towards IPM, while highly desirable and a great improvement over the prophylactic use of pesticides, does not eliminate the need for more extensive research in the following areas:

1. Understanding the total interaction of the components of the pest–crop microecosystem
2. Understanding the basic biology involved in pest–biocontrol systems
3. Understanding the plant–pest system (what differentiates a resistant host from a susceptible one?)
4. Understanding of pest resistance mechanisms
5. Simplified models for determining economic threshold sufficiently rugged to be of universal use.

The development of thresholds used in IPM requires years of research followed by care, use, and fine tuning of operational IPM programmes (Poston *et al.*, 1983). The problems of developed versus developing countries is strikingly different, as are the resources required for IPM implementation.

Although most examples cited under the IPM heading relate to insect pests, it is essential to start developing the knowledge required to consider diseases and weeds as part of the system. Factors involved in the development and implementation of IPM, together with examples, are given in numerous publications (Glass, 1975; Perkins, 1982).

The current emphasis on biological control agents (Caltagirone, 1981) will undoubtedly help to reduce pesticide input into the environment. The use of biocontrol insects in an IPM programme requires differential toxicity studies on the pesticides used to control pests and on their potential impact on the biocontrol agents. Pathogens may, in the long term, prove to be more efficient than insect parasitoids as biocontrol agents (Kurstak and Tijssen, 1982). From the point of view of potential impact on NTOs, however, one would need to have detailed knowledge regarding specificity and factors controlling infection and virulence to target pests. This will undoubtedly add to the problems already being encounterd in the registration of these materials for pest control (Summers *et al.*, 1975).

A recent publication outlines the theory and reviews the practical aspects of IPM implementation (Burn *et al.*, 1987). The editors considered that widespread application of IPM was not possible due to the lack of fundamental understanding of the interactions between pest, crop or animal, climate, and biocontrol agents.

6.7   RISK–BENEFIT ANALYSIS

In essence, a risk–benefit analysis is a process whereby a decision may be reached regarding whether the continued use of a pesticide is justified, taking to account the latest information regarding the risk. It is a method whereby existing data and information are organized and analysed. Of necessity, it involves the retrieval of all available data on the material, critical evaluation of the methodology, and verification of the data. Increasingly the process is being used by regulatory officials to reach decisions regarding continued pesticide use. Successful application of the risk–benefit analysis process requires availability of information that is, for the most part, incomplete or completely lacking. Attempting such analyses helps to identify inadequacies in databases and to pinpoint areas of particular concern. The risk assessment and benefit assessment are essentially separate processes carried out independently, and brought together for the final decision process.

6.7.1   RISK ANALYSIS

Generally, it seems to be easier to produce data for risk assessments. Partly, this may be attributed to the registration process which requires toxicological data on NTOs. In addition, the risk–benefit analysis is usually carried out in response to new toxicological or environmental concerns.

Risk analysis is dealt with in numerous publications which deal at length with the problems and processes involved in risk assessment (Lovell, 1986; Ragsdale and Kuhr, 1987; Willes *et al.*, 1985; Tardiff and Rodricks, 1988). The WHO Recommended Classification of Pesticides by hazard has gained wide acceptance, and provides a comprehensive listing of current pesticides based on the technical materials used in formulations rather than the pure active ingredient (WHO, 1988). Data sheets are published on the impact of specific pesticides on NTOs.

While there are many weak areas in the risk analysis of NTOs exposed to pesticides, exposure estimates are one of the most difficult. The need to develop new techniques and approaches and their validation has often been identified. Exposure assessment is based largely on disparate approaches using invalidated and unpublished models. The US Environmental Protection Agency's Science Advisory Board further indicated that 'biomarkers' seemed to be a research area of particular promise and was being evaluated by a National Academy of Sciences Committee. Biomarkers are defined as indicators of variation in cellular or biochemical components or processes, and in structure or function in biological systems or samples. Thus, current interest stems in part from advances in the area of biotechnology (Anonymous, 1987).

6.7.2 BENEFIT ANALYSIS

All too often, this consists of an economic benefit analysis (Krystynak, 1983; Dunnett, 1983; Stemeroff and George, 1983). Health and social benefits, while often apparent, are more difficult to document (Spindler, 1983).

The recent series published by the National Research Council of Canada (NRCC) critically reviewed the risk–benefit process. The NRCC assessed the strengths and weaknesses of available information and processes using case studies of pesticides to evaluate current measures of benefits (Roberts *et al.*, 1985b; Victor, 1985).

6.8 SUMMARY AND RESEARCH PRIORITIES

In summary, research priorities are as follows.

1. To develop an understanding of community population dynamics of the microecosystem being investigated by utilizing a multidisciplinary team approach. This is essential to establish baselines from which effects can be measured over the short and long terms. This holistic, integrated, multidisciplinary approach is essential for ecotoxicological studies requiring extrapolation of laboratory findings to the field.

2. To develop reliable, biological, biochemical, physiological, and possibly behavioural indicators of environmental pesticide impact. This is required to deal with the real-world conditions of varying levels of exposure to pesticides mixed with numerous other potential toxicants, the wide variation of climatic and geographic conditions, and inherent problems with estimation of exposure–time relationships.

3. To expand research into mode-of-action studies including secondary effects. This will indicate where adverse effects may be expected and which particular groups of organisms are particularly at risk.

4. To investigate the impact of non-active ingredients in formulations, of impurities, and of variability of active ingredients, and formulation components.

5. To determine whether cause–effect relationships can be established in the majority of cases.

6. To establish whether sublethal effects are of concern—this again requires knowledge of what we are looking for and the methodology.

7. To carry out more research on the impact of formulation types.

8. To establish whether some particular groups of pesticides merit a more detailed investigation (e.g., chitin-active materials) because of the

potential impact on NTOs (Marks *et al.*, 1982). Impact on the basic photosynthetic mechanism also would be an area of particular concern (Murthy, 1983).

9. To develop a basic understanding of the interactions between pest, crop or animal, climate, and biocontrol agents.

10. To establish the impact of changing agricultural practices (e.g., no-tillage techniques) on NTOs in relation to the increased use of pesticides necessitated by such changes.

6.9   REFERENCES

Anonymous (1987) Exposure estimates seen as weak link in EPA risk assessment. *Pest. Toxic Chem. News*, Dec. 23, pp. 5–7.

Atkins, E. L., Kellum, D. and Atkins, K. W. (1978) Encapsulated methyl parathion formulation is highly hazardous to honeybees. *Am. Bee J.* **118**, 483–485.

Beitinger, T. L. and Freeman, L. (1983) Behavioral avoidance and selection responses of fishes to chemicals. *Residue Rev.* **90**, 35–55.

Booth, G. M., Weber, D. J., Ross, L. M., Burton, S. D., Bradshaw, W. S., Hess, W. M. and Larsen, J. R. (1983) Mechanisms of pesticide resistance in non-target organisms. In: Georghiou, G. P. and Saito, T. (Eds), *Pest Resistance to Pesticides*, Plenum Press, New York, pp. 387–409.

Brown, A. W. A. (1978) *Ecology of Pesticides*, Wiley-Interscience, New York.

Burn, A. J., Coaker, T. H. and Jepson, P. C. (Eds) (1987) *Integrated Pest Management*, Academic Press, London, New York, Sydney, Tokyo, 474pp.

Butler, G. L. (1977) Algae and pesticides. *Residue Rev.* **66**, 19–62.

CPCR (1986) *Crop Protection Chemicals Reference* (2nd edn), Chemical and Pharmaceutical Press, Wiley, New York, 2030pp.

Caltagirone, L. E. (1981) Landmark examples in classical biological control. *Ann. Rev. Entomol.* **26**, 213–233.

Camper, N. D., Fleming, M. M. and Skipper, H. D. (1987) Biodegradation of carbofuran in pretreated and non-pretreated soils. *Bull. Environ. Cntam. Toxicol.* **39**, 571–578.

Coats, J. R. (Ed.) (1982) *Insecticide Mode of Action*, Academic Press, New York, London, 470pp.

Corbett, J. R., Wright, K. and Baillie, A. C. (1984) *The Biochemical Mode of Action of Pesticides* (2nd edn), Academic Press, London, New York, Tokyo, 382pp.

Croft, B. A. and Strickler, K. (1983) Natural enemy resistance to pesticides: documentation, characterization, theory and application. In: Georghiou, G. P. and Saito, T. (Eds), *Pest Resistance to Pesticides*, Plenum Press, New York, pp. 669–702.

Dempster, J. P. (1987) Effects of pesticides on wildlife and priorities in future studies. In: Brent, K. J. and Atkin, R. K. (Eds), *Rational Pesticide Use*, Cambridge University Press, Cambridge, Melbourne, New York, pp. 17–25.

Domsch, K. H., Jagnow, G. and Anderson, T. H. (1983) An ecological concept for the assessment of side effects of agrochemicals on soil microorganisms. *Residue Rev.* **86**, 66–105.

Dunnett, E. (1983) An economic assessment of the benefits of captan use in Canada. *Can. Farm Econ.* **18**, 31–40.

Edwards, C. A. and Thompson, A. R. (1973) Pesticides and the soil fauna. *Residue Rev.* **45**, 1–79.

Edwards, C. A. and Thompson, A. R. (1973) Pesticides and the soil fauna. *Residue Rev.* **45**, 1–79.

Elwood, P. C. (1986). Interpretation of epidemiological data—pitfalls and abuses. In: M. Richardson (Ed.), *Toxic Hazard Assessment of Chemicals*, The Royal Society of Chemistry, London.

Flint, M. L. and Van den Bosch, R. (1981) *Introduction to Integrated Pest Management*, Plenum Press, New York, 240 pp.

Georghiou, G. P. and Mellon, R. B. (1983) Pesticide resistance in time and space. In: Georghiou, G. P. and Saito, T. (Eds) *Pest Resistance to Pesticides*, Plenum Press, London, New York, pp. 1–46.

Giattina, J. D. and Garton, R. R. (1983) A review of the preference-avoidance responses of fishes to aquatic contaminants. *Residue Rev.* **87**, 43–90.

Glass, E. H. (1975) *Integrated Pest Management: Rationale, Potential, Needs and Implementation*. Special Publication 75-2, Entomological Society of America, Lanham, Maryland, 141pp.

Graham-Bryce, I. J. (1987) Chemical methods. In: Burn, A. J., Coaker, T. H. and Jepson, P. C. (Eds) *Integrated Pest Management*, Academic Press, London, New York, Sydney, Tokyo.

Gunther, F. A., Iwata, Y., Carman, G. E. and Smith, C. A. (1977) The citrus re-entry problem: research on its causes and effects and approaches to its minimization. *Residue Rev.* **67**, 1–139.

Gunther, F. A. (Ed.) (1980) Minimizing occupational exposure to pesticides (research conference and workshop). *Residue Rev.* **75**, 1–183.

Hart, C. W., Jr and Fuller, S. L. H. (1974) *Pollution Ecology of Freshwater Invertebrates*, Academic Press, New York.

Hartley, G. S. and Graham-Bryce, I. J. (1980) *Physical Principles of Pesticide Behaviour: the Dynamics of Applied Pesticides in the Local Environment in Relation to Biological Responses*, Academic Press, London, New York, Tokyo.

Hassall, K. A. (1982) *The Chemistry of Pesticides*, Macmillan, New York.

Hassan, S. A. (1987) Integrating chemical control with the activity of beneficial organisms. In: Brent, K. J. and Atkin, R. K. (Eds) *Rational Pesticide Use*, Cambridge University Press, Cambridge, Melbourne, New York, pp. 27–32.

Haynes, K. F. (1988) Sublethal effects of neurotoxic insecticides on insect behaviour. *Ann. Rev. Entomol.* **33**, 149–168.

Helsel, Z. R. (1987) Pesticide use in world agriculture. In: Stout, B. A. (Ed.) *Energy in World Agriculture, Vol. 2*, Elsevier, New York, pp. 179–195.

Holden, H. (1986) Risk to work forces. In: Richardson, M. L. (Ed.) *Toxic Hazard Assessment of Chemicals*, The Royal Society of Chemistry, London.

Hull, L. A., Beers, E. H. and Meagher, R. L. Jr (1985) Impact of selective use of the synthetic pyrethroid fenvalerate of apple pests and natural enemies in large-orchard trials. *J. Econ. Entomol.* **78**, 163–168.

Hull, L. A. and Starner, V. R. (1983) Impact of four synthetic pyrethroids on major natural enemies and pests of apples in Pennsylvania. *J. Econ. Entomol.* **76**, 122–130.

Hurlbert, S. H. (1975) Secondary effects of pesticides on aquatic ecosystems. *Residue Rev.* **57**, 81–148.

Hurlbert, S. H., Mulla, M. S. and Wilson, H. R. (1972) Effects of organophosphorus insecticide on the phytoplankton zooplankton, and insect populations of fresh-water ponds. *Ecol. Monographs* **42**, 269.

Jensen, A. A. (1983) Chemical contaminants in human milk. *Residue Rev.* **89**, 1–128.

Johansen, C. A. (1977) Pesticides and pollinators. *Ann. Rev. Entomol.* **1**, 51–54.

Jury, W. A., Winer, A. M., Spencer, W. F. and Focht, D. D. (1987) Transport and transformations of organic chemicals in the soil-air-water ecosystem. *Rev. Environ. Contam. Toxicol.* **99**, 119–163.

Kahn, E. (1979) Outline guide for performance of field studies to establish safe re-entry intervals for organophosphate pesticides. *Residue Rev.* **70**, 27–43.

Krenek, M. R. and King, D. N. (1987) The relative phytotoxicity of selected hydrocarbons and oxygenated solvents and oils. In: Vander Hooven, D. I. B. and Spicer, L. D. (Eds) *Pesticide Formulations and Application Systems, Sixth Volume*, ASTM Special Technical Publication 943, American Society for Testing and Materials, Philadelphia, pp. 3–19.

Krystynak, R. (1983) An economic assessment of 2,4-D in Canada: the case of grain. *Canadian Farm Economics* **18**, 7–30.

Kurstak, E. and Tijssen, P. (1982) Microbial and viral pesticides: modes of action, safety and future prospects. In: Kurstak, E. (Ed.) *Microbial and Viral Pesticides*, Marcel Dekker, New York, 720 pp.

Lal, R. and Saxena, D. M. (1980) Cytological and biochemical effects of pesticides on microorganisms. *Residue Rev.* **73**, 49–86.

Lebaron, H. M. and Gressel, J. (Eds) (1982) *Herbicide Resistance in Plants*, Wiley-Interscience, New York. 401 pp.

Liss, W. J., Gut, L. J., Westigard, P. H. and Warren, C. E. (1986) Perspectives on arthropod community structure, organization, and development in agricultural crops. *Ann. Rev. Entomol.* **31**, 455–578.

Lovell, D. P. (1986) Risk assessment—general principles. In: Richardson, M. L. (Ed.), *Toxic Hazard Assessment of Chemicals*, The Royal Society of Chemistry, London.

MacPhee, A. W., Caltagirone, L. E., van de Vrie, M. and Collyer, E. (1976) Biological control of pests of temperate fruits and nuts. In: Huffaker, C. B. and Messenger, P. S. (Eds) *Theory and Practice of Biological Control*, Academic Press, New York, 788 pp..

Marks, E. P., Leighton, T. and Leighton, F. (1982) Modes of action of chitin synthesis inhibitors. In: Coats, J. R. (Ed.) *Insecticide Mode of Action*, Academic Press, New York, London, Sydney, Tokyo, pp. 281–313.

Matthews, G. A. (1979) *Pesticide Applications Methods*, Longman, White Plains, New York, 480 pp.

McCann, A. E. and Cullimore, D. R. (1979) Influence of pesticides on the soil algal flora. *Residue Rev.* **72**, 1–31.

Melander, A. L. (1914) Can insects become resistant to sprays? *J. Econ. Entomol.* **72**, 901.

Moriarty, F. (1983) *Ecotoxicology: the Study of Pollutants in Ecosystems*, Academic Press, London.

Mulla, M. S., Majori, G. and Arata, A. A. (1979) Impact of biological and chemical mosquito control agents on non-target biota in aquatic ecosystems. *Residue Rev.* **71**, 121–173.

Mulla, M. S. and Mian, L. S. (1981) Biological and environmental impacts of the insecticides malathion and parathion on non-target biota in aquatic ecosystems. *Residue Rev.* **78**, 101–135.

Muirhead-Thomson, R. C. (1987) *Pesticide Impact on Stream Fauna with Special Reference to Macroinvertebrates*, Cambridge University Press, Cambridge, Melbourne, New York, 270pp.

Murthy, C. H. S. N. (1983) Effects of pesticides on photosynthesis. *Residue Rev.* **86**, 107–129.

Newsomc, L. D. (1975) Pest management: concept to practice. In: Pimentel, D. (Ed.), *Insects, Science and Society*, Academic Press, New York, 284pp.

Norris, L. A. (1981) The movement, persistence, and fate of the phenoxy herbicides and TCDD in the forest. *Residue Rev.* **80**, 65–131.

NRCC (1975a) *Fenitrothion: the Effects of its Use in Environmental Quality and Its Chemistry.* NRCC Report No. 14104. Associate Committee on Scientific Criteria for Environmental Quality, National Research Council of Canada, Ottawa, 162pp.

NRCC (1975b) *Endosulfan: its Effects on Environmental Quality.* NRCC Report No. 14098. Associate Committee on Scientific Criteria for Environmental Quality, National Research Council of Canada, Ottawa, 100 pp.

NRCC (1976) *Bacillus thuringiensis: its Effects on Environmental Quality.* NRCC Report No. 15385. Associate Committee on Scientific Criteria for Environmental Quality, National Research Council of Canada, Ottawa, 133pp.

NRCC (1977) *Fenitrothion: the Long-Term Effects of Its Use in Forest Ecosystems.* NRCC Report No. 16073. Associate Committee on Scientific Criteria for Environmental Quality, National Research Council of Canada, Ottawa, 628pp.

NRCC (1978a) *Ecotoxicology of Chlorpyrifos.* NRCC Report No. 16079. Associate Committee on Scientific Criteria for Environmental Quality, National Research Council of Canada, Ottawa, 314pp.

NRCC (1978b) *Phenoxy Herbicides—Their Effects on Environmental Quality.* NRCC Report No. 16075. Associate Committee on Scientific Criteria for Environmental Quality, National Research Council of Canada, Ottawa, 440pp.

NRCC (1979) *Carbofuran: Criteria for Interpreting the Effects of Its Use on Environmental Quality.* NRCC Report No. 16740. Associate Committee on Scientific Criteria for Environmental Quality, National Research Council of Canada, Ottawa, 191pp.

NRCC (1981) *Pesticide-Pollinator Interactions.* NRCC Report No. 18471. Associate Committee on Scientific Criteria for Environmental Quality, National Research Council of Canada, Ottawa, 190pp.

NRCC (1982a) *Aminocarb: the Effects of Its Use on the Forest and the Human Environment.* NRCC Report No. 18979. Associate Committee on Scientific Criteria for Environmental Quality, National Research Council of Canada, Ottawa, 253pp.

NRCC (1982b) *Effects of Propoxur on Environmental Quality with Particular Reference to Its Use for Control of Biting Flies.* NRCC Report No. 18572. Associate Committee on Scientific Criteria for Environmental Quality, National Research Council of Canada, Ottawa, 238pp.

NRCC (1982c) *Chlorinated Phenols: Criteria for Environmental Quality.* NRCC Report No. 18578. Associate Committee on Scientific Criteria for Environmental Quality, National Research Council of Canada, Ottawa, 191pp.

NRCC (1983a) *2,4-D: Some Current Issues.* NRCC Report No. 20647. Associate Committee on Scientific Criteria for Environmental Quality, National Research Council of Canada, Ottawa, 99pp.

NRCC (1983b) *Impact Assessments in Lotic Environments—Methoxychlor.* NRCC Report No. 20645. Associate Committee on Scientific Criteria for Environmental Quality, National Research Council of Canada, Ottawa, 130pp.

NRCC (1985a) *The Role of Biochemical Indicators in the Assessment of Ecosystem Health—Their Development and Validation.* NRCC Report No. 24371. Associate Committee on Scientific Criteria for Environmental Quality, National Research Council of Canada, Ottawa, 119pp.

NRCC (1985b) *Organotin Compounds in the Aquatic Environment: Scientific Criteria for Assessing Their Effects on Environmental Quality.* NRCC Report No. 22494. Associate Committee on Scientific Criteria for Environmental Quality, National Research Council of Canada, Ottawa, 248pp.

NRCC (1985c) *TPM and Bayer 78: Lampricides in the Aquatic Environment.* NRCC Report No. 22488. Associate Committee on Scientific Criteria for Environmental Quality, National Research Council of Canada, Ottawa, 184pp.

NRCC (1986) *Pyrethroids: their Effects on Aquatic and Terrestrial Ecosystems*. NRCC Report No. 24376. Associate Committee on Scientific Criteria for Environmental Quality, National Research Council of Canada, Ottawa, 330pp.

Osborn, D. (1986) Effects of pesticides on non-target organisms. In: Richardson, M. L. (Ed.) *Toxic Hazard Assessment of Chemicals*, The Royal Society of Chemistry, London, pp. 247–258.

Padhy, R. N. (1985) Cyanobacteria and pesticides. *Residue Rev.* **95**, 1–44.

Perkins, J. W. (1982) *Insects, Experts and the Insecticide Crisis*, Plenum Press, New York, 304pp.

Peakall, D. B. (1985) Behavioral responses of birds to pesticides and other contaminants. *Residue Rev.* **96**, 46–76.

Pieters, A. J. (1961). Triphenyltin hydroxide, a fungicide for the control of *Phytophthora infestans* on potatoes and some other fungicide diseases. *British Insecticide and Fungicide Conference, Brighton, Proceedings, Vol. 2*, pp. 461–470. British Cor Protection Conference, Binfield, Bracknell, Berks RG12 5QE, England.

Pimentel, D. and Levitan, L. (1986) Pesticides: amounts applied and amounts reaching pests. *Bioscience* **36**, 86–91.

Pimentel, D. and Pimentel, M. (1979) *Food, Energy, and Society*, Edward Arnold Ltd, London, 165pp.

Plapp, F. W., Jr and Wang, T. C. (1983) Genetic origins of insecticide resistance. In: Georghiou, G. P. and Saito, T. (Eds) *Pest Resistance to Pesticides*, Plenum Press, New York, pp. 47–70.

Poston, F. L., Pedego, L. P. and Welch, S. W. (1983) Economic injury levels: reality and practicality. *Bull. Entomol. Soc. Am.* **29**, 49–53.

Ragsdale, N. N. and Kuhr, R. J. (Eds) (1987) *Pesticides: minimizing the Risks*. ACS Symposium Series 336, American Chemical Society, Washington DC, 183pp.

Rajagopal, B. S., Brahmaprakash, G. P., Reddy, B. R., Singh, U. D. and Sethunathan, N. (1984) Effect and persistence of selected carbamate pesticides in soil. *Residue Rev.* **93**, 1–199.

Read, D. C. (1986) Influence of weather conditions and micro-organisms on persistence of insecticides to control root maggota *Diptera anthomyiidae* in rutabagas. *Agric. Ecosystems Environ.* **16**, 165–174.

Reynolds, E. F. (Ed.) (1987) *Pesticides: Synonyms and Chemical Names* (5th edn), Australian Government Publishing Service, Canberra, 299pp.

Rhoades, D. F. and Cates, R. G. (1976) Towards a general theory of plant antiherbivore chemistry. *Recent Adv. Phytochem.* **10**, 168–213.

Roberts, J. R., Curry, P. B., Willes, R. F., Mitchell, M. F., Narod, S. and Neri, L. C. (1985a) Epidemiologic evidence of the effects of pesticides on human health in Canada. Monograph II, *Strengths and Limitations of Benefit–Cost Analyses Applied to the Assessment of Industrial Organic Chemicals Including Pesticides*. NRCC Report No. 22852. Associate Committee on Scientific Criteria for Environmental Quality, National Research Council of Canada, Ottawa.

Roberts, J. R., Lloyd, K. M., Stemeroff, M., Stephenson, G. R., Sutton, R. F., Ellis, C. R., Edgington, L. V. and Payandeh, B. (1985b) Evaluation of the biological and economic benefits of pesticide use. Monograph V, *Strengths and Limitations of Benefit–Cost Analyses Applied to the Assessment of Industrial Organic Chemicals Including Pesticides*. NRCC Report No. 23988. Associate Committee on Scientific Criteria for Environmental Quality, National Research Council of Canada, Ottawa.

Smith, T. M. and Stratton, G. W. (1986) Effects of synthetic pyrethroid insecticides on non-target organisms. *Residue Rev.* **97**, 93–120.

Spencer, E. Y. (1982) *Guide to Chemicals Used in Crop Protection* (7th edn) Research Branch, Agriculture Canada, Ottawa.

Spindler, M. (1983) DDT: health aspects in relation to man and risk/benefit assessment based thereupon. *Residue Rev.* **90**, 1–34.

Stemeroff, M. and George, J. A. (1983) *The Benefits and Costs of Controlling Destructive Insects on Onions, Apples and Potatoes in Canada, 1960–80*, Entomological Society of Canada, Ottawa, 96pp.

Summers, M., Engler, R., Falcon, L. and Vail, P. (1975) *Baculoviruses for Insect Pest Control: Safety Consideration*, American Society for Microbiology, Washington DC, 186pp.

Swain, T. (1977) Secondary compounds as protective agents. *Ann. Rev. Plant Physiol.* **28**, 479–501.

Symons, P. E. K. (1977) Dispersal and toxicology of the insecticide fenitrothion; predicting hazards of forest spraying. *Residue Rev.* **68**, 1–36.

Tardiff, R. G. and Rodricks, J. V. (Eds) (1988) *Toxic Substances and Human Risk: Principles of Data Interpretation*, Plenum Press, New York, 460pp.

Tsukamoto, M. (1983) Methods of genetic analysis of insecticide resistance. In: Georghiuo, G. P. and Saito, T (Eds) *Pest Resistance to Pesticides*, Plenum Press, New York, pp. 71–98.

Tu, C. M. and Miles, J. R. W. (1975) Interactions between insecticides and soil microbes. *Residue Rev.* **64**, 17–65.

Van den Bosch, R., Messenger, P. S. and Gutierrez, A. P. (1982) *An Introduction to Biological Control*, Plenum Press, New York, 247pp.

Vander Hooven, D. I. B. and Spicer, L. D. (Eds) (1987) *Pesticide Formulations and Application Systems, Sixth Volume*, ASTM Special Technical Publication 943, American Society for Testing and Materials, Philadelphia, 186pp.

Victor, P. (1985) Evaluation of costs associated with human health impacts. Monograph IV, NRCC Associate Committee on Scientific Criteria for Environmental Quality, *Strengths and Limitations of Benefit–Cost Analyses Applied to the Assessment of Industrial Organic Chemicals Including Pesticides*. NRCC Report No. 22489, National Research Council of Canada, Ottawa.

Vouk, V. B., Butler, G. C., Upton, A. C., Parke, D. V. and Asher, S. C. (Eds) (1987) *Methods for Assessing the Effects of Mixtures of Chemicals*. SCOPE 30, IPCS Joint Symposia 6, SGOMSEC 3, John Wiley & Sons, Chichester, New York, 894pp.

WHO (1988) *The WHO Recommended Classification of Pesticides by Hazard and Guidelines to Classification 1988–1989*, World Health Organization, Geneva.

Willes, R. P., Mitchell, M. F., Curry, P. B. and Roberts, J. R. (1985) Extrapolation of toxicological data from laboratory studies to the human situation. Monograph III, NRCC Associate Committee on Scientific Criteria for Environmental Quality, *Strengths and Limitations of Benefit–Cost Analyses Applied to the Assessment of Industrial Organic Chemicals Including Pesticides*. NRCC Report No. 23909, National Research Council of Canada, Ottawa.

Williams, I. H., Pepin, H. S. and Brown, M. J. (1976) Degradation of carbofuran by soil microorganisms. *Bull. Environ. Contam. Toxicol.* **15**, 244–249.

Worthing, C. R. (1987) *The Pesticide Manual* (8th edn), British Crop Protection Council, London.

7 Methods to Evaluate Exposures to Pesticides

D. STEPHEN SAUNDERS
RJR Nabisco, Bowman Gray Technical Center, North Carolina, USA

7.1 INTRODUCTION

The use of pesticides in industrialized and developing nations has led to concern over the effects of pesticide exposures on humans and other NTOs. There is little doubt that such exposures can result in illness or death. The World Health Organization (WHO) has estimated that approximately 500 000 human poisonings occur each year worldwide (WHO, 1981) and the number of fatalities has been estimated at greater than 10 000 per year (Loevinsohn, 1987). Although epidemiological data indicate that the primary hazards of exposures to pesticides are acute toxic reactions, these exposures have also been implicated as a possible risk factor for cancer in agricultural workers (American Medical Association, 1988).

The goal of this chapter will be to examine existing methods and approaches for assessment of exposure of humans and other NTOs to pesticides. In general, there are three principal sources of human exposure to pesticides—occupational (including agricultural), non-occupational (for example non-commercial treatments of dwellings and workplaces, home gardening, etc.), and dietary, that is indirect exposure of the population through the use of pesticides on agricultural commodities. Each of these sources of exposure will be discussed separately, and the methods for assessing each type of exposure will be examined.

7.2 OCCUPATIONAL EXPOSURES TO PESTICIDES

The major types of occupational exposures, in terms of the magnitude and frequency of exposure, are agricultural (mixers, loaders, applicators, and harvesters), professional pesticide applicators who treat dwellings and workplaces, and workers in pesticide manufacturing plants. In general, these

Methods to Assess Adverse Effects of Pesticides on Non-target Organisms
Edited by R. G. Tardiff
©1992 SCOPE Published by John Wiley & Sons Ltd
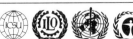

types of exposures are regulated by national agencies, who set permissible limits on exposure and determine whether a particular use has an adequate margin of safety for the worker.

Two principal approaches are currently employed for evaluating occupational exposures to pesticides—passive dosimetry and biological monitoring. A third area of monitoring is 'physiological monitoring', and involves the observation of exposed populations for changes in biological/physiological parameters. Each approach has significant strengths and weaknesses, and no single approach will provide a complete estimate of exposure.

7.2.1   PASSIVE DOSIMETRY

The most common passive type of method used to estimate occupational exposure is a combination of patches on the skin and clothing and hand washes to estimate dermal exposure, and air sampling to estimate inhalation exposure (USEPA, 1987a; Reinert et al., 1986; Durham and Wolfe, 1962). In general, absorbent patches are placed on the skin in sufficient number and location as to estimate total dermal exposure. Patches are also frequently placed on the outside of garments to assess the effectiveness of protective clothing. After exposure to the pesticide under conditions of field use, the patches are removed and analysed for pesticide content. Exposure to the hands can be estimated by swabbing, hand washes, or absorbent gloves. Since the major portion of occupational pesticide exposure occurs to the hands, the method of assessment of this type of exposure is critical to the overall estimate of exposure. No single technique is fully satisfactory for determining exposures to the hands, as washing will not recover residues that are absorbed into skin (Wester and Maibach, 1985), and absorbent gloves may significantly overestimate exposure to the hands, because the gloves absorb or trap more pesticide than would be found in contact with bare skin (Reinert et al., 1986; Davis et al., 1983).

A variety of techniques exist for measuring inhalation exposure, ranging from modified respirators, which contain an absorbent material, to powered air sampling devices placed near the breathing zone of the monitored individual (Lewis, 1976). The choice of a method by which to estimate inhalation exposure will depend in large part on the physical–chemical nature of the specific pesticide and the specific activity of the monitored individual.

7.2.2   BIOLOGICAL MONITORING

This approach involves the direct measurement of pesticides and/or metabolites in blood, urine, and occasionally tissues (Coye et al., 1986a; Reinert et al., 1986). It is, therefore, theoretically possible to estimate the actual absorbed dose, providing that sufficient information on the pharmacokinetics of the specific chemical is available.

Another common approach in this area is to monitor some physiological or biochemical parameter as an index of exposure, for example measurement of decreases in serum or erythrocyte acetylcholinesterase activity after exposure to organophosphate insecticides. Although frequently referred to as 'biological monitoring', this approach might be more correctly categorized as 'physiological monitoring' or 'health surveillance', since a response rather than actual biological dose is measured. For example, measurement of serum (pseudo-) cholinesterase activity is a common method for estimating exposure to organophosphate insecticides. Even though one may infer exposure by this technique, it is difficult to estimate the dose that an individual has received, and one could not identify the specific chemical involved by this technique alone. In addition, because of the wide variability in blood cholinesterase activity among humans, the utility of this technique depends on accurate pre-exposure baseline measurements in the monitored individual.

Other physiological techniques that have been used to assess pesticide exposure include monitoring of peripheral blood for chromosomal abnormalities and assessment of pupillary reflexes. Immunological techniques such as enzyme-linked immunosorbent assays (ELISA) hold promise as reliable, rapid, and inexpensive methods for 'real-time' personal monitoring of pesticide exposures under field conditions (Hammock et al., 1987; Mumma and Brady, 1987). Although widely used in laboratories for many years, recent technical advances in this area have resulted in products with potential application for monitoring field exposure. Such techniques may be particularly useful in developing countries or rural areas where the sophisticated laboratory equipment necessary for chemical measurements of pesticides is not readily accessible. At least one such product has been developed for paraquat and parathion ('QUIK-CARD', Granite Division, Environmental Diagnostics, Inc., Burlington, North Carolina, USA). The card contains an indicator which will change colour in the presence of the particular chemical, and is a rapid, semi-quantitative method for screening exposures to these two highly toxic pesticides. In addition to monitoring personal exposure, immunological techniques may also provide economical methods for monitoring field residues to prevent worker re-entry hazard, and to monitor agricultural runoff so as to prevent surface water contamination.

7.2.3 PASSIVE DOSIMETRY VERSUS BIOLOGICAL MONITORING

The major advantage of passive techniques is that the contribution of inhalation and dermal routes, and of the different areas of the body to total dermal exposure, can be independently estimated (Reinert et al., 1986). In addition, activities which produce a high potential for exposure can be identified. Over time, a database can be developed that will allow prediction of exposure under a given set of conditions. The major disadvantage of this technique is that the actual dose is unknown, and assumptions must be made to estimate dermal penetration and extrapolate from patches to total body surface area. In addition, patch measurements seem to have inherent limitations in terms of reproducibility (Fenske *et al.*, 1987).

Biological monitoring has the advantage of potentially allowing for the measurement of the actual dose of a pesticide. The disadvantages of this type of approach are that some knowledge of the metabolism and pharmacokinetics of the pesticide is required, and it is generally not possible to distinguish between discrete work activities as sources of exposure. Even when pharmacokinetic data are known, extrapolations to estimate exposure can be confounded by extraneous variables such as concomitant drug or chemical exposure (Borm and de Barbanson, 1988).

Physiological monitoring and health surveillance suffer from similar limitations, in that it is not possible to quantify the dose or identify discrete work activities that produce exposures. The most relevant types of measurements generally require that a pre-exposure baseline be established and the exposure monitored through sequential measurements (Richter *et al.*, 1986).

None of these techniques alone can provide a complete estimate of exposure, and the use of any of these methods to estimate exposure will require certain assumptions. Combining passive dosimetry and biological monitoring, although costly in terms of resources and time, may provide the best overall estimate of occupational exposure and thereby potential risk (Chester *et al.*, 1987; Grover *et al.*, 1986; Carmen *et al.*, 1982; Leavitt *et al.*, 1982).

7.2.4 METHODS FOR REDUCING OCCUPATIONAL PESTICIDE EXPOSURE

In general, absorption through the skin is the most significant route of occupational exposure to pesticides, at least during outdoor operations (USEPA, 1987b; Grover *et al.*, 1986; Leavitt *et al.*, 1982; Atallah *et al.*, 1982). Of all areas of the skin, the hands generally receive the greatest exposure for most occupational activities involving pesticides. Depending on the specific pesticide and occupational activity, estimates of exposure through the hands range from 25 to 98 per cent of total dermal exposure (USEPA, 1987a; Reinert *et al.*, 1986; Grover *et al.*, 1986; Putnam *et al.*, 1983; Leavitt *et al.*, 1982). Therefore, by simply instituting the use of protective gloves that are impermeable to the pesticide, exposure can be greatly reduced. Other types of protective clothing such as long-sleeve shirts, pants, head gear and face shields may also significantly reduce exposure (Putnam *et al.*, 1983; Atallah *et al.*, 1982; Davies *et al.*, 1982). In indoor operations, such as greenhouse pesticide applications, and for outdoor applications of certain chemicals, the inhalation route of exposure may be most significant, since for many chemicals the rate of absorption through the lung is likely to be higher than the rate of absorption through the skin, even though the total dermal dose is higher (Fenske *et al.*, 1987). The use of a respirator in addition to other protective gear would be indicated in those situations.

Although protective clothing can greatly decrease dermal exposure to a pesticide, care must be taken to launder clothing properly to prevent saturation of the clothing material with a pesticide and subsequent chronic dermal exposure. In addition, the type of clothing material seems to have an effect on pesticide retention. For most situations, cotton material appears to be desirable in terms of protective efficacy and ease of cleaning balanced against the need for prevention of heat stress in the wearer (Chiao-Cheng et al., 1988; Davies et al., 1982). Washing the skin after pesticide exposure may not fully remove the chemical, reiterating the need to prevent exposure through appropriate protective measures (Wester and Maibach, 1985).

The level of occupational exposure is also directly dependent on the type of activity involved. For example, individuals who direct aerial spray operations from the ground (so-called 'flaggers' or 'flagmen'), may receive a dermal dose of pesticide that is several thousand times higher than other workers, such as mixer-loaders or applicators (Atallah et al., 1982). The use of a mechanical device would eliminate the need for this type of exposure.

The method of mixing or applying the pesticide also has a significant effect on the level of exposure to the mixer/loader/applicator and other NTOs. Pouring rather than pumping a pesticide formulation from a mixing tank into the application apparatus (i.e. open versus closed systems) can greatly increase exposure. Depending on the specific chemical and type of activity, the use of a wettable powder as compared to an emulsifiable concentrate may also increase exposure to the worker due to the generation of dusts which may be inhaled by the worker or drift onto clothing and other areas (Putnam et al., 1983). Similarly, the use of closed-cab ground application systems can greatly limit exposure to the applicator (Cowell et al., 1987; Carmen et al., 1982). Airblast or aeroplane spraying operations have the greatest potential for drift of the pesticide away from the application area, resulting in exposures in areas where pesticide application was not intended. Thus, minimization of this type of application in favour of ground-based methods can also reduce the extent of inadvertent exposure to NTOs. In terms of long-term impact on worker health, reduction of exposures through engineering controls may prove superior to personal protective measures.

7.3 NON-OCCUPATIONAL PESTICIDE EXPOSURES

Although a significant effort has been devoted to the quantification of occupational exposures, particularly in the agricultural sector, relatively little information exists on the overall level of pesticide exposure in the general population. In the US, attempts are under way to evaluate incidental homeowner exposures to pesticides through the EPA's Non-Occupational Pesticide Exposure Study (NOPES) (USEPA, 1987b). The monitoring methods for this study involve the use of personal air monitors, analysis of drinking water, and gloves (to assess dermal hand exposures) in cases where household applications of pesticides were involved (Lewis *et al.*, 1988; Lewis, 1988; USEPA, 1987b). Although the data from the full study are still being analysed, the results of the pilot study suggest that incidental pesticide exposures in and around the home (at least in the US) are below the threshold of toxicological concern. Limited experimental data in this area also suggest that normal homeowner use of pesticides produces exposures well below those encountered in agricultural uses (Weisskopf *et al.*, 1988; Everhart and Holt, 1982). The use of highly persistent organochlorine insecticides in dwellings and on food has created a great deal of interest in many countries regarding the body burden of these chemicals in the general population. In the US, the National Health and Nutrition Examination Survey (NHANES II) evaluated adipose and blood samples for residues of pesticides and other substances. More than 90 per cent of the adipose samples had detectable residues of DDT, chlordane, heptachlor epoxide, dieldrin, BHC, and HCB, which exist in equilibrium with fluid compartments. The median concentrations of these compounds in serum ranged from 1.4 p.p.b. for oxychlordane and *trans*-nonachlor to 11.8 p.p.b. for DDE (Murphy and Harvey, 1985; Murphy *et al.*, 1983).

Evaluation of human adipose tissue for mirex, an organochlorine insecticide used in the southern US to control fire ants, indicated that about 10 per cent of the population in that region would be predicted to carry residues of mirex of about 0.3 p.p.m. in body fat (Kutz *et al.*, 1985). Compilations of data for tissue and/or serum residues of organochlorine compounds suggest that levels are quite variable from region to region, and definite trends in the human body burden over time are difficult to establish. The variation in detected residue levels may be the result of differences in analytical techniques among laboratories, but undoubtedly also reflects variations in usage among the different regions. In the US, data compiled from sampling of adipose tissues obtained over the years 1970–1977 indicated that total adipose DDT + metabolite levels have been declining, from around 8 p.p.m. in 1970 to around 4 p.p.m. in 1977. However, the frequency of detection of DDT and/or its metabolites in adipose tissue remained constant over these years at 100 per cent. Chlordane, heptachlor, *trans*-nonachlor, and dieldrin concentrations remained fairly constant, although at much lower concentrations than for DDT (around 0.1 p.p.m.). As for DDT, the frequency of detection of these other organochlorine compounds approached 100 per cent in most cases. Experimental studies in man, and computer modelling of residues suggest that adipose concentrations of these compounds should slowly decline over time in the absence of further usage. Obviously, in areas where these compounds are still used, no reductions would be expected (Strassman and Kutz, 1981; Matsumara, 1985).

One area of concern related to the persistence of these compounds in the human body has been the transfer of organochlorine insecticides (and other persistent chemicals such as PCBs) to the infant via the placenta and breast milk. Lipophilic pesticides such as the organochlorines will transfer from adipose tissue to milk fat during lactation, and the levels in either medium are comparable (Travis *et al.*, 1988; Skaare *et al.*, 1988). These insecticides can potentially translocate to the fetus also, as evidenced by chemical residues detected in cord blood (Skaare *et al.*, 1988). Although it is generally difficult to identify the source of exposure, at least one report has correlated the use of chlordane in termite treatments of dwellings with the appearance of chlordane in human milk (Taguchi and Yakushiji, 1988).

Monitoring of adipose tissue or other biological samples from humans provides valuable information regarding the total exposure of the population to certain pesticides; however, it is not possible to determine the route or circumstance by which that exposure occurred. These data illustrate the need for managing and assessing exposures as they occur, since residues may persist in the environment, food chain, and human body long after the use of the chemical has been discontinued.

7.4 DIETARY EXPOSURES TO PESTICIDES

In terms of the number of people potentially exposed to pesticides, the dietary route is the most significant route of exposure, even though the magnitude of such exposure is generally lower than that resulting from occupational or household use of pesticides. Virtually everyone receives at least occasional low doses of pesticide via the diet. The entry of pesticides into the diet results primarily from the use of these chemicals in agricultural production, but may also result from treatments of warehouses, food-processing and food-preparation facilities, and households. A variety of methods exist for estimating dietary exposures to pesticides; however, all existing methods are hampered by the relative lack of accurate data on residues of pesticides in food at the time of consumption.

In the US, dietary exposure estimates are derived from the EPA Tolerance Assessment System (TAS). This system is a computerized database that contains consumption estimates derived from the 1977–1978 USDA Nationwide Food Consumption Survey. The TAS can estimate exposures to the average population, or to any of 22 subgroups of that population based on age, sex, ethnicity, geographic region, or season of the year. Any valid residue estimate can be used to estimate exposure (Saunders, 1987; Saunders and Petersen, 1986).

Historically, estimation of dietary exposure in the US was based on an estimate of residue in food, called the 'tolerance'. The tolerance is actually an enforcement value, and represents the upper limit of residue that is permitted on a crop as it enters commerce. (The tolerance is similar in concept to the maximum residue limit, MRL, used by the WHO/FAO for recommendation to the CODEX.) By definition, the residues on food at the time of consumption will be less than the tolerance or MRL value, and in fact data submitted to the EPA generally demonstrate that actual residue values in food as eaten are far below the tolerance value. When actual residue levels are used to estimate exposure, the calculated dietary risk for a particular chemical may be several orders of magnitude less than that calculated from tolerances (Petersen and Chaisson, 1988; Saunders, 1987).

For this reason, the EPA has developed the concept of 'anticipated residue', which may be operationally defined as any residue value other than a tolerance which is used for purposes of calculating exposure and estimating risk. In practice, this value may be calculated by applying correction factors to the tolerance to account for the per cent of crop treated with a chemical (generally less than 100 per cent of a crop is treated with any single chemical), by using field-trial data to calculate an average field residue, and by applying processing factors to the mean field residue (preferably) or to the tolerance if adequate field-trial data are not available to estimate a valid mean (Saunders, 1987). Processing factors can take into account activities such as washing, peeling, canning, and cooking, which will generally decrease residues of pesticide in food at the time that it is consumed. If the application of appropriate factors still results in an unacceptable level of exposure, monitoring studies are conducted to determine the actual levels of chemical present in representative foods at the consumer level.

For most chemicals, the effects that may be of potential human health concern are identified in chronic feeding studies conducted in experimental animals. In assessing dietary exposures to these chemicals, the appropriate measure is an estimate of the average daily intake of the chemical. However, certain pesticides, notably some carbamate insecticides, are acutely toxic, and do not have chronic toxicity *per se*. In these cases, the relevant measure of dietary exposure is not average daily intake, but rather the maximum amount that an individual can consume in a single day. The TAS can calculate this value by determining the distribution of single-day exposures. In this manner, the regulator can determine whether a portion of the population will be at risk due to acute dietary exposure to the pesticide. As was discussed previously, tolerances, anticipated residues, and/or monitoring data can be used to calculate acute dietary exposures.

WHO is currently in the process of developing a computerized model for predicting dietary exposures to pesticides. This model will be based on Food and Agricultural Organization food consumption estimates (called 'food balance sheets') and will be used by the WHO/FAO Joint Meeting on Pesticides Residues (JMPR) to assess the impact of MRLs on established ADIs. This proposed system will also have the capability of applying processing and/or production factors to the MRL when calculating potential dietary exposures (WHO, 1988). Upon completion, this system will provide most nations with a rapid and simple method for screening dietary exposures and identifying sources of potential concern relative to the diet. However, since the FAO food balance sheets are based on gross estimates of food consumption for the population as a whole, this technique does not permit estimation of food consumption or dietary pesticide to subgroups of potential concern such as infants and children.

A research product of this investigation will be a compilation of food consumption data on a worldwide basis, which may also be useful for estimates of dietary pesticide exposure in many countries.

At the present, a comprehensive compilation of pesticide residues in food does not exist, and it has only been in recent times that various efforts have commenced to address this issue. One source of such data in the US has been the FDA Total Diet Study (Gartrell et al., 1986). Although limited by the number of samples analysed, this study does provide a useful indication of pesticide residues in the diet. The study has consistently shown over the past several years that concentrations for most pesticides are quite low (the majority of composite averages are between 0.1 and 10 p.p.b.). When compared to the acceptable daily intakes (ADIs) for pesticides established by USEPA or WHO, the calculated exposures do not appear to represent an appreciable risk.

Monitoring for pesticide residues in food is the most desirable method of generating data for estimating dietary pesticide exposures, as this approach is likely to provide the most accurate estimate of residues in food at the time of consumption. Unfortunately, this type of data is expensive and time-consuming to generate. One approach that has been used in the US to increase the efficiency of this type of data collection has been the Surveillance Index, developed by the FDA to target chemicals for monitoring that are likely to pose a significant health threat based on their toxicities, use patterns, or potential for high dietary exposure (Reed, 1985). A similar ranking method has been proposed for monitoring the intake of toxicants via seafood (Brown et al., 1988).

An area of potential exposure to pesticides that is of concern to many nations is the contamination of drinking water by pesticides and/or other chemicals (WHO, 1987). Indeed, contamination of drinking water supplies with a xenobiotic toxicant has been implicated or suspected in several episodes of disease (Rajput et al., 1987; Armstrong et al., 1984). Many countries have initiated programs to monitor the quality of drinking water and to identify regions which have been contaminated (Cohen et al., 1987). An accurate assessment of dietary pesticide exposure should include an estimate of the contribution of drinking water to the total dietary burden of pesticides.

7.5   DISCUSSION

In terms of the magnitude of potential exposures to the individual, it is clear that occupational exposures should be of greatest concern, and that exposures in this area must be carefully monitored to prevent serious disease. The risks from these types of exposures have been well documented by epidemiological reports of illness in agricultural workers (Edmiston and Maddy, 1987; Xue, 1987; Saunders et al., 1987; Coye et al., 1986b).

Many of the existing methods can estimate exposure; however, calculations of dose are difficult. A better understanding of the metabolism and pharmacokinetics of pesticide absorption (dermal, oral, and inhalation) and elimination would allow better estimation of actual doses, and, therefore, better risk management. Although some efforts have been made in this direction (Shehata-Karam et al., 1988; Wester and Maibach, 1985; Wester et al., 1983), the database is not large in terms of the number of different chemicals evaluated. For many chemicals, it may be necessary to extrapolate from experimental animal data in order to estimate human dose.

Construction of models of exposure may provide a valuable tool for predicting and managing occupational (or other types) of exposure, and alleviating the great expense of conducting studies for each chemical under each set of potential uses and exposure conditions. Research efforts in this area suggest that this approach holds promise (e.g. Chester and Hart, 1986; Nigg et al., 1984), but more research is needed to develop models that may be applied under more than a single set of conditions.

With respect to non-occupational exposures, existing data are scanty. Studies such as the EPA's NOPES are very useful as a means for estimating the total burden of pesticides that is likely to occur in the general population as a result of incidental household pesticide exposure. Additional studies of this type are desirable on an international basis, particularly in areas where the level of exposure may be high due to local pest pressures or agricultural practices.

Dietary exposures to pesticides remain an area of significant concern to many people, although evidence for adverse health effects resulting from exposure to low levels of pesticides in the diet is generally lacking. In fact, it has been suggested that natural constituents of food may actually present more of a hazard than pesticides or other chemical contaminants in food (Ames et al., 1987). The expansion of monitoring efforts such as the FDA Total Diet Study to provide better statistical representation and reliability would yield much useful information, and allow better estimation of the potential health effects of pesticides in the diet.

Although most calculations of dietary exposures have focused on estimates that are population-based average exposures, concern has been expressed over the potential effects of pesticide exposure in infants and children. These two subgroups are of particular interest, because they may be more sensitive to some toxic effects (e.g., lead) and because children and infants are well known to consume more food relative to body weight than adults. Therefore, if residue levels are constant, children and infants will receive a higher dose of pesticides in the diet—in fact, 2–5 times higher, depending on the crops involved (Saunders, 1987). In addition, ingestion of household dust may also represent a significant route of pesticide exposure for small children (Lewis, 1988). These phenomena raise an interesting and important question: how should the data from chronic feeding studies conducted in experimental animals be extrapolated to derive estimates of risk in infants and children? This is an area that requires more research, in terms of both the extrapolation of long-term animal toxicity studies to pesticide exposures in children, and the identification of effects to which infants and children may be uniquely susceptible.

In summary, occupational pesticide exposures seem to present the greatest risk in terms of the magnitude of individual exposure, and attention should be focused on that area to reduce individual risks. In addition, adequate methods must exist to allow regulatory agencies to protect the quality of the food supply, as is rightly demanded by the public. However, it is important that the data derived from the various exposure methodologies be viewed objectively and that national priorities and resources be focused on those areas that represent the most significant hazard.

7.6 RECOMMENDATIONS

1. Occupational exposures can be reduced through changes in application methodology. Specifically, ground-based applications rather than airblast or airborne applications should be used; and high-exposure occupations such as flagging should be eliminated by the substitution of mechanical devices. In addition, further advances in protective clothing and the use of closed application systems should be advocated.
2. The development of immunoassay methods, which hold the promise of providing rapid and inexpensive methods for monitoring exposures, should be encouraged. These techniques will be most useful in rural areas where access to sophisticated laboratory equipment is limited. In addition, further development and refinement of methodologies for assessing occupational exposure are desirable.
3. A better understanding of the manner in which pesticides are metabolized and excreted in humans is desirable. Such knowledge will permit better extrapolations of toxicity data from experimental animals to man, and allow for a better understanding of the significance of exposures to pesticides in man.
4. Improved methods are necessary on an international scale to provide developing nations with the capability of screening dietary exposures and identifying sources of potential hazard in the diet. The effort currently in progress at the WHO is a promising first step in that direction. In addition, better monitoring of residues as they occur in food and water at the time of consumption is necessary so that adequate data are available to correctly assess dietary risk.
5. Finally, more attention should be given to the effects of pesticide exposures on subgroups, such as infants and children, who are known to be exposed to relatively higher concentrations of pesticides through dietary and household exposures. Data on the specific effects of such exposures in these two important groups is relatively lacking.

7.7 REFERENCES

American Medical Association, Council of Scientific Affairs (1988) Cancer risk of pesticides in agricultural workers. *J. Am. Med. Assoc.* **260**, 959–966.

Ames, B. N., Magaw, R. and Gold, L. S. (1987) Ranking possible carcinogenic hazards. *Science* **236**, 271–280.

Armstrong, C. W., Stroube, R. B., Rubio, T., Siudyla, E. A. and Miller, G. B. (1984) Outbreak of fatal arsenic poisoning caused by contaminated drinking water. *Arch. Environ. Health* **39**, 271–279.

Atallah, Y. H., Cahill, W. P. and Whitacre, D. M. (1982) Exposure of pesticide applicators and support personnel to *O*-ethyl-*O*-(4-nitrophenyl)phenylphosphonothioate (EPN). *Arch. Environ. Contam. Toxicol.* **11**, 210–225.

Borm, P. J. A. and de Barbanson, B. (1988) Bias in biologic monitoring caused by concomitant medication. *J. Occup. Med.* **30**, 214–223.

Brown, H. S., Goble, R. and Tatelbaum, L. (1988) Methodology for assessing hazards of contaminants in seafood. *Reg. Toxicol. Appl. Pharmacol.* **8**, 76–101.

Carmen, G. E., Iwata, Y., Pappas, J. L., O'Neal, J. R. and Gunther, F. A. (1982) Pesticide applicator exposure to insecticides during treatment of citrus trees with oscillating boom and air-blast units. *Arch. Environ. Contam. Toxicol.* **11**, 651–659.

Chester, G. Hatfield, L. D., Hart, T. B., *et al.* (1987) Worker exposure to, and absorption of, cypermethrin during aerial application of 'ultra low volume' formulation to cotton. *Arch. Environ. Contam. Toxicol.* **16**, 69–78.

Chester, G. and Hart, T. B. (1986) Biological monitoring of a herbicide applied through backpack and vehicle sprayers. *Toxicol. Lett.* **33**, 137–149.

Chiao-Cheng, J. G., Regan, B. M., Bresee, R. R., Meloan, C. E. and Kadoum, A. M. (1988) Carbamate insecticide removal in laundering from cotton and polyester fabrics. *Arch. Environ. Contam. Toxicol.* **17**, 87–94.

Cohen, S. Z., Eiden, C. and Lorber, M. N. (1987) Monitoring ground water for pesticides in the U.S.A. *Schriftenr. Ver. Wasser Boden Lufthyg. (Ger.)* **68**, 265–295.

Cowell, J. E., Danhaus, R. G., Kuntzman, J. L., *et al.* (1987) Operator exposure from closed system loading and application of alachlor herbicide. *Arch. Environ. Contam. Toxicol.* **16**, 69–78.

Coye, M. J., Lowe, J. A. and Maddy, K. J. (1986a) Biological monitoring of agricultural workers exposed to pesticides. I. Cholinesterase activity determinations. *J. Occup. Med.* **28**, 628–636.

Coye, M. J., Barnett, P. G., Midtling, J. E., *et al.* (1986b) Clinical confirmation of organophosphate poisoning of agricultural workers. *Am. J. Ind. Med.* **10**, 399–409.

Davies, J. E., Freed, V. H., Enos, H. F., *et al.* (1982) Reduction of pesticide exposure with protective clothing for applicators and mixers. *J. Occup. Med.* **24**, 464–468.

Davis, J. E., Stevens, E. R. and Staiff, D. C. (1983) Potential exposure of apple thinners to azinphosmethyl and comparison of two methods for assessment of hand exposure. *Bull. Environ. Contam. Toxicol.* **31**, 631–638.

Durham, W. F. and Wolfe, H. R. (1962) Measurement of the exposure of workers to pesticides. *Bull WHO* **26**, 75–91.

Edmiston, S. and Maddy, K. T. (1987) Summary of illnesses and injuries reported in California by physicians in 1986 as potentially related to pesticides. *Vet. Human Toxicol.* **29**, 391–397.

Everhart, L. P. and Holt, R. F. (1982) Potential benlate exposure during mixer/loader operations, crop harvest, and home use. *J. Agric. Food Chem.* **30**, 222–227.

Fenske, R. A., Hamburger, S. J. and Guyton, C. L. (1987) Occupational exposure to fosetyl-Al fungicide during spraying of ornamentals in greenhouses. *Arch. Environ. Contam. Toxicol.* **16**, 615–621.

Gartrell, M. J., Craun, J. C., Podrebarac, D. S. and Gunderson, E. L. (1986) Pesticides, selected elements, and other chemicals in adult total diet samples, October 1980–1982. *J. Assoc. Off. Anal. Chem.* **69**, 146–161.

Grover, R., Cessna, A. J., Muri, N. I. *et al.* (1986) Factors affecting the exposure of ground-rig applicators to 2,4-D dimethylamine salt. *Arch. Environ. Contam. Toxicol.* **15**, 677–686.

Hammock, B. D., Gee, S. J. Cheung, P. Y. K., Miyamoto, T., Goodrow, M. H., *et al.* (1987) Utility of immunoassay in pesticide trace analysis. In: Greenhalgh, R. and Roberts, T. R. (Eds) *Pesticide Science and Biotechnology*, Blackwell Science, Oxford, pp. 309–316.

Kutz, F. W., Straussman, S. C., Stroup, C. R., Carra, J. S., Leininger, C. C., Watts, D. L. and Sparacino, C. M. (1985) The human body burden of mirex in the Southeastern United States. *J. Toxicol. Environ. Health* **15**, 385–394.

Leavitt, J. R., Gold, R. E., Holcslaw, T. and Tupy, D. (1982) Exposure of professional pesticide applicators to carbaryl. *Arch. Environ. Contam. Toxicol.* **11**, 57–62.

Lewis, R. G. (1976) Sampling and analysis of airborne pesticides. In: Lee, R. E., Jr. (Ed.) *Air Pollution from Pesticides and Agricultural Processes*, CRC Press, Cleveland, Ohio, pp. 51–94.

Lewis, R. G. (1988) *Human Exposure to Pesticides Used in Air and Around the Household.* Report prepared for the Task Force on Environmental Cancer and Heart and Lung Disease, Working Group on Exposure, US Environmental Protection Agency, Office of Research and Development, Environmental Monitoring Systems Laboratory, Research Triangle Park, North Carolina.

Lewis, R. G., Bond, A. E., Johnson, D. E. and Hsu, J. P. (1988) Measurement of atmospheric concentrations of common household pesticides: a pilot study. *Environ. Monit. Assess.* **10**, 59–73.

Loevinsohn, M. E. (1987) Insecticide use and increased mortality in rural Phillipines. *Lancet* **8546**, 1359–1362.

Matsumara, F. (1985) Insecticide residues in man. In: Matsumura, F. (Ed.) *Toxicology of Insecticides* (2nd edn), Plenum Press, New York, London, pp. 547–568.

Mumma, R. O. and Brady, J. F. (1987) Immunological assays for agrochemicals. In: Greenhalgh, R. and Roberts, T. R. (Eds) *Pesticide Science and Biotechnology*, Blackwell Science, Oxford, pp. 309–316.

Murphy, R. S., Kutz, F. W. and Strassman, S. C. (1983) Selected pesticide residues or metabolites in blood and urine specimens from a general population survey. *Environ. Health. Perspect.* **48**, 81–86.

Murphy, R. and Harvey, C. (1985) Residues and metabolites of selected persistent halogenated hydrocarbons in blood specimens from a general population survey. *Environ. Health Perspect.* **60**, 115–120.

Nigg, H. N., Stamper, J. H. and Queen, R. M. (1984) The development and use of a universal model to predict tree crop harvester pesticide exposure. *Am. Ind. Hyg. Assoc. J.* **45**(3), 182–186.

Petersen, B. and Chaisson, C. (1988) Pesticides and residues in food. *Food Technol.* **42**(7), 59–64.

Putnam, A. R., Willis, M. D., Binning, L. K. and Boldt, P. F. (1983) Exposure of pesticide applicators to nitrofen: influence of formulation, handling systems, and protective garments. *J. Agric. Food Chem.* **31**, 645–650.

Rajput, A. H., Uitti, R. J., Stern, W., *et al.* (1987) Geography, drinking water chemistry, pesticides and herbicides and the etiology of Parkinson's disease. *Can. J. Neurol. Sci.* **14**, 414–418.

Reed, D. V. (1985) Chemical contaminants monitoring—the FDA surveillance index for pesticides: establishing food monitoring priorities based on potential health risk. *J. Assoc. Off. Anal. Chem.* **68**(1), 122–124.

Reinert, J. C., Nielsen, A. P., Lunchik, C., Hernandez, O. and Mazzetta, D. M. (1986) The United States Environmental Protection Agency's guidelines for applicator exposure monitoring. *Toxicol. Lett.* **33**, 183–191.

Richter, E. D., Rosenvald, Z., Kaspi, L. and Gruener, N. (1986) Sequential cholinesterase tests and symptoms for monitoring organophosphate absorption in field workers and in persons exposed to pesticide spray drift. *Toxicol. Lett.* **33**, 25–32.

Saunders, D. S. and Petersen, B. P. (1986) *Introduction to the Tolerance Assessment System*, US Environmental Protection Agency, Office of Pesticide Programs, Residue Chemistry Branch, Washington DC.

Saunders, D. S. (1987) *Briefing paper on the Tolerance Assessment System for Presentation to the FIFRA Scientific Advisory Panel*, US Environmental Protection Agency, Office of Pesticide Programs, Residue Chemistry Branch, Washington, DC.

Saunders, L. D., Ames, R. G., Knaak, J. B. and Jackson, R. J. (1987) Outbreak of Omite-CR-induced dermatitis among orange pickers in Tulare County, California. *J. Occup. Med.* **29**, 409–413.

Shehata-Karam, H., Monteiro-Riviere, N. A. and Guthrie, F. E. (1988) *In vitro* penetration of pesticides through human newborn foreskin. *Toxicol. Lett.* **40**, 233–239.

Skaare, J. U., Tuveng, J. M., and Sande, H. A. (1988) Organochlorine pesticides and polychlorinated biphenyls in maternal adipose tissue, blood, milk, and cord blood from mothers and infants living in Norway. *Arch. Environ. Contam. Toxicol.* **17**, 473–478.

Strassman, S. C. and Kutz, F. W. (1981) Trends of organochlorine pesticide residues in human tissue. In: Khan, M. A. Q. and Stanton, R. H. (Eds), *Toxicology of Halogenated Hydrocarbons: Health and Ecological Effects*, Pergamon Press, New York, pp. 38–49.

Taguchi, S. and Yakushiji, T. (1988) Influence of termite treatment in the home on the chlordane concentration in human milk. *Arch. Environ. Contam. Toxicol.* **17**, 65–71.

Travis, C. C., Hattermer-Frey, H. A. and Arms, A. D. (1988) Relationship between dietary intake of organic chemicals and their concentrations in human adipose tissue and breast milk. *Arch. Environ. Contam. Toxicol.* **17**, 473–478.

USEPA (1987a) *Pesticide Assessment Guidelines. Subdivision U. Applicator Exposure Monitoring*, US Environmental Protection Agency, Office of Pesticide Programs, Exposure Assessment Branch, Washington, DC.

USEPA (1987b) *Non-Occupational Pesticide Exposure Study (NOPES)—Phase II: Jacksonville, Florida, Summer, 1986*, Interim report, US Environmental Protection Agency, Office of Research and Development, Environmental Monitoring System Laboratory, Research Triangle Park, North Carolina.

Weisskopf, C. P., Sieber, J. N., Maizlish, N. and Schenker, M. (1988) Personal exposure to diazinon in a supervised pest eradication program. *Arch. Environ. Contam. Toxicol.* **17**, 201–212.

Wester, R. C. and Maibach, H. I. (1985) *In vivo* percutaneous absorption and decontamination of pesticides in humans. *J. Toxicol. Environ. Health* **16**, 25–37.

Wester, R. C., Maibach, H. I., Bucks, D. A. W. and Guy, R. H. (1983) Malathion percutaneous absorption and repeated administration to man. *Toxicol. Appl. Pharmacol.* **68**, 116–119.

WHO (1981) Pesticide deaths. What's the toll? *Ecoforum* **6**, 10.

WHO (1987) *Drinking-Water Quality. Guidelines for Selected Herbicides*, Environmental Health Series #27, World Health Organization, Regional Office for Europe, Copenhagen, Denmark.

WHO (1988) *Guidelines for Predicting Dietary Intake of Pesticide Residues* (prepared by the joint UNEP/FAO/WHO Food Contamination Monitoring Programme in collaboration with the Codex Committee on Pesticide Residues), World Health Organization, Geneva.

Xue, S. Z. (1987) Health effects of pesticides: a review of epidemiologic research from the perspective of developing nations. *Am. J. Ind. Med.* **32**, 269–279.

8 Role of Evaluative Models to Assess Exposures to Pesticides

D. CALAMARI and M. VIGHI
University of Milan, Institute of Agricultural Entomology, Italy

8.1 INTRODUCTION

For many years the information on the environmental distribution and fate of chemical substances was acquired largely in retrospect from empirical observations after large-scale monitoring efforts with an enormous number of chemical analyses. This retrospective approach left wide margins for error in the environmental management of chemical substances, and the possibility of large-scale undesirable effects remained largely uncontrolled. It is sufficient to note the widespread distribution of organochlorine pesticides and their detection in areas very far from the application zones, and the presence of herbicides in groundwater used for human consumption.

One way to face the problem might have been to model the environmental distribution of individual substances. In the sixties, the modelling era started when technical facilities made the solution of complex numerical calculations easier; but after an initial period of euphoria, complex models were considered much less applicable and useful than expected. For example, large-scale models such as that of Randers (1973) worked for DDT, but only with large quantities of input data; their predictive capability was therefore very limited.

In the early seventies, several groups of scientists began thinking in predictive terms. Moreeover, legislative mandates, such as the Toxic Substance Control Act (USEPA, 1978) in the US and the Directive on Dangerous Substances (EEC, 1979) in Europe, gave a strong impetus to the predictive approach. Initially, several investigators advanced the hypothesis that one could predict the behaviour of a new chemical by comparing properties measured in a laboratory with those of compounds for which more environmental data were available. The concept of environmental chemodynamics was then proposed as a holistic approach for the comprehensive understanding of the behaviour of chemical substances in the environment.

Methods to Assess Adverse Effects of Pesticides on Non-target Organisms
Edited by R. G. Tardiff
©1992 SCOPE Published by John Wiley & Sons Ltd
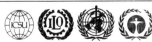

Contemporary management of chemical substances assesses the hazard as one step needed for a comprehensive risk assessment of potentially dangerous chemicals. In essence, a hazard assessment is a comparison of the no-observed-effect level and the expected environmental concentration. For making such an evaluation, the prediction of exposure has become a key issue in research on specific substances.

8.2 DEVELOPMENT OF EVALUATIVE MODELS

To predict environmental distribution and fate of chemicals, Baughman and Lassiter (1978) introduced the concept of an evaluative model with the aim of developing a quantitative approach for exposure estimation. According to these authors, evaluative models 'incorporate the dynamics of no specific environment but are based on the properties of stylized environment or hypothetical pollutants for which we specify (rather than measure) inputs'.

In the ensuing years, many publications appeared on the same subject (see, for example, Haque, 1980; Neely, 1980; Hutzinger, 1980, 1982; Gunther, 1983; Neely and Blau, 1985; Sheehan et al., 1985; GSF, 1985). The Organization of Economic Cooperation and Development, within the framework of its Chemical Group and Management Committee in the Hazard Assessment Project, prepared a report on the practical approaches for the assessment of environmental exposure (OECD, 1986).

Several authors produced simple evaluative models (Mackay, 1979; Neely, 1979; Roberts and Marshall, 1980; Frische et al., 1982). A 'fugacity' model was proposed to calculate the relative amount of a substance that would ultimately partition into each environmental compartment (Mackay and Paterson, 1982). In these models, no attempt was made to simulate the precise or actual environmental conditions; but they were intended to allow the prediction of the potential distribution of the chemical compounds.

The most relevant possibilities for application of the results of such types of models were, according to Calamari and Vighi (1988), the following:

1. Preliminary screening of the environmental behaviour of a number of chemicals,
2. Indications of the partition and affinity for the main environmental compartments,
3. Identification of the compartments where high levels are more likely to be present, and of the matrices where the transformation processes are more likely to be relevant,
4. Information to assist with the planning of laboratory or field experiments and/or monitoring campaigns,
5. Data for preliminary hazard assessment.

Fugacity models of increasing complexity were produced by Mackay and others (Mackay and Paterson, 1982; Mackay *et al.*, 1983) and laboratory and field studies were undertaken to clarify fully the concept of fugacity and to identify the value and limitations of such an approach, the areas of applicability, and the predictive capability of evaluative models.

In the following sections the fugacity approach will be described, because the experience of the authors deals mainly with this kind of model; various evaluative models of comparable applicability have been developed recently, but are not discussed here.

8.3 THE FUGACITY MODEL

8.3.1 CONCEPT AND APPLICATION

The concept of fugacity was introduced by Lewis at the beginning of this century as a criterion for equilibrium between phases. Fugacity can be regarded as the tendency of a chemical substance to escape from a phase. It has units of pressure, and can be linearly related to concentration (Mackay and Paterson, 1982).

The relation between fugacity (f) and concentration (C) for a given phase (or environmental compartment) can be written as:

$$f = \frac{C}{Z} \tag{8.1}$$

where Z is a 'fugacity capacity constant' depending, at a given temperature and pressure, on the nature of the substance and of the environmental compartment under examination. Z quantifies the capacity of a given phase or compartment for fugacity.

Each substance tends to accumulate in compartments where Z is high and where high concentrations can be present with relatively low fugacities. Where a chemical is introduced in a multicompartment system, the fugacity at equilibrium is equal in all media, but concentrations are different functions of the different capacities. To evaluate equilibrium concentrations on a comparative basis and express them in commonly accepted units, the concept of 'unit of world' was then introduced (Mackay, 1979). This is a hypothetical model environment that includes the main environmental compartments at defined volumes.

If one can find Z values for a substance for each environmental phase, the distribution of the substance at equilibrium can be easily calculated. The highest concentrations will correspond to the highest values of Z. To obtain Z values for the different environmental compartments, it must be noted that in the atmosphere, fugacity can be considered in general as equivalent to the partial pressure (P) for the vapour phase of a chemical. Concentration (C) is related to partial pressure through the gas law:

$$PV = nRT \tag{8.2}$$

$$C = \frac{n}{V} = \frac{P}{RT} = \frac{f}{RT} \tag{8.3}$$

From equation (8.1) it follows that

$$C = fZ = \frac{f}{RT} \tag{8.4}$$

Thus,

$$Z = \frac{1}{RT} \tag{8.5}$$

For all other compartments, one must remember that in a multicompartment system at equilibrium,

$$f_1 = f_2 = \ldots f_i \tag{8.6}$$

where f_i is the fugacity of a substance for the compartment i. Considering two compartments i and j, from equation (1),

$$f_i = f_j = \frac{C_i}{Z_i} = \frac{C_j}{Z_j} \tag{8.7}$$

$$\frac{Z_i}{Z_j} = \frac{C_i}{C_j} = K_{ij} \tag{8.8}$$

where K_{ij} is the partition coefficient between the two phases. From equation (8.8).

$$Z_i = K_{ij} * Z_j \tag{8.9}$$

Therefore, one can easily calculate Z for each compartment, if one knows the partition coefficient between two phases and the Z values for one of the two compartments. For example, for water,

$$Z_w = K_{wa} * Z_a \tag{8.10}$$

where K_{wa} is the partition coefficient between water and air. It follows that

$$Z_w = \frac{C_w}{C_a} * \frac{1}{RT} \tag{8.11}$$

From equation (8.3),

$$Z_w = \frac{C_w RT}{P} * \frac{1}{RT} = \frac{C_w}{P} = \frac{1}{H} \qquad (8.12)$$

where H is the Henry's law constant.

Through this procedure, one can easily include new environmental compartments in the original 'unit of world'.

8.3.2   APPLICATIONS

In a series of papers, the concept of fugacity and its potential to describe environmental distribution and fate phenomena were explored and explained. Fugacity, which at the beginning was no more than a simple definition of 'escaping tendency', has been and could be used for different purposes.

The first application could be in the prediction of environmental distribution with a fixed scenario (e.g., the standard 'unit of world') to compare different substances and rank them on the basis of their affinity for a certain compartment. Fugacity can be used, for example, to select which of a number of herbicides with similar agronomical performances has the lowest affinity for the water compartment, providing a basis for minimization of the probability of water contamination.

Some of the essential aspects of the environmental distribution and fate of cypermethrin (Bacci *et al.*, 1987) have been elucidated by means of a combination of evaluative models and a few *ad hoc* experiments in a simulation chamber. The experiments produced results that had been predicted by the fugacity model. In fact, according to its physical and chemical properties, cypermethrin should have strong soil affinity, be practically non-volatile in air, unable to reach water, and unable to accumulate in plants. Degradation occurred in soil over a period of time comparable with that previously reported.

Although evaluative models are not intended for prediction of detailed fate in a specific environment, one can vary the standard scenario to improve the simulation and obtain an enhanced understanding of the behaviour of a single molecule (e.g., a unit of world in interstitial water to mimic fate in a cultivated field, or the removal of the soil compartment to simulate a lake, etc.).

The mass balance concept and biogeochemical approach should be considered for a complete understanding of the behaviour of a chemical in an environment; therefore, these types of simulations can be of great help for the preparation of monitoring campaigns or large-scale field experiments. Clark *et al.* (1988) discussed the utility of such an approach in relation to a monitoring program to identify persistent and biocumulative contaminants such as chlorinated hydrocarbons. From a theoretical example, they stated that, if reliable bioconcentration relationships exist between water, fish, birds, and bird eggs, it could be more convenient routinely to analyse a few eggs instead of high numbers of samples from any media or organisms with lower and more variable concentration levels.

The fugacity approach was applied to evaluative models, laboratory experiments, and field work to understand mechanisms regulating environmental distribution and fate of a pesticide under specific conditions and to define acceptable loads in a given territory. In the watershed of Lake Chiusi (Sienna, Italy), an area of about 100 ha of clay soil was studied after treatment with a single dose of atrazine (Bacci *et al.*, 1990). The fugacity model was adapted to the specific environmental system (watershed plus lake) considering the differences at various times (rainfall, growing of crops, etc.). Laboratory experiments were performed to evaluate degradation in conditions comparable to those existing in the examined system. Concentrations of atrazine were measured at various times in different media, and compared with those calculated by the model. A good agreement was shown between the prediction of the model and the measured values (Table 8.1). Moreover, advection by runoff was demonstrated as the only route of transport of atrazine from the terrestrial to the aquatic environments.

Table 8.1. Comparison of predicted and measured levels of atrazine (from Vighi and Calamari, 1990) in environmental compartments of the Lake Chiusi area at different times after treatment

Time (days)	Soil		Lake water		Lake sediments	
	Predicted	Observed	Predicted	Observed	Predicted	Observed
0	401	—	62	66*	5	—
90	104	—	—	46	—	—
130	54	42	—	32	—	—
180	26	20	—	25	—	1.8
230	11	9	—	21	—	—

*Calculated from the loss rate constant

This integrated approach allows the estimation of the acceptable load of atrazine in fields during 'medium' rainfalls to obtain acceptable levels of the herbicide in lakes whose water is used for drinking purposes (Vighi and Calamari, 1989).

Besides the practical and concrete applications of the fugacity approach already cited, other potential implications have been suggested by Clark *et al.* (1988). These authors proposed that by converting disparate concentration units related to various media into one common unit (e.g., fugacity in Pa), it is reasonably easy to evaluate the significance of various concentrations in different environmental compartments (i.e., a trend for bioaccumulation). In case of equifugacity in a medium, an equilibrium status or a rapid exchange among compartments could be recognized. The same type of calculation (concentration expressed as fugacity) could identify hot spots and clean areas.

8.3.3   PROBLEMS AND CONSTRAINTS IN THE USE
OF THE FUGACITY MODEL

A limitation inherent in the original form of the fugacity model is the absence in the unit world for biota other than aquatic animals. Terrestrial plants are a very important component due to their biomass and to the possibility of transfer of contaminants to higher levels, including man, of the trophic chain.

On the other hand, as has been previously emphasized, the inclusion of a new compartment into the model is conceptually an easy task, requiring only the calculation of the Z value once partition coefficients are known.

A wide range of literature is available on bioconcentration factors for aquatic animals, whereas very scanty information exists for terrestrial plants. This situation can explain why these species have not been included in the standard form of the model. The inclusion of plant biomass in the fugacity model was attempted by Calamari et al. (1987). Three equations have been used relating accumulation in roots and in the stem with the log of the octanol–water partition coefficient, log K_{ow} (Briggs et al., 1982, 1983) and accumulation in foliage with the Henry's law constant, utilizing data reported by Bacci and Gaggi (1987). By means of the resulting bioaccumulation factors, terrestrial plants have been included as a sum of three separate compartments (namely roots, stem, and foliage).

To produce a theoretical validation of the consistency of the improved model, the hypothesis was proposed that bioaccumulation in foliage depends on log K_{ow} and H. This hypothesis has been successively confirmed by Travis and Hattemer-Frey (1988), who used the same data from Bacci and Gaggi (1987) and found that the logarithm of the bioconcentration factor is directly related to log K_{ow} and inversely to log H. Thus, an improved equation for bioaccumulation in foliage, based on new experimental data, has been proposed by Bacci et al. (1990).

Major problems in the use of the fugacity model can derive from the lack of availability and the poor quality of basic data on the physico-chemical properties of the molecules. Theoretically, the only data essential to apply the fugacity model are water solubility and vapour pressure. Even for these elemental properties, much uncertainty exists. In the most frequently consulted reference books, such as The Pesticide Manual (Worthing and Walker, 1987), data are often expressed in vague terms or are not available at all (e.g., solubility in water: 'negligible'; vapour pressure: 'less than . . .'). A recent review (Suntio et al., 1988) of Henry's law constants for pesticides demonstrates that data in the literature are often conflicting and that the selection of the most reliable data is a very vexing task.

All other parameters needed for the fugacity model (octanol–water partition coefficient, soil sorption coefficient, bioconcentration factors, etc.) could be obtained, in theory, by means of property-to-property equations (e.g., from solubility). Nevertheless, the applicability of property-to-property equations has been shown to be relatively limited and to have great potential for error, particularly in the calculation of K_{ow}, a key property in each type of evaluative model.

A more reliable approach is the calculation of K_{ow} by means of the fragment constants method (Hansch and Leo, 1979) or other comparable techniques. Computer programs exist for the calculation of log K_{ow} by means of this method. Recently the US Environmental Protection Agency has modified these programs for the personal computer (USEPA, 1987).

Many authors consider the fragment constants method the best way to obtain reliable values for log K_{ow}; in some cases, this method is even preferred to experimental measurements. Nevertheless, for very complex chemicals (such as many pesticides and drugs) and in particular for values of log K_{ow} values and other basic physico-chemical data must be carefully examined before use.

8.3.4   WIDENING THE FUGACITY CONCEPT

In addition to the previously discussed limitations of these models, another relevant constraint is the absence of any indication of the time scale for the attainment of equilibrium. A second observations is that, for the same system

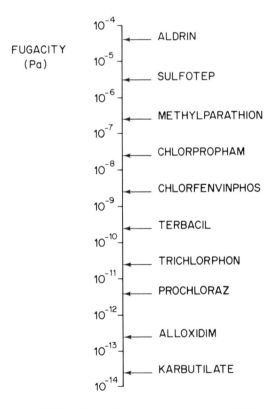

Figure 8.1. Range of variability of fugacity values for some pesticides at equilibrium after an emission of 100 moles into the system; physico-chemical data taken from Worthing and Walker (1987) and from Suntio *et al.* (1988)

of reference (i.e., the standard 'unit of world'), fugacities varied over a range of several orders of magnitude even if one considers pesticides alone (Figure 8.1).

Accordingly, based on these two observations, an attempt was made to explore whether a difference in the fugacity could also be an indication of a potential difference in mobility among molecules. Fugacity by definition is not an intrinsic property of the molecule, since it depends on the compartments of the environmental system and the relative concentrations in the various phases of the system besides the characteristics of the molecule.

In a dynamic system, fugacity is not constant, but varies with time and concentration. However, if the parameters of the system (i.e., standard unit of world) and the time (i.e., initial condition or equilibrium condition) are fixed, fugacity can be considered independent of the system and, therefore, an 'intrinsic' property of the molecule.

If one considers the fugacity at equilibrium in the standard unit of world, it can be observed that sometimes different molecules may show similar distribution in the environmental compartments, notwithstanding different fugacity values.

As an example, Table 8.2 shows the physico-chemical properties needed for the application of the fugacity model to four pesticides (part A) and the percentage distribution and fugacity in the standard unit of world (part B). The percentage distribution of the four molecules is very similar in all compartments, with the exception of air, while fugacity ranges over about three orders of magnitude.

Considering the relation between concentration and fugacity ($C = fZ$) and that Z for the air compartment is independent of the characteristics of the molecule ($Z_a = 1/RT$), one concludes that it is impossible to obtain similar concentrations in air with different fugacities.

In compartments other than air, partition is regulated by log K_{ow} or other partition coefficients directly related to it (soil sorption coefficients, bioconcentration factors, etc.). These coefficients are practically identical for the molecules considered here. In Figure 8.2, data from Table 8.2 for sulfotep and chlorfenvinphos are graphically presented; in each box, representing an environmental compartment, a similar distribution can be observed. When the system is at equilibrium, by definition the same quantities of the substance move in and out from each compartment. The total mass transport in a fixed unit of time is different for the two chemicals and depends on their escaping tendencies. This is shown in Figure 8.2, where escaping tendency (fugacity) is represented as a vector. If we consider two molecules having different fugacities but similar equilibrium distributions in the standard unit of world, one could expect that, by placing the same quantity in the same compartment, the mass transfer in a fixed time should be different for the two chemicals due to differences in fugacity.

A numerical example for the two molecules examined is shown in Figure 8.2. Placing the same quantity (e.g, 100 moles) into the same compartment (e.g., water), one can calculate the initial fugacity from equations (8.1) and (8.12):

Table 8.2. Physico-chemical properties needed for the application of the fugacity model to four pesticides (part A); percentage-distribution and fugacity in the standard unit of world (part B)

		Sulfotep	Parathion methyl	Chlorpropham	Chlorfenvinphos
A	Molecular weight	322	263	214	360
	Solubility (g/l)	0.025	0.037	0.158	0.129
	Vapour pressure (Pa)	0.0226	3×10^{-3}	1.6×10^{-3}	1×10^{-4}
	log K_{ow}	3.0	3.0	3.1	3.1
	H (Pa m^3/mol)	0.29	0.021	2.1×10^{-3}	2.8×10^{-4}
B	Air	7.5	0.6	0.06	7.4×10^{-3}
	Water	75.1	80.8	77.5	77.5
	Soil + Sediment + SS	17.3	18.5	22.4	22.4
	Biota	5.3×10^{-3}	5.7×10^{-3}	6.6×10^{-3}	6.7×10^{-3}
	f(Pa)	3.1×10^{-6}	2.5×10^{-7}	2.4×10^{-8}	3.1×10^{-9}

SS = suspended solids

$$f = \frac{C_w}{Z_w} = C_w H \tag{8.13}$$

It follows that values of 4.1×10^6 and 3.9×10^4 can be calculated for sulfotep and chlorfenvinphos, respectively. This means that the former exerts an escaping tendency from water to all other compartments about a thousand times higher than the latter. In other words, the higher the fugacity, the shorter the time needed for the attainment of equilibrium. This intuitive statement is also supported by the fact that fugacity is expressed in units of pressure (i.e, lower pressure, lower mobility).

Unfortunately, if this is true, it can be proposed only on a qualitative basis, and the role of fugacity as a mobility parameter cannot at present be quantified. There is a need for experimental work to confirm this hypothesis and eventually to define the relationship between fugacity and rate of transport.

8.4   CONCLUSIONS

Ideally, evaluative models should allow calculation of the potential exposure concentration in each ecosystem; however, this is still a distant prospect. This paper has presented some positive achievements in the use of evaluative models. Recently, other evaluative models, based on simple physico-chemical properties, have been developed, such as those proposed by Rao *et al.* (1985) to predict the potential for groundwater contamination from pesticides. Jury *et al.* (1987) indicate that further development of integrated models will provide an interesting

129

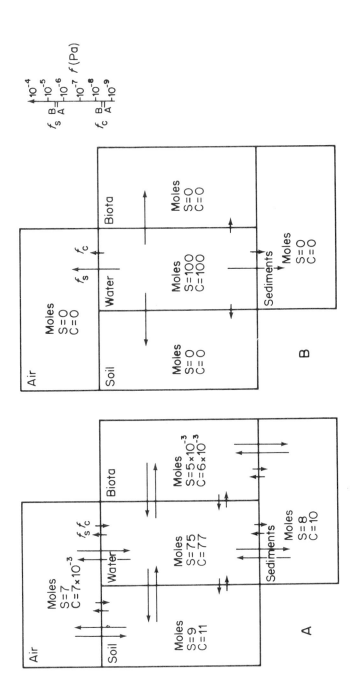

Figure 8.2. Illustration of equilibrium distribution for sulfotep (S) and chlorfenvinphos (C) in 'unit of world'; fugacities shown as vectors

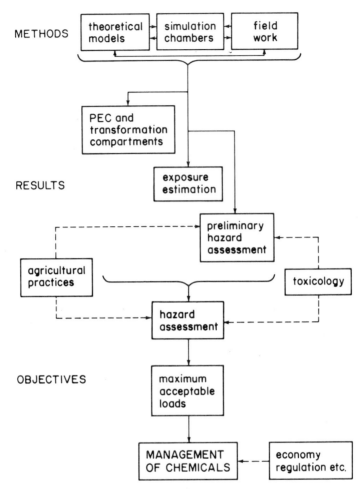

Figure 8.3. Overall research strategy on valuative models for the environmental management of pesticides

methodology to understand and quantify transport and transformation pathways of organic chemicals in the environment.

The scientific community has a general interest in this subject, as evidenced by the number of references in the joint report, this paper, and in specialized publications, such as the proceedings of a workshop on environmental modelling for priority setting among existing chemicals (GSF, 1985). Figure 8.3, from Calamari and Vighi (1988), illustrates a strategy of the use of an evaluative model to minimize the impact of pesticides on the environment. The overall strategy is aimed predominantly at developing predictive systems to confidently calculate the potential exposure in various compartments of the ecosystem. Recently, this field of investigation has increased exponentially, and offers great promise for future research in environmental sciences.

8.5 REFERENCES

Bacci, E., Calamari, D., Gaggi, C. and Vighi, M. (1987) An approach for the prediction of environmental distribution and fate of cypermethrin. *Chemosphere* **16**, 1373–1380.

Bacci, E. and Gaggi, C. (1987) Chlorinated hydrocarbons vapours and plant foliage: kinetics and applications. *Chemosphere* **16**, 2515–2522.

Bacci, E., Renzoni, A., Gaggi, C., Calamari, D., Franchi, A., Vighi, M. and Severi, A. (1990) Models, field studies, laboratory experiments: an integrated approach to evaluate the environmental fate of atrazine (*s*-triazine herbicide). In: Paoletti, M. G., Stinner, B. R., and Lorenzoni, G. G. (Eds) *Agricultural Ecology and Environment: Proceedings of an International Symposium, Padova, Italy, 5–7 April, 1988*, Elsevier, Amsterdam.

Baughman, G. L. and Lassiter, R. R. (1978) Prediction of environmental pollution concentration. In: Cairns, J., Dickson, K. L., and Maki, A. W. (Eds) *Estimating the Hazard of Chemical Substances to Aquatic Life*, ASTM Special Technical Publication 657, American Society for Testing and Materials, Philadelphia, pp. 35–54.

Briggs, G. G., Bromilow, R. H. and Evans, A. A. (1982) Relationship between lipophilicity and root uptake and translocation of non-ionized chemicals by barley. *Pest. Sci.* **13**, 492–500.

Briggs, G. G. Bromilow, R. H., Evans, A. A. and Williams, M. (1983) Relationships between lipophilicity and the distribution of non-ionized chemicals in barley shoots following uptake by roots. *Pest. Sci.* **14**, 492–500.

Calamari, D. and Vighi, M. (1988) Experiences on QSARs and evaluative models in ecotoxicology. *Chemosphere* **17**, 1539–1549.

Clark, T., Clark, K., Paterson, S., Mackay, D. and Norstrom, R. J. (1988) Wildlife monitoring, modelling, and fugacity. *Environ. Sci. Technol.* **22**, 120–127.

EEC (1979) Council directive 79/831. *Off. J. Europ. Commun.* L**259**, 10pp.

Frische, R., Esser, G., Schoenborn, W. and Kloepffer, W. (1982) Criteria for assessing the environmental behaviour of chemicals: selection and preliminary quantification. *Ecotoxicol. Environ. Saf.* **6**, 283–293.

GSF (1985) *Environmental Modelling for Priority Setting among Existing Chemicals*, Workshop, 11–13 November 1985, Munchen-Neuherberg Gesellschaft fur Strahlen und Umweltforschung mbH, Munchen.

Gunther, F. A. (Ed.) (1983) Residues of pesticides and other contaminants in the Total Environment. *Residue Rev.* **85**, 1–307.

Hansch, C. and Leo, A. J. (1979) *Substituent Constants for Correlation Analysis in Chemistry and Biology*, John Wiley, New York.

Haque, R. (Ed.) (1980) *Dynamics, Exposure and Hazard Assessment of Toxic Chemicals*, Ann Arbor Science, Ann Arbor, Michigan.

Hutzinger, O. (Ed.) (1980) *The Handbook of Environmental Chemistry. Reaction and Processes*, Vol. 2, Part B, Springer-Verlag, Berlin, Heidelberg, New York.

Jury, W. A., Winer, A. M., Spencer, W. F. and Focht, D. D. (1987) Transport and transformations of organic chemicals in the organic chemicals in the soil–air–water ecosystem. *Rev. Environ. Contam. Toxicol.* **99**, 119–164.

Lyman, W. J., Reehl, W. F. and Rosenblatt, D. H. (1982) *Handbook of Chemical Property Estimation Methods*, McGraw-Hill, New York.

Mackay, D. (1975) Finding fugacity feasible. *Environ Sci. Technol.* **13**, 1218–1223.

Mackay, D., Joy, M. and Paterson, S. (1983) A quantitative water, air, sediment interaction (QWASI) fugacity model for describing the fate of chemicals in lakes. *Chemosphere* **12**, 981–997.

Mackay, D. and Paterson, S. (1982) Fugacity revisited. *Environ. Sci. Technol.* **16**, 654–660.

Mackay, D., Paterson, S. and Joy, M. (1983) A quantitative water, air, sediment interaction (QWASI) fugacity model for describing the fate of chemicals in rivers. *Chemosphere* **12**, 1193–1208.

Neely, W. B. (1979) A preliminary assessment of the environmental exposure to be expected from the addition of a chemical to a simulated aquatic ecosystem. *Int. J. Environ. Studies* **13**, 101–108.

Neely, W. B. (1980) Chemicals in the environment. *Distribution, Transport, Fate Analysis*, Marcel Dekker, New York, Basel.

Neely, W. B. and Blau, G. E. (Eds) (1985) *Environmental Exposure from Chemicals*, Vol. I, CRC Press, Boca Raton, Florida.

OECD (1986) *Hazard Assessment Project*, report of workshop on practical approaches for the assessment of environmental exposure, ENV/CHEM/CM/86.8.

Randers, J. (1973) DDT movement in the global environment. In: Meadows, D. L. and Meadows, D. H. (Eds) *Toward Global Equilibrium*, Wright-Allen Press, Cambridge, Mass., pp. 49–83.

Rao, P. S. C., Hornsby, A. G. and Jessup, R. E. (1985) Indices for ranking the potential for pesticide contamination of groundwater. *Proc. Soil Crop Sci. Soc.* **44**, 1–24.

Roberts, J. R. and Marshall, W. K. (1980) Retentive capacity: an index of chemical persistence expressed in terms of chemical-specific and ecosystem-specific parameters. *Ecotoxicol. Environ. Saf.* **4**, 158–171.

Sheehan, P., Korte, F., Klein, W. and Bourdeau, P. (Eds) (1985) *Appraisal of Tests to Predict the Environmental Behaviour of Chemicals*, SCOPE 25, John Wiley & Sons, Chichester, New York, Brisbane, Toronto, Singapore.

Suntio, L. R., Shiu, W. Y., Mackay, D., Seiber, J. N. and Glotfelty, D. (1988) Critical review of Henry's law constant for pesticides. *Rev. Environ. Contam. Toxicol.* **103**, 1–59.

Travis, C. C. and Hattemer-Frey, H. A. (1988) Uptake of organics by aerial plant parts: a call for research. *Chemosphere* **17**, 227–283.

USEPA (US Environmental Protection Agency) (1978) Toxic Substances Control Act; chemical information rules. *Fed. Reg.* **43**, 11318.

USEPA (1987) *Graphical Exposure Modelling System (GEMS), Personal Computer Version*, PC CHEM, US Environmental Protection Agency, Environmental Criteria and Assessment Office, Research Triangle Park, North Carolina 27711.

Vighi, M. and Calamari, D. (1989). Evaluative models and field work in estimating the exposure. In: Sommerville, L., and Walker, R. (Eds) *Pesticide Effect on Terrestrial Wildlife*, Taylor & Francis, New York.

Worthing, C. R. and Walker, S. B. (1987) *The Pesticide Manual: A World Compendium* (8th edn), The British Crop Protection Council, Thornton Heath, UK.

9 Exposure Assessment Models: Accuracy and Validity

J. R. ROBERTS
Revenue Canada, Ottawa, Ontario, Canada

9.1 INTRODUCTION

The critical step in establishing the impacts of toxicants is the characterization of the exposure encountered by non-target organisms such as humans. This is equally true whether approaching the problem through epidemiological or classical toxicity studies. In either case, it is inadequate to show only that an exposure exists; it is also necessary to establish the nature and magnitude of the exposure and how this correlates with the response of organisms to such exposures. Often, so many toxicants are present in the environment and they have such similar effects that valid estimations of the types of potential hazards cannot be made from the simple demonstration that a toxicant is present. Evaluations of the magnitude of the impacts, if any, are even more remote.

The conundrum faced by the environmental health scientist is in obtaining valid exposure profiles for the thousands of chemicals currently used in society. Each compound is likely to have hundreds of distinct exposure profiles related to a multiplicity of uses. It is impractical to establish these profiles directly through studies of ambient pollutant concentration except for the most important cases, particularly those which appear to have major human health consequences. Even in these cases, retrospective exposure profiles cannot be established from the direct measurement of ambient pollutant concentrations, a condition that significantly hampers any evaluation.

Over the last decade, environmental scientists and toxicologists have turned to predictive models to obtain the needed information on exposure profiles. Regulatory agencies and industry are developing environmental fate and exposure models to be used in support of regulated activities. The objective of all such exercises is similar—the integration of mathematical descriptions of the major processes affecting the fate of chemicals through the use of computer technology so that the user can easily examine how a chemical will behave in

Methods to Assess Adverse Effects of Pesticides on Non-target Organisms
Edited by R. G. Tardiff
© 1992 SCOPE Published by John Wiley & Sons Ltd

various environmental situations (e.g., Neely and Mackay, 1982; Burns *et al.*, 1981; Di Toro *et al.*, 1982; Neely and Blau, 1985; Neely and Oliver, 1986; Oliver and Laskowski, 1986; Wood, 1986; NRCC, 1981a; Asher *et al.*, 1985). The agencies hope eventually to make decisions based on predictions of the persistence and fate of chemicals in the environment.

Predictions by these models are based on the physical and chemical properties of a chemical and on measured parameters describing the specific environment of interest. The proponents of their use argue that models provide a feasible alternative to costly field monitoring programs. These models range from relatively simple ones such as the 'fugacity' and 'persistence' models (NRCC 1981a) to highly complex ones such as the 'unified transport', or 'UTM-tox', model (Patterson, 1986) or the exposure model incorporated into NRCC's general model of Roberts and co-workers describing the economic impacts of pesticides (Mitchell *et al.*, 1987). The reader may refer to the articles of Imboden (1988), Mackay (1979), and NRCC (1981a) for general introductions to modelling concepts.

The problem today is not the lack of models, computing capacity, or an understanding of the mathematics of programming techniques; the software exists to permit any scientist with a rudimentary understanding of computers to generate exposure profiles.

The issue is the validity and usefulness of the generated predictions. Functionally different models can give very similar results in some cases and drastically different predictions in others. For example, both the fugacity and persistence models can give either very similar or dissimilar predictions about the fate of chlorobenzenes, depending on the constraints and conditions employed (Asher *et al.*, 1985). Sabijic (1987) has expressed the problem most directly:

> ... In general, models are used in sciences to represent, explain, predict or estimate phenomena of interest. They are simply approximations to reality primarily developed for the purpose of prediction. Thus the real value of a model is neither related to the type and size of the model nor to its results for the training data set, but rather its ability to correctly handle new situations . . . bad models are as readily available as the good ones. Moreover, desktop computers and modern software allow people with modest or no statistical backgrounds to construct and 'test' elaborate formal models. In addition, microcomputers enable us to abuse models at superhuman speed and to produce enormous volumes of questionable numerical results. . . .

To understand the source of the problem, one must understand how exposure models are constructed; their sensitivity depends on the nature of the construction; and the basic underlying assumptions used to approximate the environmental processes that govern the fate of pollutants released into the environment.

Specifically, the exposure models currently used are constructed of individual models of the input, transport, and removal processes impacting on the fate of a chemical, as well as a model of the environment in which the chemical is ultimately to be distributed. The usefulness of each of these models is dependent on our ability to develop correlations between the nature of chemicals, their mobility, and their persistence in a given matrix. The hypothetical model of the environment, sometimes called the 'environmental system', is first created by describing several environmental 'compartments' considered to have distinct, uniform characteristics, such as pH, percentage of organic matter, or temperature (Figure 9.1). The 'discharge', 'loading', or 'emission' rates of a chemical are then described by discrete models. Finally, mathematical relationships are developed to describe the intercompartmental transfer and removal processes that influence the dynamics of a chemical. If the description of the processes is accurate, only then is the construct a good model. This is true regardless of the appearance of the output. This is the central most important factor often overlooked by many inexperienced users of exposure models. Complex models can almost always be adjusted to mimic observed pollution patterns. In spite of the apparent success of a model, the predictions are only as valid as the submodels that are incorporated into the construct used to predict exposure profiles. Additionally, since each submodel must be calibrated for the characteristics of a pollutant and an ecosystem, predictions will be inadequate unless the input parameters (e.g., Table 9.1) utilized to calibrate the submodels are themselves adequate.

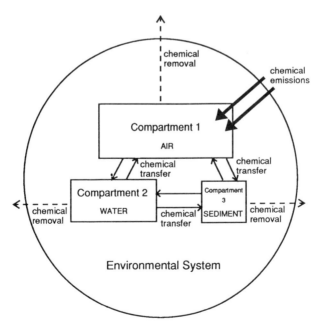

Figure 9.1. Basic design of a simple environmental model

This paper examines the level of validation and usefulness of key submodels of the processes, the environmental systems, and ultimately, the macromodels constructed on the basis of this knowledge.

A critical point to be examined in evaluating the usefulness of models is the degree to which submodels permit extrapolations from one chemical to another or from one environmental system to another. Additionally, these submodels are only useful to the regulator if the properties characterizing the chemicals and the environmental systems are available. With respect to this issue, the availability of the appropriate information on chlorobenzenes will be examined. Chlorobenzenes are chemicals that have received the attention of industrial chemists for decades, and their usage is common. Their properties have been extensively catalogued, and the usefulness of these data for modelling indicates that the data required are available for use in establishing regulations.

Table 9.1. Common parameters used in exposure models of a chemical's fate in the environment

Purpose	Parameter
Characterization of environment	Month
	Latitude
	Water temperature
	Water depth
	Water volume
	Light attenuation in water
	Sediment weight
	Organic content of sediment
	Concentration of suspended solids
	Number of fish
	Average fish weight
	Chemical emissions
Pollutant characterization	Melting point
	Molecular weight
	Vapour pressure
	Water solubility
	Octanol–water partition coefficient
	Fraction of chemical biodegradable by fish
	Quantum yield and extinction coefficients for 290–400 nm
Process description	Hydrolysis rate constant
	Photodegradation rate constant
	Volatilization rate constant
	Biodegradation rate constants for sediments and suspended solids
	Partition coefficients between water and each compartment
	Transfer rate constants between water and each compartment

In summary, central issues in determining the usefulness of these models are the following:

1. Are the processes that govern a chemical's fate adequately characterized in the models?
2. Does the integration of the processes provide realistic predictions of a chemical's fate?
3. Does sufficient information exist on the physical and chemical properties of the chemicals to provide input for the models?

9.2 VALIDATION OF KEY SUBMODELS OF PROCESSES

Once a pollutant enters an aquatic environment, its concentration is influenced by the rate at which it is lost to the atmosphere through volatilization and to sorptive pools such as suspended organic matter, flora, and sediments. Additionally, advective and degradative processes can attenuate the concentrations. The accuracy of all aquatic models is dependent on the accuracy of the submodels of these processes.

9.2.1 VOLATILIZATION

Extensive work has been carried out to develop a model of the volatilization process for dissolved organic pollutants by Mill *et al.* (1982), Spacie *et al.* (1977), Liss and Slater (1974), and Mackay and Yeun (1983). While the model is conceptually well established, its usefulness is dependent on the availability of accurate determinations of the Henry's law constants of the chemicals, as well as the exchange coefficients at the air–water interface. These latter coefficients reflect the depth of the heterogeneous layers at this interface and hence the level of turbulence and the velocity of the wind. The variability induced in the predictions of exposure profiles by these factors may be between one and two orders of magnitude (NRCC 1981a).

In the case of the Henry's law constants, there is a paucity of measurements for most pollutants of interest. Measured constants are not available for the chlorobenzenes. Thus, the constants are conventionally estimated from measurements of a chemical's liquid vapour pressure and solubility in water. In the case of solids, the liquid vapour pressure must be estimated from the solid's vapour pressure, thereby compounding errors. The accuracy of extrapolations from the crystal state to the liquid state for the solids is not established. Another problem in the case of chlorobenzenes is that there are few determinations of their vapour pressures in the 10–20° range, and further extrapolations are required. Asher *et al.* (1985) found that vapour pressures reported for chlorobenzenes normally vary by less than 20–50 per cent and that errors in the reported solubilities may generally be a greater limitation on the

Table 9.2. Variation in physical-chemical properties among chlorobenzenes (Asher *et al.*, 1985)

	Dichlorobenzenes range (% increase)	*Trichlorobenzenes* range (% increase)	*Tetrachlorobenzenes* range (% increase)
Vapour pressure (mm Hg)	1.478–1.82 (23.1)	0.323–0.389 (19.7)	0.0272–0.071 (161)
Water solubility (mg/l)	89.67–124.1 (38.4)	6.59–34.57 (424)	0.595–4.31 (624)

use of the submodel. For the highly lipophilic chemicals such as the tetra- and penta-chlorobenzenes, the variation in water solubility can be in the range of 500–1000 per cent (Table 9.2), significantly hampering any attempt to predict distributional patterns (Asher *et al.*, 1985).

Besides the problems presented by the lack of precision in the parameters used to characterize the chemicals, the influence of natural surfactants on volatilization rates has not been established. Mackay and Shiu (1977) have shown that even low concentrations of dissolved surfactants can significantly increase the solubility—and hence potentially decrease volatilization rates—in natural systems as compared with pure water. Today's models assume that the rate of volatilization is unaffected. Thus, while the submodel for volatilization is good at the conceptual level, its use to produce accurate predictions is hampered by very fundamental problems with the data needed for its accurate use.

9.2.2 SORPTION

The major sinks for the highly chlorinated hydrocarbons are the sorptive matrices in aquatic environmental systems. Algae, suspended solids, and sediment serve as major pools in such sinks. The validity of predicted time-dependent exposure profiles of such chemicals can be highly dependent on the accuracy of estimates of the rate of transfer of a chemical in and out of these compartments.

Assuming that the processes are diffusion controlled and surface-area dependent, as in the persistence model (NRCC, 1981a), one concludes that the time it takes for equilibrium to be achieved is solely dependent on the desorption soil rate constant and inversely related to the water–soil sorption equilibrium constant. If this is correct, situations will occur in which it takes years for equilibrium to be reached in the sediments and suspended solids. For example, using the persistence model, 2,3,7,8-tetrachlorodibenzo-*p*-dioxin (TCDD) is predicted to take years to reach equilibrium in these matrices (NRCC, 1981b). On the other hand, the fugacity model of Mackay assumes that equilibrium will be reached in hours (Asher *et al.*, 1985). Significantly different exposure profiles (Figure 9.2) will thus be produced depending on which model is used. There is no clear choice between the models. The error that might be introduced in the exposure profiles by use of the incorrect submodel for volatilization can invalidate use of the model in non-equilibrium situations.

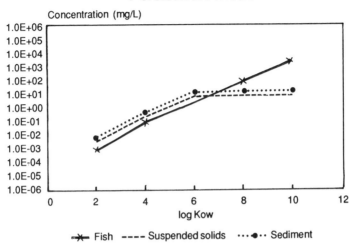

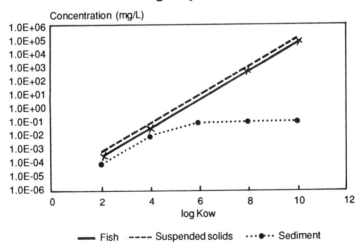

Figure 9.2. Predicted concentrations of a hypothetical compound in sediments, suspended solids, and fish when varying log K_{ow} (Asher *et al.*, 1985)

Models for the desorption process are not validated. However, when equilibrium is assumed in the models, the tacit assumption today is usually that both sorption and desorption processes are described by simple first-order kinetics and that equilibrium is rapidly achieved. For example, this is the assumption used when relations between a chemical's octanol–water partition coefficient and its partition coefficient with organic matter (e.g., Karickhoff *et al.*, 1979; Sabijic, 1987) are utilized to describe the partitioning of pollutants between water, sediment, and suspended solids of an environmental system. This is clearly not the case. Empirically determined isotherms for sorption demonstrate that other more complex relations are needed to describe the process. Explicitly, sorptive–desorptive processes can involve multiple phases, some of which may be 'bound' (e.g., Khan, 1980; Selvakumar *et al.*, 1988). An additional question raised by the existence of multiple phases is whether each phase is equally available to organisms that ingest contaminated sediments or suspended solids. Today's models cannot provide valid exposure profiles in such situations.

The octanol–water partition coefficient (K_{ow})/soil sorption coefficient relationship is often used to provide gross predictions of the influence of these sinks on the concentration of organic pollutants in the water phase at equilibrium. The field validation of these relationships is often difficult, and in the case of chlorobenzenes, not possible (Asher *et al.*, 1985). Asher *et al.* concluded in the study of chlorobenzenes that the variation in the empirically determined octanol–water partition coefficients was sufficient to mask any variation among isomers in exposure profiles (Table 9.3). In the case of these chemicals, this fact severely limits the usefulness of the predictions, since the toxicity of chlorinated aromatics reflects the specific isomeric structure of the compound ingested. In general, these relations provide the basis for only gross submodels of the sorption phenomenon. Their utilization in models of environmental systems has to be done with great care to avoid overestimation of the results. This is in part due to the fact that few studies report the organic content of the suspended solids and sediments and in part because the size of the sediment layer in equilibrium with the water column is unknown.

Table 9.3. Range of reported experimental 1-octanol–water partition coefficients for some industrial organic chemicals

Compound	Range of K_{ow}
Toluene	2.11–2.80
3,4,5-trichlorophenol	3.60–4.41
Pentachlorophenol	3.32–5.86
Trichloroethene	2.29–3.30
Benzene	1.56–2.15
Naphthalene	3.01–4.70
Chlorobenzene	2.18–3.79
Pentachlorobenzene	4.88–5.69
Hexachlorobenzene	4.13–7.42
2,2'-dichlorobiphenyl	4.04–5.00
2,4,5,2',4',5'-hexachlorobiphenyl	6.34–8.11
p,p'-DDT	3.98–6.36
Aldrin	5.52–7.40

The values given to these parameters can significantly influence the results (Asher *et al.*, 1985). For example, the sediment compartments of the fugacity and persistence models vary by as much as 1000 times in commonly used configurations, and the variation in the predicted exposure patterns for the two models can be extremely wide (Figure 9.2). The variation reflects the fundamental differences in the way the sorptive processes are treated and not in the way the characteristics of the chemicals are treated. Presently, the correct choice cannot be made.

One major issue faced in developing exposure profiles is the validity of models for the bioconcentration of organic pollutants by aquatic plants. Under some conditions, aquatic plants can serve as major sorptive pools for industrial pollutants; and these pools can represent significant exposure vectors for benthic organisms, fish, and other animals that feed upon them. Today, predictions can usually be based only on empirically determined evaluations of accumulation rates that are valid only under the specific conditions encountered in the environmental system in which the measurements were made. Hence, the handling of these compartments with current models requires decisions about their importance.

9.2.3 BIOCONCENTRATION IN FISH

Possibly the best models for any of the processes are those for the accumulation of organic pollutants in fish. These can be either highly sophisticated models based on the energy requirement of the fish (Norstrom *et al.*, 1976) or relatively simple correlative relations of bioconcentration factors with the octanol–water partition coefficient of the chemicals (e.g., Veith *et al.*, 1979). The level of

Table 9.4. Variations in predicted bioconcentration factors of chlorobenzenes due to the range in reported octanol–water partition coefficients

Chlorobenzene	Range of maximum BCF, from log K_{ow}	Range of minimum BCF, predicted BCF
Mono-	2.46–2.84	25–522
1,2-di-	3.34–3.59	138–2251
1,3-di-	3.38–3.62	149–2381
1,4-di-	3.35–3.59	140–2251
1,2,3-tri-	3.88–4.27	396–8502
1,2,4-tri-	3.93–4.27	437–8502
1,3,5-tri-	4.15–4.49	672–13082
1,2,3,4-tetra-	4.41–5.05	1118–39133
1,2,3,5-tetra-	4.46–5.05	1233–39133
1,2,4,5-tetra-	4.52–5.52	1387–98177
Penta-	4.88–5.79	2805–166535
Hexa-	5.00–7.42	3548–404600114

laboratory validation of these correlations is good for compounds with octanol–water coefficients of less than about 10. The difficulty is the magnitude of the variation in the octanol–water partition coefficients (Table 9.4), which can lead to considerable uncertainty in the predictions. In the case of chlorobenzenes, this factor can range from a low of at least 160 per cent to a high of 10 000 per cent for hexachlorobenzene. The variation completely masks the prediction of isomeric patterns of bioaccumulation. The actual bioaccumulation factors observed in field studies and those predicted by these correlations can be surprisingly divergent in practice, as evidenced by measurements of chlorobenzenes in water and fish in Lake Ontario (Table 9.5). The divergence is far in excess of that expected to arise from the variation in octanol–water partition coefficients and seems likely to reflect analytical problems in the measurement of the contaminants in the field.

9.2.4   DEGRADATION

Ultimately, the exposure profile reflects not only the tendency of the chemical to migrate from compartment to compartment, but also its susceptibility to degrade in the various matrices in which it is sequestered. Important degradative processes include photolysis, hydrolysis, and microbial degradation. Unless the impacts of these processes can realistically be included in the models, the validity of the prediction is suspect.

The removal rate constants used in models today may be drawn either from values measured directly in the laboratory or the field, or they may be calculated using published mathematical descriptions and correlations that may be part of the computer programs. Problems exist with both approaches. Using empirical data is a problem because of the sparseness of reliable data on the kinetics of chemicals in the environment and the variability of the data when they are available. Furthermore, when data are collected, the rate constants are derived from widely differing environmental or laboratory conditions. The problem is that such data are often valid only for the particular environmental system or laboratory study in which they were determined. Thus, the data cannot be used to describe other environmental situations.

The problem with using predictive equations is that, with the exception of the equations for estimating primary photodegradation and hydrolysis (NRCC, 1981a; Smith *et al.*, 1979), none of the relationships have been adequately validated. Even in the cases of photolysis and hydrolysis, the role of sensitizers, such as humic compounds, and natural catalysts lessen the value of any predictive relation. Furthermore, in the case of photolysis, key parameters such as quantum yields and spectra relevant to the aqueous environment are frequently missing. For example, measurements of quantum yields of primary photodegradation of chlorobenzenes under conditions relevant to an environmental analysis could not be found. A reliable estimate of the quantum yield of 1,2,4-trichlorobenzene in 2-propanol at 300 hm and in the presence of oxygen was reported by Akermark

Table 9.5. Measured and predicted bioconcentration factors (BCF) for several chlorobenzenes from Lake Ontario

Chlorobenzene	BCF Predicted	BCF Measured
Mono-		
1,2-di-	138	143
1,3-di-	17	—
1,4-di-	158	63
1,2,3-tri-	396	5000
1,2,4-tri-	463	5000
1,3,5-tri-	699	10000
1,2,3,4-tetra-	1118	24000
1,2,3,5-tetra-	1414	—
1,2,4,5-tetra-	1387	17000
Penta-	3155	27000
Hexa-	5248	1270000

et al. (1976); therefore, it is necessary to start arbitrarily with this value to model other polychlorobenzenes (Asher *et al.*, 1985).

The possible role of sensitizers in their own photodegradation has not been examined and, even for these relatively well-characterized chemicals, cannot be quantified. All the predictions reflect arbitrary choices. The rate of biodegradation is determined by many environmental and chemical variables, which are little understood for quantitative prediction (e.g., Lyman *et al.*, 1982). While anaerobic habitats generally retard biodegradation, the degradation of certain compounds, such as some chlorinated hydrocarbon pesticides (e.g., DDT), is enhanced (Hill and McCarty, 1967; Lyman *et al.*, 1982).

Variations in the rate may also be caused by the rate of growth, rate of death, or debilitation of the microbial population. The viability of the population is difficult to determine unless respirometry or similar techniques are employed (Lyman *et al.*, 1982). The use of such techniques is the exception in field studies, but not in laboratory studies. Other environmental variables not already mentioned that affect the biodegradation rate include light, pH, temperature, moisture, oxygen availability, and salinity. Variability in rates may also be due to inter- and intra-species interactions and to previous history, spatial distribution, and enzymatic make-up of the microbial population (Lyman *et al.*, 1982; Bartholomew and Pfaender, 1983).

Comprehensive integrated predictive models of these processes do not exist. Consideration of microbial processes in current models requires the acceptance of highly arbitrary decisions about the rates appropriate for a specific environmental situation. The empirical studies available commonly relate specifically to the conditions of the study; the correctness of the use of such results in other situations is not established. For example, the biodegradation rate constants used by Asher *et al.* (1985) for the chlorobenzenes were estimated on the basis of the values from Bartholomew and Pfaender (1983) for monochlorobenzene and 1,2,4-trichlorobenzene in water. Based on the report of Marinucci and Bartha (1979) that the degradation rate of 1,2,3-trichlorobenzene was one-half to one-third that of 1,2,4-trichlorobenzene, the value for 1,2,3-trichlorobenzene was then arbitrarily set at one-third of the reported value of 1,2,4-trichlorobenzene by Asher *et al.* (1985).

More controlled and standardized research using direct analytical techniques (e.g., chromatography, radiotracers, spectrometry) is needed to obtain reliable degradation rate constants and to establish patterns of degradation. Recommendations for the standardization of methodology and analytical techniques for basic biodegradation studies are outlined in Lyman *et al.* (1982). Examination of the degradation of a mixture of compounds would be helpful in establishing relative rates and patterns of microbial degradation.

9.3 VALIDATION OF EXPOSURE MODELS FOR ECOLOGICAL SYSTEMS

Validation has been defined as the testing of the 'agreement between the behaviour of the model and the real system' (Mihram, 1973). It is thus a functional aspect of modelling, because it describes how well the model provides a useful level of convergence between predicted and observed patterns of behaviour. The ease with which this analysis can be done depends upon the system or real world being modelled. If considerable theory exists on how a system's behaviour should vary under extreme conditions, experiments can be designed to test the theory, and validation is relatively straightforward. It becomes far more difficult when knowledge of the system is limited or when there appear to be several feasible explanations for the observed behaviour. In such cases, apparent convergence between field observations and predictions can be artifacts of the choice of input parameters.

The difficulty is that the sensitivity of the models to inaccuracies in the submodels and to inaccuracies in their integration is highly dependent on the environmental systems themselves. For example, if photolysis is the dominant removal process postulated in a model, the accuracy of the submodel and hence the full model will only be tested when significant quantities of a chemical partition in favour of other compartments. At the process level, field measurements in any two connected compartments may be sufficient to test model predictions of partitioning or degradation. This is true when two processes dominate.

To validate the integration of the processes at the environmental system level, measurements in all major compartments of the model may conceivably be necessary. It cannot be assumed that if the field data fit the predicted results for two compartments, they will fit the predictions for other compartments.

In addition, to prove that the fit of one field test to the predicted results is not likely to change, several independent tests are required. If the predicted behaviour consistently fits results from several field studies, the model may be an adequate description of the real world for predictive purposes. This does not necessarily mean that the model is correct; however, such models are useful within the defined limits.

Good validation studies require a thorough understanding of the sensitivity of the model's prediction to the character of the environmental system. Only from this knowledge can true tests be designed that actually estimate whether the model is accurate under sensitive conditions. In the development of the fugacity and persistence models (particularly the latter), numerous field studies have been examined to determine the fit of predictions (NRCC, 1981a; Asher et al., 1985). Fits could normally be achieved by adjusting parameters within the legitimate scope, given the accuracy of the measurements and the descriptions provided of the systems. However, this does not mean that the models are valid. The process models themselves are not validated, and a model's validation cannot be better than this level of validation. The 'fits' often reflect arbitrary but judicious choices of characteristics of the system, such as the depth and nature of the sediment layer, and the role of aquatic flora or sinks.

9.4 CONCLUSIONS

The implications of the above observations in the assessment of exposure are the following.

1. It is unlikely that generic models of complex environmental systems will have the precision necessary for the prediction of exposure patterns in widely different ecosystems and for chemicals with widely differing properties.

2. Models of environmental systems must depend largely on empirical determinations of the descriptive processes. Hence, the results will be highly system-specific. This makes their use unreliable in predicting patterns in highly differing ecosystems. On the other hand, good models can be established for a specific ecosystem, if sufficient effort is focused on characterizing the processes.

3. Studies on models of the processes rather than models of environmental systems are undoubtedly the most important step in expanding our predictive capabilities.

4. Model validation is dependent on carefully designed field experiments which examine pollutant levels under conditions producing significantly different exposure patterns.

5. There is a role for standard models of troublesome situations for comparative purposes. Such models can provide tests of the usefulness of the

databases and provide a basis for the prediction of patterns from one chemical to another.

6. Models have roles as tools for assessing the limits and the implications of hypotheses about the impact of ecosystem structure and process descriptions on exposure profiles.

Before modelling techniques for predicting exposure profiles can be of general use to regulators, more attention will need to be paid to developing good models of the critical processes. Explicitly, the current focus on the concepts of modelling rather than the details of the models is relatively unproductive.

9.5 REFERENCES

Akermark, B., Baeckstrom, P., Westlin, U. E., Gothe, R. and Wachtmeister, C. A. (1976) Photochemical dechlorination of 1,2,4-trichlorobenzene. *Acta Chem. Scand.* **B30**(1), 49–52.

Anders W., Doucette, W. and Deckhut, R. M. (1987) Methods for estimating solubilities of hydrophobic organic compounds: environmental modeling efforts. *Adv. Chem. Series* **216**, 3–26.

Asher, S. C., Lloyd, K. M., Mackay, D., Paterson, S. and Roberts, J. R. (1985) *A Critical Examination of Environmental Modeling—Modeling the Environmental Fate of Chlorobenzenes Using the Persistence and Fugacity Models*, NRCC Report No. 23990, National Research Council of Canada, Ottawa, 203pp.

Bartholomew, G. W. and Pfaender, F. (1983) Influence of spatial and temporal variations on organic pollutant biodegradation rates in an estuarine environment. *Appl. Environ. Microbiol.* **45**(1), 102–109.

Burns, L. A., Cline, D. M. and Lassiter, R. R. (1981) *Exposure Analysis Modeling Systems (EXAMS): User Manual and System Documentation*, US Environmental Protection Agency, Environmental Research Laboratory, Athens, Georgia.

Di Toro, D. M., O'Connor, D. J., Thomann, R. V. and St. John, J. P. (1982) Simplified model of the fate of partitioning chemicals in rivers and streams. In: Dickson, K. L., Maki, A. W. and Cairns, J. (Eds) *Modeling the Fate of Chemicals in the Aquatic Environment*, Ann Arbor Science Publishers, Ann Arbor, Michigan, p. 165.

Hill, D. W. and McCarty, P. L. (1967) Anaerobic degradation of selected chlorinated hydrocarbon pesticides. *J. Water Pollut. Control Fed.* **39**, 1259–1277.

Imboden, D. M. (1986) Mathematical modeling of the behavior of organic micropollutants in the aquatic environment. *Commission of European Communities* **1986**, 460–464.

Karickhoff, S. W., Brown, D. S. and Scott, T. A. (1979) Sorption of hydrophobic pollutants on natural sediments. *Water Res* **13**, 241–248.

Khan, S. U. (1980) *Pesticides in the Soil Environment*, Elsevier, New York, 140pp.

Liss, P. S. and Slater, P. G. (1974) Flux of gases across the air–sea interface. *Nature (Lond.)* **247**, 181–184.

Lyman, W. J., Reehl, W. F. and Rosenblatt D. H. (Eds) (1982) *Handbook of Chemical Property Estimation Methods, Environmental Behavior of Organic Compounds*, McGraw-Hill, Toronto, 977pp.

Mackay, D. and Shiu, W. Y. (1977) Aqueous solubility of polynuclear aromatic hydrocarbons. *J. Chem. Eng. Data* **22**, 399–402.

Mackay, D. and Paterson, S. (1981) Calculating fugacity. *Environ. Sci. Technol.* **15**(9), 1006–1014.

Mackay, D. and Yeun, A. T. K. (1983) Mass transfer coefficient correlations for volatilization of organic solutes from water. *Environ. Sci. Technol.* **17**, 211–217.

Mackay, D. (1979) Finding fugacity feasible. *Environ. Sci. Technol.* **13**(10), 1218–1223.

Marinucci, A. C. and Bartha, R. (1979) Biodegradation of 1,2,3- and 1,2,4-trichlorobenzene in soil and in liquid enrichment culture. *Appl. Environ. Microbiol.* **38**(5), 811–817.

Mihram, G. A. (1973) Some practical aspects of the verification of validation of simulation models. *Oper. Res. Quart.* **23**(1), 17–29.

Mill, T., Mabey, W. R., Bomberger, D. C., Chou, T. W., Hendrey, D. G. and Smith, J. H. (1982) *Laboratory Protocols for Evaluating the Fate of Organic Chemicals in Air and Water*, Report No. EPA-600/3-82-022, US Environmental Protection Agency, Environmental Research Laboratory, Athens, Georgia, 338pp.

Mitchell, M. F., Vavasour, E., Curry, P. B. and Roberts, J. R. (1987) Quantitative estimation of the risk to humans resulting friom exposure to chemicals. Monograph VI, *Strengths and Limitations of Benefit–Cost Analyses Applied to the Assessment: Industrial Organic Chemicals Including Pesticides*, NRCC Report No. 24465, National Research Council of Canada, Ottawa, 90pp.

Neely, W. B. and Oliver, G. R. (1986) A chemical runoff model. In: Cohen, Y. (Ed.) *Pollutants in a Multimedia Environment. Proceedings of a Workshop on Pollutant Transport and Accumulation in a Multimedia Environment*, Plenum, New York, pp. 133–148.

Neely, W. B. and Mackay, D. (1982) Evaluative models for estimating environmental fate. In: Dickson, K. L., Maki, A. W. and Cairns, J. (Eds) *Modeling the Fate of Chemicals in the Aquatic Environment*, Ann Arbor Science, Ann Arbor, Michigan, p. 127.

Neely, W. B. and Blau, G. E. (1985) Introduction to environmental exposure from chemicals. In: Neely, W. B. and Blau, G. E. (Eds) *Environmental Exposure from Chemicals*, CRC Press, Boca Raton, Florida, pp. 1–11.

Norstrom, R. J., McKinnon, A. E. and deFreitas, A. S. W. (1976) A bioenergetics-based model for pollutant accumulation by fish. Simulation of PCB and methylmercury residue levels in Ottawa River yellow perch (*Perca flavescens). J. Fish. Res. Board Can.* **33**, 248–267.

NRCC (1981a) *A Screen for the Relative Persistence of Liphophilic Organic Chemicals In Aquatic Ecosystems. An Analysis of the Role of a Simple Computer Model in Screening*, NRCC Report No. 18570, National Research Council of Canada, Ottawa, 300pp.

NRCC (1981b) *Polychlorinated Dibenzo-p-Dioxins: Criteria for Their Effects on Man and His Environment*, NRCC Report No. 18574, National Research Council of Canada, Ottawa, 248pp.

Oliver, R. G. and Laskowski, D. A. (1986) Development of environmental scenarios for modeling the fate of agricultural chemicals in soil. *Environ. Toxicol. Chem.* **5**, 225–232.

Patterson, M. R. (1986) Unified transport model for organics. In: Patterson, M. R. (Ed.) *Pollutants in a Multimedia Environment. Proceedings of a Workshop on Pollutant Transport and Accumulation in a Multimedia Environment*, Plenum, New York, pp. 93–115.

Sabijic, A. (1987) Nonempirical modeling of environmental distribution and toxicity of major organic pollutants. In: Kaiser, K. L. (Ed.) *QSAR in Environmental Toxicity, Vol. II*, Reidel Holland, Dordrecht, and Kluwer Academic Publications, Norwell, Massachusetts, pp. 309–332.

Selvakumar, G. A., Rodrigo, A. M. and Chan, P. (1988) Binding characteristics of hazardous organic substances to clay soils. In: Bell, J. M. (Ed.) *Proceedings of the 42nd Industrial Waste Conference, 1987, Purdue University*, Lewis Publishers, Boca Raton, Florida, pp. 775–780.

Smith, J. H., Mabey, W. R., Bohonos, N., Hold, B. R., Lee, S. S., Chou, T. W., Bomberger, D. C. and Mill, T. (1979) *Environmental Pathways of Selected Chemicals in Freshwater Systems. III. Laboratory Studies*, Report No. EPA-600/7-78-074, US, Environmental Protection Agency, Environmental Research Laboratory, Athens, Georgia.

Spacie, A., Hamelink, J. L. and Waybrant, R. C. (1977) Application of an evaporative loss model to estimate the persistence of contaminants in lentic environments. In: Mayer, F. L. and Hamelink, J. L. (Eds) *Aquatic Toxicology and Hazard Evaluation*, ASTM Special Technical Publication 634, American Society for Testing and Materials, Philadelphia, pp. 214–227.

Veith, G. C., Defoe, D. L. and Bergstedt, B. V. (1979) Measuring and estimating the bioconcentration factor of chemicals in fish. *J. Fish. Res. Board Can.* **36**, 1040–1048.

Wood, W. (1986) Use of exposure models to support TSCA priority setting. In: *Environmental Modeling for Priority Setting among Existing Chemicals*, Workshop, 11–13 November 1985, Gesellschaft fur Strahlen und Umweltforschung MbH, Munchen, pp. 429–436.

10 Assessment of Acute Toxicity of Pesticides on Humans and Domestic Animals

J. DOULL

University of Kansas Medical Center, Kansas, USA

The general approach for evaluating the potential adverse effects of pesticides in non-target species was established over four decades ago by Lehman, Fitzhugh and Nelson at the Food and Drug Administration which was responsible at that time for regulating pesticides in the US. This approach, which was similar to that used for drugs, involved a case-by-case comparison of the risk–benefit ratio for each pesticide.

The evaluation of risk was based primarily on two types of toxicity studies in animals:

1. Acute studies which included LD_{50} determinations coupled with a description of the symptoms or adverse effects
2. Chronic studies which were multidose one- to two-year rodent studies.

The intent of this approach was to identify all of the potential adverse effects that could be produced by either acute or chronic exposure to the pesticide and to determine the exposure dose of the pesticide required to produce all such effects.

Subchronic (90-day) studies were utilized to establish the dose levels for the chronic studies; additional kinetic, metabolism, and mechanism-of-action studies were carried out, if needed, to characterize the toxicity of the pesticide.

Both the acute and chronic data were then used to establish a threshold for the adverse effects of the pesticide; and, in most cases, the tolerances and other regulatory positions were established by dividing the lowest threshold by an appropriate safety factor. This approach, which was subsequently adopted as the acceptable daily intake (ADI) method for food additives, was and is used both in the US and abroad for regulating pesticides as well as other classes of chemicals.

Methods to Assess Adverse Effects of Pesticides on Non-target Organisms
Edited by R. G. Tardiff
© 1992 SCOPE Published by John Wiley & Sons Ltd

During the subsequent two decades preceding the creation of the EPA and the transfer of the major responsibility for regulating pesticides from FDA to EPA, several additions to the toxicity testing requirements were made to evaluate the hazard of pesticides. The discovery of organophosphate (OP) insecticide potentiation by Frawley at the FDA led to a requirement for testing of all new OP insecticides for such synergistic effects, and a leghorn chicken test was also required for all new organophosphate insecticides to detect any delayed neuromuscular effects of these agents. The thalidomide episode stimulated the development of teratology as a part of the toxicologic testing procedures; and growing concern over other types of feto-toxicity stimulated the development of multi-generation protocols for evaluating fertility, postnatal and other reproductive effects of pesticides. Methods to detect and evaluate the genotoxic effects of pesticides were stimulated by the studies of Bruce Ames and his associates. Significant developments occurred in the areas of neurotoxicology, behavioural toxicology, and in immunotoxicology; but these have not yet resulted in validated protocols, and thus they have not been incorporated into regulatory requirements for pesticides. Although these changes in toxicological methodology provided a broader database for predicting potential adverse effects in non-target species, the basic approach in pesticide regulation continues to rely on both acute and chronic data for hazard evaluation and for the setting of pesticide tolerances.

The current approach to pesticide regulation differs from this earlier approach in two ways. First, it is focused on the chronic effects of pesticides rather than on the acute effects, and, second, it is focused on a single chronic effect— cancer. Emergency room physicians who treat pesticide poisoning have pointed out that it is the acute effects of pesticides that are responsible for most of the actual morbidity and mortality associated with most types of pesticide poisoning, and they argue that we should be more concerned about the acute effects which are 'real-world' than the cancer risks which are largely hypothetical. Further, the current protocol used for chronic studies on pesticides is based on the National Cancer Institute/National Toxicology Program Oncogenicity Bioassay rather than on the more holistic procedure which was previously required by FDA. The NCI/NTP protocol was designed to serve as a screening test for carcinogenicity, and, consequently, is neither adequate nor appropriate as a bioassay for chronic toxic effects other than cancer.

Another major difference between the current approach and the previous 'FDA' approach for evaluating the adverse effects of pesticide exposure involves the way in which toxicity data are interpreted. In the current system, the carcinogenicity data from the chronic rodent studies is extrapolated using mathematical models which provide a numerical estimate of the upper bound of the cancer risk, and these numbers (Q_1*values are then used for a variety of regulatory purposes. In essence, this approach substitutes mathematical guidelines for the scientific judgement that was the key element in the 'FDA' approach.

Since the basic purpose of conducting toxicity studies is to provide an accurate prediction of the potential adverse effects of a chemical in non-target as well as in the test species, we need to ask whether the methodology that we use both for testing and for interpreting the test results is yielding answers that protect both the environment and public health. Based on the arguments presented in the preceding discussion, it is likely that our predictions regarding the adverse effects of pesticides on humans would be improved if they included a greater emphasis on the acute effects and on the non-cancer chronic effects of pesticide exposure.

Protocols for detecting both acute and chronic neurotoxicity and the behavioural effects of pesticides (including specific tests for neuronal dysfunction) should be a part of the requirements for pesticide registration. Recent workshops devoted to these areas (LSRO report to FDA on 'Predicting Neuro-toxicity and Behavioral Dysfunction from Preclinical Toxicologic Data' and the 'Workshop on the Effects of Pesticides on Human Health which was organized by the Task Force on Environmental Cancer, Heart and Lung Disease) have recommended methods and test batteries that would detect sensory, motor, autonomic, cognitive and behavioural dysfunction.

Another area that would be of direct benefit to the medical personnel responsible for treating pesticide exposure in humans is the development of antidotal and symptomatic treatment for the various classes of pesticides. Although we have more specific antidotes available to treat pesticide poisoning than for any other single class of acute poisons, the number of antidotes is small for non-insecticidal pesticides, and these cases must be treated symptomatically. The current acute toxicity protocols do not currently provide the kind of clinical information needed in such cases.

Endocrine- and immunologic-related adverse effects of pesticides are another example of an area where we need toxicologic testing methods that will detect both acute and chronic toxicity and provide a reliable basis for predicting human effects.

Before we add new protocols to the current methodology, however, we need to evaluate the answers provided by our current methodology. The two scientific disciplines which contribute most directly to the evaluation of cancer and all other human health hazards that may result from exposure to pesticides and all other toxic chemicals are epidemiology and toxicology. When these disciplines function in this 'watch-dog' role, both have the same goal: to gather sufficient information about the potential adverse effects of exposure to the chemical so that we can reliably predict both the type of adverse effects that may occur and the exposure conditions likely to produce each of these anticipated adverse effects.

Although the primary difference between these two disciplines is the subjects (i.e., epidemiologists use humans, whereas toxicologists use rodents), there are also major differences in how we approach the problem, the techniques we use to generate the data and how we use these data to predict the hazards. Each starts and ends at the same place, but each discipline gets there by a different path.

It should be pointed out, however, that there is no disagreement between epidemiologists and toxicologists as to the priority of human data over rodent data. Toxicologists recognize that in those situations where we have sufficient human data, there is no need to do any type of toxicity studies unless we are predicting for environmental or non-human effects. The main reason why toxicology rather than epidemiology serves as the basis for most regulatory decisions involving cancer and other adverse health effects is that human data are insufficient for most chemicals for which estimates of safe exposures are needed. In addition, there are ethical constraints, particularly with chemicals which are not drugs, that often preclude the type of epidemiologic studies we need to make reliable predictions about risks to humans.

Since it is obvious that we will need to continue to rely on the toxicity database for making hazard or risk predictions, it is important that in addition to searching for new methods for obtaining and interpreting the toxicology data, we also ask whether our current approach is giving us correct answers.

One approach to the question of whether risk assessment methods based on the results of oncogenicity studies in rodents are giving us the right answers is to compare the predictions from the epidemiologic studies with those from the toxicity database. When we do this for those agents for which we have predictions from both sources, there are only a few discrepancies. We do not have animal data demonstrating that asbestos causes mesothelioma or lung tumours and only limited evidence that arsenic and benzene cause cancer in rodents, although the human evidence for these chemicals is clearly sufficient to establish causation. More recently, epidemiologists have concluded that the herbicide 2,4-D causes non-Hodgkins lymphoma in exposed farmers and that alcohol ingestion causes cancer of the oesophagus, liver, and possibly breast; but neither of these chemicals produces cancer in rodents. Although it has been argued that the epidemiologic evidence in these cases is weak since it is based on an association rather than on a cause–effect link, these findings are of particular concern to toxicologists since they are not like asbestos, where our failure to produce lung tumours can be attributed to the lack of a good animal model and to inadequate testing. We now have 18-negative rodent studies for ethanol, and the 2,4-D oncogenicity study was considered by the EPA FIFRA Science Advisory Panel to be an excellent study. Neither 2,4-D nor ethanol is mutagenic; and acetaldehyde which is the primary metabolite of ethanol in both rodents and man is also not mutagenic, although it did produce lung tumours in an inhalation study in rats. While it is reassuring to find that, in most cases, the toxicologic data supports the epidemiologic predictions, it is also clear that the exceptions must be investigated and resolved to maintain the credibility of the animal tests as reliable predictors of cancer and other adverse effects of chemicals in humans.

We also need to look at the exceptions in the reverse situation in which the toxicity data are positive, but the epidemiology findings are negative. Such exceptions can occur if the test species is more susceptible to the tumourigenic effects of a chemical than the target species; e.g., it has been suggested that the liver tumours produced by the halogenated hydrocarbons are illustrative of this situation. Many of the pesticides and solvents in this group, such as chlordane, heptachlor, trichloroethylene, and methylene chloride, produce liver tumours in rodents, but epidemilogic studies generally do not support these findings.

It can be argued, of course, that the epidemiologic studies are inadequate, and that is certainly true for some of these agents; it can also be argued that, in these cases, the rodent studies are over-predicting the cancer risk for man. The $B_6C_3F_1$ mouse which is widely used as a rodent test species does have a high incidence of liver tumours, and it has been suggested by the International Agency for Research on Cancer (IARC, Lyon, France) that when positive results are found only in mice and not in other species that such results should not be used as a basis for a regulatory action. Similar arguments have been made regarding the increased incidence of thyroid tumours in rats exposed to goitrogens such as the sulfonamides. In this case the mechanism by which the thyroid tumours are produced appears to have a clear threshold, and it has been recommended by an EPA Working Group that such agents be regulated on the basis of a no-observed-effect level (NOEL) approach rather than with the conventional cancer models.

Another example of a case where rodent tests appear to be giving incorrect answers, or at least over-predicting the human risk, is the production of kidney tumours in the male rat by gasoline, p-dichlorobenzene, limonene, and tetrachloroethylene. The mechanism by which these agents cause kidney tumours in male rats appears to involve conjugation with an α-2u-globulin and the formation of hyaline droplets in the P2 segment of tubule. Since these droplets are not found in female rats or other species including humans, it is argued that male rat kidney tumours produced through this mechanism are not predictive for human carcinogenesis. On the basis of this argument and the lack of positive genotoxicity evidence for p-dichlorobenzene, the EPA halogenated organics subcommittee of the SAB has recommended that the classification for this agent be downgraded from B2 to C in the new drinking water regulations for p-dichlorobenzene. During the past few months, the EPA has held workshops on the predictive value of mouse liver tumours, rat kidney tumours, and thyroid tumours induced by various goitrogens, and on the use of pharmacokinetic parameters in risk assessment. Some of the recommendations from these workshops are likely to be incorporated in the new Cancer Assessment Guidelines being developed by EPA.

One of the most common complaints about the use of mathematical models in risk assessment is that these models ignore the relevant biology. Partly in response to this criticism, a NAS/NRC committee has issued a report which presents methods for incorporating pharmacokinetic data in risk assessment. When recommendations of this committee were applied to the risk assessment of methylene chloride, the predicted carcinogenic risk was reduced by a factor of 7. Another approach that is receiving considerable current attention is to identify and quantify all uncertainties that exist in the mathematical modelling process, so that we can design and carry out the research needed to substitute hard data for these uncertainties. The procedures should improve both the relevance and the accuracy of the model-based approach. We must also consider the more basic issue, which is whether there is sufficient scientific or biologic justification for extrapolating the results of our high-dose rodent studies to the low doses needed for prediction.

As was pointed out previously, the current protocol for conducting chronic toxicity studies is based on the NCI oncogenicity bioassay, which was a screening test designed primarily to answer two qualitative questions: Is the chemical oncogenic? What kind of tumours are produced? When this program was transferred to NTP, some additional features were added to make it more like the conventional chronic toxicity study, and an effort was made to obtain an indication of dose–response relationsips. Basically, however, it is still a screening test for oncogenesis, and the manipulation of these data with sophisticated mathematical models which generate finite risk estimates does not alter the quality of the input. The idea that these models somehow generate quantitative data which is valid far beyond the range of the actual data may well be an illusion; in any event, it is an idea that needs to be rigorously tested. At the same time, we need to re-examine the protocols that we use to generate the cancer data in animals to determine whether we can develop procedures that will provide quantitative information that can be used either on a stand-alone basis or as input for the extrapolation models.

Many of these issues are being considered by various scientific and regulatory groups both in the US and in other countries, and some of the issues may be addressed in legislative proposals to revise the laws under which pesticides are regulated (e.g., HR 4737, HR 4739, and the Pesticide Reform Bill). In this process of seeking remedies for actual or perceived deficiencies in the scientific methodology used to identify and quantify the hazards of pesticide exposure, we need to remember that the major problem is not methodological, but is rather the lack of data on which to base the prediction.

11 Assessment of Chronic Effects of Pesticides on Humans

R. KROES and E. M. DEN TONKELAAR
National Institute of Public Health and Environmental Hygiene, Bilthoven, The Netherlands

11.1 INTRODUCTION

'Pesticides' is the umbrella term for chemicals or biologicals effective in the control of pests. This activity may involve unwanted growth and/or infestation of bacteria, fungi, insects, or other organisms in materials. The compounds can be divided into agricultural chemicals, household chemicals, veterinary products, wood preservatives, disinfectants, and preservatives in end-products. Agricultural chemicals may be used on non-nutritional crops such as flowers, bulbs, trees and garden plants, or on nutritional crops used for human or animal consumption. Household chemicals may be used outside or inside buildings, on curtains, or in wallpapers or textiles. Veterinary pesticides are used to prevent or control the growth or existence of unwanted organisms in stables, animal rooms, or on small or large domestic animals. Wood preservatives are used outside or inside buildings and sometimes even in packaging materials used for food products. Disinfectants are mainly used in industrial or medical environments, but they may also be used in materials that come into contact with food. This also holds true for preservatives in end-products, e.g., when applied in paper coatings used for packaging. Furthermore, such preservatives are used in paints, pastes, glues, textiles, or cutting oils. In some countries, some categories of chemicals are not included in regulations; this is particularly true for wood preservatives, disinfectants, and preservatives.

The widespread use of pesticides gives ample possibilities for such substances to come in contact with the environment, man, and animals, either incidentally or intentionally, acutely or chronically, depending on their use, their persistence, and their migrating properties.

Methods to Assess Adverse Effects of Pesticides on Non-target Organisms
Edited by R. G. Tardiff
©1992 SCOPE Published by John Wiley & Sons Ltd

Humans can be exposed to pesticides occupationally when producing or applying a substance, as users of the product, or as consumers of food or liquids containing residues. Whereas in the first case people may be aware of a possible exposure to the substance, in the third they may be completely unaware of the exposure, which is usually at low levels. In addition, people may inadvertently and unknowingly be exposed to products used in buildings or equipment.

Since pesticides by nature are used in concentrations sufficiently high to have detrimental effects on biological organisms, they are at the same time a serious threat to living organisms that were not intended to be controlled. In this way, pesticides can be compared with drugs: their biological activity is a prerequisite for use. At the same time, this means that the 'margin of safety' between wanted and unwanted adverse effects may be small in contrast with, for example, food additives.

Variations in the use of pesticides forces regulatory bodies to consider such variations carefully with respect to required testing. If a substance is used only on non-nutritional crops, contamination of food products is unlikely and one will focus attention mainly on such acute aspects as acute oral, dermal, or inhalation toxicity, skin and eye irritation, and sensitization.

On the other hand, if the use of such a substance gives rise to residues in food or to contamination of a food product, subchronic oral toxicity testing is certainly indicated. In most cases, chronic toxicity testing (including carcinogenicity, mutagenicity, and reproductive toxicity) is warranted to predict possible effects, especially when humans are exposed repeatedly. This chapter focuses primarily on the assessment of chronic adverse effects of pesticides, although prescreen procedures used to make more appropriate use of chronic toxicity bioassays will be discussed as well.

11.2 STRATEGIES IN CHRONIC TOXICITY TESTING

Toxicology includes both the gathering of data in biological systems and the interpretation and evaluation of those data to predict possible risk for humans. Currently toxicity testing has become quite a rigid procedure. Standardized protocols inhibit the real goal of toxicity testing: to obtain as complete as possible an understanding of the mechanisms of toxicity at the tissue, cellular and subcellular levels (i.e., 'receptor' toxicology) (Kroes and Feron, 1984).

The main goal in toxicity testing is the identification and proper description of adverse effects a pesticide may produce, and in addition, knowledge concerning the dose–response relationships for such effects. Moreover, information with respect to the mechanism of action should ideally be obtained as well. The two aims in toxicity testing—obtaining a toxicity profile and the establishment of a safe dose—are complementary and not interchangeable, since different goals and different methodologies may be involved (Doull, 1984).

Among regulatory bodies, a reasonable agreement exists concerning the basic pattern of toxicity testing, although a divergence of philosophy is apparent: for some, a cookbook approach specifies that all substances should be subject to the same pattern of tests; for others, a more flexible approach requires the generation of only those data needed to adequately estimate the potential risks of exposure to a chemical. The latter approach is to be preferred.

Toxicity tests are presently carried out according to consensus guidelines as adopted by the Organization for Economic Cooperation and Development (OECD, 1981). These procedures are helpful in providing an efficient and cost-effective means of testing for toxicity.

The scope of toxicology has broadened considerably, especially over the past decade (Doull, 1984; Conning, 1986; Kroes and Feron, 1990). The firmly rooted conventional approach based on empirical observations—i.e., quantification of biological effects with no elucidation of mechanisms—has resulted in studies which are costly and consume many research resources, yet provide no insight into the causal role of chemicals in possible disease.

The basic questions remain how to predict long-term effects on the basis of results of relatively short-term observations, and how to extrapolate data from laboratory animals to humans. These questions can only be answered if more attention is given to pharmacokinetic and pharmacodynamic studies, which provide insight into absorption, distribution, metabolism, and tissue concentration at target site. Ideally, comparative information between humans and laboratory animals on target tissues and pharmacokinetic aspects should be made available; however, such data generally become available only after accidental exposure. Comparative studies on cell or tissue cultures of humans and laboratory animals may add to a better prediction of the possible hazard to humans.

When long-term exposure of humans to pesticides is anticipated, acute and subchronic toxicity testing is not generally considered to be sufficient; in that case, chronic toxicity testing may be necessary, as well as studies for such specific toxic responses as carcinogenicity, reproduction, neurotoxicity, behavioural toxicity, and immunotoxicity. The results of acute and subchronic tests should be thoroughly evaluated to determine which special studies to undertake.

Chronic oral exposure of humans to pesticides can be expected when residues of agricultural pesticides remain in food after application on crops or reach the food through environmental pathways.

When substances are used as household chemicals inside buildings and long-standing inhalation exposure can be expected, subchronic inhalation studies may be pertinent; likewise, if their use gives rise to detectable residues in food, chronic oral testing may be warranted.

Similarly, subchronic dermal testing may be indicated when the use of chemicals in clothing textiles would lead to longstanding dermal exposure. Chronic oral toxicity testing may also be required for veterinary pesticides in those cases where their use leads to detectable residues in meat, meat products, milk, or eggs. The same holds for wood preservatives, disinfectants, or preservatives that reach food items in finite amounts. Depending on the results of short-term testing studies and the intended use of a pesticide, studies for carcinogenicity, reproductive toxicity, neurotoxicity, or behavioural toxicity may be performed as well.

It will never be possible to describe beforehand which procedure should be followed and which tests should be performed. Toxicologists should be as flexible as possible in their way of thinking and their approach to conducting toxicity studies. Their main goal, however, should be to gather as much information as possible concerning the toxicity profile, the dose–response relationship, and the mechanisms of action involved to make the most reliable hazard assessment and safety evaluation.

11.2.1   TOXICITY TESTING: CURRENT STATUS AND PERSPECTIVES

The basic package required for toxicity testing generally includes acute, subchronic and chronic toxicity testing and special studies, as noted previously. Considerable changes in the methods used for investigation have been made in the last decades. Parallel with increasing insight into physiology, biochemistry, and morphology, many new parameters have been introduced to study the functional state of the organism, organs, and organelles. An increasing number of parameters is studied, and several parameters are examined frequently in long-term experiments. Likewise, extensive gross and microscopic examinations are being performed on a greater number of organs and tissues. One wonders if this increase in parameters studied provides more relevant information. A lack of balance still seems to exist in the parameters required for general toxicity testing; while much emphasis is being placed on functional tests for liver and kidney, far less attention is being paid to other targets such as the endocrine, cardiovascular, and central nervous systems.

11.2.2   BASIC REQUIREMENTS FOR CHRONIC TOXICITY TESTS

In toxicity testing, the important factors are the chemical, route of exposure, selection of dose, selection and care of animals, caging, diet, temperature, humidity, parameters studied, data acquisition, presentation of results, and overall evalution and presentation. The *Principles and Methods for Evaluating Toxicity of Chemicals* (WHO, 1978), *Principles for the Safety Assessment of Food Additives and Contaminants in Food* (WHO, 1987), *Principles for the Toxicological Assessment of Pesticide Residues in Food* (WHO, 1990), and the critical appraisal in *Long-Term and Short-Term Assays for Carcinogens* (Montesano *et al.*, 1986) provide a wealth of relevant information.

For long-term toxicity studies or special toxicity studies, one should determine detailed physico-chemical properties, and the administered dose or exposure concentration of the test chemical. Throughout the study, all efforts should be made to provide accurate evidence of exposure. Selection of animals is extremely important (WHO, 1978; Fox *et al.*, 1979; Montesano *et al.*, 1986), but probably the most important criterion is knowledge of and experience with the test animal used.

The importance of diet as a major environmental variable in toxicity testing has been fully recognized in the last decade. The type, composition, and contaminant concentration may influence the health of animals and thus the effects of chemicals measured in tests. Different levels of macro- and micro-nutrients may profoundly influence results; high fat may change biotransformation enzyme activities and is associated with high incidence of certain tumours; low fat affects palatability (Kroes and Feron, 1990). High protein may influence the sensitivity to pesticides, whereas it may simultaneously increase spontaneous renal disease (Feldman *et al.*, 1982). The acid–base balance of a diet may also affect the results of a toxicity study, especially when substances involved cause an acidic or basic load to the body (Kroes and Feron, 1990). Reduced food intake may strongly influence toxicity, as demonstrated by paracetamol, whose hepatotoxicity was reduced considerably with the reduction of food intake. Finally, careful monitoring of contaminants in the diet and drinking water (pesticides, mycotoxins, trace minerals, nitrosamines, and other suspect chemicals) is essential and should not be omitted. Other environmental variables should be controlled as adequately as possible.

Unfortunately, insufficient knowledge still exists on the influence of the number of variables such as light/dark cycle and noise, which may change circadian rhythm and biochemical functions and thus modify toxic responses (Fox *et al.*, 1979).

As noted previously, parameters required for chronic toxicity testing may not have the desired balance. The increase in number of parameters has falsely introduced a feeling of confidence. Re-evaluation of the relevance of parameters used and consideration of new parameters to be included will be necessary in the coming decade.

11.2.3 CHRONIC TOXICITY TESTING

Prescreens for chronic toxicity testing are usually the acute and the subchronic repeated-dose studies performed on a substance of interest. These studies may provide information on the dose regimen to be used, the possible targets involved, the parameters to be studied, and the precautions to be taken. Retrospective studies have been performed to investigate whether certain ratios can be estimated in dose patterns between acute and subchronic and between acute and chronic studies (Weil and McCollister, 1963; Layton *et al.*, 1987). These studies suggest the existence of some relationship between the no-observed adverse-effect level (NOAEL) in subchronic studies and chronic studies. If the NOAEL of an adequately performed subchronic study is divided by a factor

5–10, one has an approximate estimate of the chronic NOAEL. Similarly, retrospective calculations were made comparing even LD_{50} to a chronic NOAEL, indicating a ratio varying for 1×10^3 to 1×10^4. Table 11.1 provides estimated conversion factors among the LD_{50}, the NOAEL of a subchronic or chronic study, and the acceptable daily intake (ADI). Such conversion factors are of course arbitrary, especially when derived from values, such as the LD_{50}, obtained from acute toxicity studies. Therefore, they should be taken with great caution when used as a guide to establish an approximate estimate for a dose range in the design of chronic toxicity studies.

Table 11.1. Estimated conversion factors between an LD_{50}, the NOAEL of a subchronic or chronic toxicity study, and the ADI

LD_{50}	NOAEL (subchronic)	NOAEL (chronic)	ADI
100 000–5 000 000	300–1000	100	1

Chronic toxicity studies today vary in duration (6–24 months) in different countries and incorporate different requirements (Patrick, 1983). For some time, a debate has existed on whether the design for chronic toxicity testing, excluding testing for carcinogenicity, should have a duration of more than 6 months. In a retrospective analysis by Lumley and Walker (1985), the pathological findings (except for carcinogenicity) after 6 months of treatment were not different from those after longer exposures; hence, the safety assessment for these compounds would have been unchanged by the longer duration of exposure.

This conclusion has been questioned by Frederick (1986). He investigated 11 drugs for which toxicity data from studies of duration of less than one year and greater than one year existed and noted that pathological lesions were observed in the longer duration studies that were not uncovered in the studies of less than one year; these lesions occurred at doses 10–200 times the proposed maximal human dose for drugs. It is doubtful whether such prolonged studies would have affected the setting of the NOAEL. Therefore, a duration of 6 months for chronic toxicity tests may be adequate; for some compounds, where toxicokinetic findings indicate that a steady-state will not exist before the end of the treatment, longer duration may be necessary.

Chronic toxicity testing in the future should focus more on establishing a dose-response relationship for the mechanism of toxicity. This approach may necessitate the use of additional groups of test animals subject to interim sacrifice to obtain additional relevant information, such as the presence of the parent substance or its metabolites at the target site and in blood, for subsequent comparison with findings from low-dose studies in human volunteers.

With the existence of subchronic toxicity data in both sexes, the value of continuing to test both sexes of experimental animals in chronic tests has been questioned. Restricting a study to one sex when no sex-related differences in toxicity are likely offers the opportunity to add satellite groups to obtain relevant information. Parameters indicative for cardiovascular, endocrine, behavioural, or gastrointestinal function may be highly useful for safety evaluation, whereas some traditional parameters in blood and urine and some morphological parameters should be included only if they are relevant. For instance, morphological examination should perhaps be eliminated for organs that do not show evidence of change by gross examination, function tests, and organ weight at levels of exposure causing other toxicity.

Chronic toxicity testing of the future should be accompanied by *in vitro* studies using cells and tissues relevant to the target organ toxicity of the compound or its metabolite(s). Such *in vitro* studies may provide useful insight into the possible mechanisms of toxicity. In conclusion, chronic toxicity testing of pesticides should be made more tailor-made than it is today. The duration of the study may vary according to the pharmacokinetic data available and the design of the study may differ according to the results obtained in subchronic testing. The number of animals used, one or both sexes, the parameters, the number of groups, satellite groups, interim kills, all may differ according to the results obtained in acute and subchronic testing and according to the aim to be achieved. Comparative *in vitro* studies in both tissues and cells of experimental animals and humans, may complete the studies and provide optimal information for safety assessment and effect prediction.

11.2.4 CARCINOGENICITY TESTING OF PESTICIDES

A highly pertinent issue when pesticide exposure to humans is expected to be long term is carcinogenicity. Recently, the carcinogenicity of pesticides was evaluated by the National Research Council (1987), especially with respect to the health risks of residues in foods. This report has been the subject of considerable debate, since the risk assessment procedures used may have been inappropriate for the substances considered. Nevertheless, the possible continuous exposure of humans to small amounts of pesticides as residues in food is a major reason for conducting carcinogenesis studies.

The identification of potential carcinogenesis by using *in vitro* methods has been ameliorated considerably in the last ten years. Recently, Ashby and Tennant (1988) concluded that chemicals that were likely to cause cancer by attacking DNA can be identified with some precision in short-term studies. Their findings that a correlation of more than 90 per cent exists between structural analysis of a chemical's reactive site and the Ames *Salmonella* assay confirm the existence of at least two groups of chemical carcinogens: those that are genotoxic and those that cause cancer in other ways (non-genotoxic compounds), as was earlier claimed by a number of authors (Kroes, 1979; Weisburger and Williams, 1980; Grice, 1984).

Thus, in carcinogenicity studies, one can make fruitful use of short-term *in vitro* tests for genotoxicity (Grice, 1984; Montesano *et al.*, 1986). Such *in vitro* tests contain two components: the cell, plant, or microbe in which genetic change is expressed; and an appropriate metabolic activation system. Endpoints are point mutations, chromosome breaks, deletions or transpositions, sister chromatid exchanges, and unscheduled DNA repair.

Since genotoxicity tests show significant differences in response for the varous carcinogens, their utility for carcinogen prescreening is restricted to the qualitative detection of genotoxic activity, thus predicting, but certainly not defining, carcinogenicity (Kroes, 1987).

A considerable proportion of genotoxic substances are not carcinogenic in animal assays, due in part to poor absorption of the chemical or in part to efficient detoxification *in vivo*. Therefore, a strong need exists for appropriate, validated short-term *in vivo* tests for genotoxicity. Positive findings in such *in vivo* tests might make long-term assays for the identification of carcinogens superfluous in the future (Ashby and Tennant, 1988). Only limited bioassays (for example, studies only in one sex or one strain of animals) might be needed for further characterization, unless quantitative risk assessment procedures are needed.

Long-term carcinogenicity studies, however, may still be necessary for those substances which have genotoxic properties *in vitro*, but may not be active in short-term *in vivo* studies. If the absence of carcinogenicity is confirmed for a large number of compounds, it may be appropriate to rely solely on short-term *in vitro* and *in vivo* studies for those substances having genotoxic potential *in vitro*.

Non-genotoxic carcinogens are characterized by a variety of biological properties that are believed to underlie their carcinogenicity. Examples are non-specific stimulation or inhibition, modulation of immune response, hormone balance, or nutritional factors (Kroes, 1979; Weisburger and Williams, 1980; Grice 1984). When non-genotoxic mechanisms are suspected, attempts should be made to obtain more pertinent information concerning the mechanism of action. Although short-term *in vitro* tests have been suggested to determine specific promoting properties (Brookes, 1981; Williams, 1981; Trosko *et al.*, 1982; Yamasaki 1984), they still lack sufficient validation to be used in safety assessment. Limited *in vivo* bioassays (Williams and Weisburger, 1983) may provide adequate quantitative information relevant for safety evaluation.

The non-genotoxic nature of substances has been claimed to be indicative of the existence of thresholds (Weisburger and Williams, 1980; Kroes, 1979, 1987; Ames, 1987). In the future, it might be accepted that non-genotoxic substances do not have to be investigated in long-term bioassays for carcinogenicity, depending on results and anticipated use. If, for example, anticipated use of a non-genotoxic substance is at levels where human exposure is far below (i.e., one thousandth or less) a NOEL, carcinogen bioassays are considered by some to be superfluous (Feron and Kroes, 1986).

In performing carcinogenicity studies, the design and test methods are of primary importance in obtaining results suitable for safety assessment. The conduct of such studies has been extensively described (OECD, 1981; USEPA, 1985; Montesano *et al.*, 1986). The combined chronic toxicity/carcinogenicity study (Test 453, OECD, 1981) has become quite popular in the last decade.

In conclusion, testing of carcinogenic properties of pesticides is important in those cases where continuous exposures to small quantities in humans can be expected. The use of appropriate prescreen procedures is advocated, especially when they might make further testing unnecessary, thereby diminishing the number of animals used. Under some conditions, it might be appropriate not to perform carcinogenicity studies when non-genotoxic substances are involved and when anticipated exposure in humans is at levels far below the NOEL established in adequately performed toxicity tests.

11.3 OTHER SPECIAL STUDIES

Reproduction is a vital function; therefore, in those cases where pesticide exposure can be expected, studies on fertility, reproduction and pre- and post-natal development are needed. For many compounds, these studies have been performed rather infrequently despite the relative importance of this type of toxicity. In a safety evaluation of 51 chemicals it appeared that in 70% of the substances studied reproductive and developmental toxicity were more sensitive than, or equally sensitive to, the conventional measures used in subchronic toxicity studies (Koëter, 1983). *In vivo* and *in vitro* pilot studies have been suggested as a prescreen, but better validation should first be obtained. As a cost-effective measure, selective fertility and reproductive parameters should be included in the subchronic study.

Recently, a report became available from a workshop where the so-called Chernoff/Kavlock preliminary developmental toxicity test was evaluated (Hardin *et al.*, 1987). The test was found to be highly reliable in correctly identifying developmentally toxic chemicals for 165 chemicals. It was suggested that a negative finding in a properly conducted Chernoff/Kavlock test could be sufficient basis to determine that conventional teratology tests in the same species were not warranted. Although teratogenic properties may certainly be manifest in those exposed at high levels, it is believed that, at lower levels, thresholds exist for such phenomena (Wilson, 1977; Ames, 1987). Thus, the primary aim in reproduction studies will be the exclusion of teratogenic properties at levels 100 or more times greater than the anticipated human exposure.

Despite voluminous literature on reproductive toxicology, it was recently acknowledged that, although the correlation of reproductive effects among species is imprecise, adverse effects in experimental animals should be presumed to indicate a potential risk to human reproduction (Kimmel and Kimmel, 1986).

With respect to other special toxicity studies, the basis of knowledge about immuno-, neuro- and behavioural toxicity begins with a thorough toxicological characterization of the compound in subchronic studies.

The immune system can be influenced by chemicals in a variety of ways. Careful analysis of lymphoid organs for alterations in weight, morphology, cell count, and cellular function in classical toxicity testing may lead to suspicion of immuno-modulating potential. Such findings can then be confirmed and further characterized using a selected battery of presently available, validated assays, although there still exists a need for further development of assays in the rat, the animal of choice in chronic toxicity testing.

For neurotoxicity and behavioural toxicity, careful evaluation of the results of classic toxicity tests may shed light on such properties. For neurotoxicity, chemical structure and the half-life may prompt investigation of this phenomenon in chronic toxicity assays. Experienced personnel may be able to detect otherwise barely recognizable signs which may be indicative of neurotoxicity or behavioural disturbances. The possible behavioural effects of chemicals may be studied, where appropriate, in chronic toxicity studies by adding satellite groups that can be examined by established, validated methods.

11.4 ASSESSMENT OF ADVERSE EFFECTS OF MIXTURES

Pesticides are usually used as formulations in combination with other ingredients, often termed 'inert'. When the toxicity of an active ingredient has been characterized, the further testing of formulations is usually restricted to acute studies. Combinations of pesticides in one formulation may necessitate chronic testing. In 1981, the Joint Meeting on Pesticide Residues (JMPR) concluded that, when combinations were used at concentrations or doses equal to the NOAEL, only additive effects may be expected.

No single approach exists to assess adverse effects of mixtures. Since this issue is very complex and since only limited data are available about the approaches and limitations of testing mixtures, it is of extreme importance to use experience and knowledge in a flexible way. The type of the mixture, known or anticipated interactions among the components, and other information influence how a mixture should be tested and evaluated.

In general, the toxicity testing of mixtures is not essentially different from that performed for individual compounds, although special considerations should be given to sample selection and collection, storage and stability of the mixture, possible interaction between components, characterization, and bioavailability (USEPA, 1986; Montesano et al., 1986; Vouk et al., 1987).

Short-term assays may well be used to evaluate the potential health hazard of complex mixtures. Special problems in testing may be anticipated, such as changing pH or osmolarity of the media occasioned by the necessary high concentrations, since the effective concentration of any one compound is diluted by the accompanying compounds. Short-term tests may give relevant information to be used if chronic/carcinogenicity tests seem warranted.

11.5 ASSESSMENT OF ADVERSE EFFECTS OF BIOLOGICALS

Currently, there is a tendency to replace chemical pesticides with biological agents. Experience already exists with several bacteria, viruses, and fungi potentially usable as insecticides. No traditional procedures can be used for the assessment of their safety. Besides data on acute and subchronic toxicity, data on the ability of organisms to survive and multiply in the mammalian organism are particularly important. Bacteria can be studied *in vivo* in subchronic experiments, and viruses in cell culture. Moreover, information about the natural occurrence of these organisms is very important.

Biotechnology products are usually treated as chemicals and are routinely tested. Purity of the products and their immunogenic nature are of primary concern. Focus should be directed at the possibility that contaminants will be introduced inadvertently during fermentation or isolation. Although not pertinent to chemical pesticides, a biotechnology product's homology to native molecules is important, since slight changes in amino acid sequences may result in changes in the three-dimensional structure, thus changing its antigenicity.

11.6 ADVERSE EFFECTS IN HUMANS

Ideally humans should never experience adverse effect of pesticides; however, this ideal situation will probably never occur. First, occupational exposure in production or application may take place, not because safety rules are absent, but rather because safety precautions are not perfect. Second, pesticides are effective poisons which can be misused for suicide or homicide. Third, exposure of humans to residues of pesticides considered as safe, takes place every day.

Results from studies in humans exposed occupationally, accidentally, or via residues seem relevant to human risk assessment. Most likely, the best information from acute and subchronic exposure may be obtained from case studies. Epidemiological investigations are difficult to perform, except for those that can be designed in occupational settings; even they, however, have the intrinsic problem that humans in occupational settings are usually exposed to more than one chemical, thus making the interpretation of results rather difficult. Negative epidemiological findings may, however, provide some assurance that precautions have been effective.

Epidemiological studies in the general population exposed to pesticide residues in food seem infeasible and not worthwhile because their sensitivity is insufficient to find effects, should any be present. More use, however, could be made of information from poison control centres, where patients accidentally exposed to relatively high single doses may provide information concerning uptake and excretion and may in addition provide information on metabolism and blood concentrations.

11.7 EXTRAPOLATION AND SAFETY ASSESSMENT

The evaluation of results of toxicity tests, including extrapolation to humans, is the cornerstone of safety assesment. The result of animal experiments should be weighed against the significance for people, since any animal model may be considered unsatisfactory because of existing species differences. We must rely on animal experimentation as long as results of more advanced methods such as *in vitro/in vivo* comparisons, physiologically-based pharmacokinetic modelling, and human volunteer studies are not available.

As a prologue to extrapolation and safety assessment, all chemical-biological data derived from toxicity studies should be evaluated and, if available, information on molecular or cellular mechanisms of toxicity is extremely relevant. In the extrapolation from laboratory animals to humans, one is faced with the following aspects: interspecies variation; intraspecies variation; extrapolation from high to low dose and experimental limitations (i.e., failure to detect certain effects in mammals).

In the fifties, the concept of an acceptable daily intake (ADI) was developed. The ADI is the daily intake that appears to be without appreciable risk during an entire lifetime, based on the facts known about a chemical. The ADI is expressed in mg/kg of body weight (b.w.), and is estimated from toxicity data by a WHO panel of experts or by national authorities. In the case of pesticides, this evaluation is done by the WHO/FAO Joint Meeting on Pesticide Residues. Assuming that a biological threshold is likely for non-carcinogenic effects, the safety assessment is made by establishing the NOAEL (expresed in mg/kg b.w.) from animal experimentation. This NOAEL is then divided by a safety factor to compensate for the factors influencing extrapolation, thus predicting a safe level for humans.

Assuming that interspecies variation and intraspecies variation would each not exceed one order of magnitude, a 'worst case' approach yields a factor of 100 (i.e., 10×10) to be used as a reasonable margin of safety between the NOAEL in animals and the acceptable intake in man. This concept, now in use for almost forty years, has been shown to be sufficiently safe.

Recently, the validity of the use of a safety factor of 100 has been debated. For several reasons the factor of 100 may be high, since no evidence exists that the sensitivities of inter- and intra-species variability are related; thus, the worst-case approach may be overly conservative. Correspondingly, present-day toxicity testing is considerably advanced, and one can justifiably conclude that NOAELs found today will certainly be lower than those found in studies carried out decades ago.

One is, however, faced with an intake of a relatively substantial number of chemicals in small amounts; information on such interactions as inhibition, additivity, and synergism from combined exposures is scarce. Furthermore, a serious drawback in the procedure described above is that it takes no account of the dose–response relationship: where a steep curve may not necessitate the use of a safety factor of 100, a very shallow curve may need a margin of that magnitude. Therefore, better methods for determining allowable daily intakes should be developed.

For pesticides, however, a conservative approach seems realistic, as long as such a procedure is not applied too rigidly.

11.8 MRLs AND THE PREDICTION OF DIETARY INTAKE

Proposals for maximum residue limits (MRLs) on food crops are based in part on good agricultural practices. For residues of a pesticide on various crops to be judged acceptable, the total intake should not be higher than the ADI. However, predicting the true intake is often difficult. Calculation of the theoretical maximum daily intake provides a gross overestimation of true intake, because of uncertainties due to the variability in average daily food consumption, unaccounted reductions in pesticide content during food preparation and the assumption that residues are always present at the maximum level. Consequently, a joint FAO/WHO consultation has recently adopted guidelines for estimating dietary intake of pesticide residues (WHO, 1987–1989).

Using these guidelines, one identifies a theoretical maximum daily intake (TMDI), and an estimated maximum daily intake (EDMI) defined as a prediction of the maximum daily intake of a pesticide residue. The EDMI is derived from the assumption of average daily food consumption per person and the maximum residues on the edible portion of the commodity, corrected for the reduction in concentration of residues from food preparation, commercial processing, and cooking of the commodity. Both the TMDI and the EDMI are expressed as milligrams of the residue per person.

Finally, an estimated daily intake (EDI) is defined as a prediction of the daily intake of a pesticide residue, based on the most realistic estimation of residue levels in food and the best available food consumption data for a specific population.

Whereas TMDIs and EMDIs can be calculated grossly on international levels, EDIs can only be calculated at a national level, thus refining the system of setting maximum residue levels (MRLs). More research is needed to calculate with improved accuracy the likely intake of residues. The establishment of MRLs, as performed by the Codex Committee on Pesticide Residues, is a sensible international approach to this situation. From a public health perspective, it is reassuring to know that actual intakes of all pesticides (as measured in market-basket and total-diet studies) is much lower than the established ADIs.

11.9 REFERENCES

Ames, B. N. (1987) Six common errors relating to environmental pollution. *Reg. Toxicol. Pharmacol.* 7, 379–383.
Ashby, J. and Tennant, R. W. (1988) Chemical structure, Salmonella mutagenicity and extent of carcinogenicity as indicators of genotoxic carcinogenesis among 222 chemicals testing in rodents by the US NCI/NTP. *Mut. Res.* 204, 17–115.
Brookes, P. (1981) Critical assessment of the value of *in vitro* cell transformation for predicting *in vivo* carcinogenicity of chemicals. *Mutat. Res.* 86, 233–242.
Conning, D. M. (1986) Toxicology—the next decade. *Arch. Toxicol.*, Suppl. 9, 222–224.
Doull, J. (1984) The past, present and future of toxicology. *Pharmacol. Rev.* 36, 15S–18S.

Feldman, D. B., McConnell, E. E. and Knapka, J. J. (1982) Growth, kidney disease, and longevity of Syrian hamsters (*Mesocricetus auratus*) fed varying levels of protein. *Lab. Anim. Sci.* **4**(32), 613–618.

Feron, V. J. and Kroes, R. (1986) The long-term bioassay for identifying carcinogens: some controversies and suggestions for improvements. *J. Appl. Toxicol.* **6**, 307–311.

Fox, J. H., Thibert, P., Arnold, D. L., Krewski, D. R. and Grice, H. C. (1979) Toxicology Studies II: the laboratory animal. *Food Cosmet. Toxicol.* **17**, 661–675.

Grice, H. C. (1984) *Current Issues in Toxicology: Extrapolation of Toxicity Data*, Springer-Verlag, Berlin, Heidelberg, New York, Tokyo.

Hardin, B. D., Becker, R. A., Kavlock, J., Seidenberg, J. M. and Chernoff, N. (1987) Overview and summary: workshop on the Chernoff/Kavlock preliminary developmental toxicity test. *Teratogen. Carcinogen. Mutagen.* **7**, 119–127.

Kimmel, C. A. and Kimmel, G. L. (1986) Interagency Regulatory Liaison Group workshop on reproductive toxicity risk assessment. *Environ. Health Perspect.* **66**, 193–221.

Koëter, H. W. B. M. (1983) Relevance of parameters related to fertility and reproduction in toxicity testing, *Am. J. Ind. Med.* **4**, 81–86.

Kroes, R. (1979) Animal data, interpretaton and consequences. In: Emmelot, P. and Kriek, E. (Eds) *Environmental Carcinogenesis*, Elsevier/North Holland, Amsterdam, pp. 287–302.

Kroes, R. (1987) Contribution of toxicology towards risk assessment of carcinogens. *Arch. Toxicol.* **60**, 224–228.

Kroes, R. and Feron, V. J. (1984) General toxicity testing: sense and non-sense, science and policy. *Fund. Appl. Toxicol.* **4**, 298–308.

Kroes, R. and Feron, V. J. (1990) Toxicity testing: strategies and conduct. In: Clayton, D. and Munro, D. (Eds) *Progress in Predictive Toxicology*, Elsevier, Amsterdam.

Layton, D. W., Mallon, B. J., Rosenblatt, D. H. and Small, M. J. (1987) Deriving allowable daily intakes for systemic toxicants lacking chronic toxicity data. *Reg. Toxicol. Pharmacol.* **7**, 96–112.

Lumley, C. E. and Walker, S. R. (1985) The value of chronic animal toxicity studies of pharmaceutical compounds: a retrospective analysis. *Fund. Appl. Toxicol.* **5**, 1007–1024.

Montesano, R., Bartsch, H., Vainio, H., Wilbourn, J. and Yamasaki, H. (Eds) (1986) *Long-Term and Short-Term Assays for Carcinogens: A Critical Appraisal*, IARC Scientific Publications No. 83, International Agency for Research on Cancer, Lyon.

National Research Council (1987) *Regulating Pesticides in Food: the Delaney paradox*, National Academy Press, Washington, DC.

OECD (Organisation for Economical Cooperation and Development) (1981) *OECD Guidelines for Testing of Chemicals*, OECD, Paris.

Patrick, C. P. (1983) Harmonization of toxicological testing in chemical safety evaluation. *Chem. Ind.* **1983**, 55–59.

Trosko, J. E., Yotti, L. P., Warren, S. T. Tsushimoto, S. C. and Chang, G. (1982) Inhibition of cell–cell communication by tumor promotors. *Carcinog. Compr. Surv.* **7**, 565–585.

USEPA (US Environmental Protection Agency) (1986) Guidelines for the health risk assessment of chemical mixtures. *Fed. Reg.* **51**, 34014–34025.

Vouk, V. B., Butler, G. C., Upton, A. C., Parke, D. V. and Asher, S. C. (Eds) (1987) *Methods of Assessing the Effects of Mixtures of Chemicals*, SCOPE 30/SGOMSEC 3, John Wiley & Sons, Chichester.

Weil, C. S. and McCollister, D. D. (1963) Relationship between short- and long-term feeding studies in designing an effective toxicity test. *J. Agric. Food Chem.* **11**, 486–491.

Weisburger, J. H. and Williams, G. M. (1980) Chemical carcinogens. In: Doull, J., Klaassen, C. C. and Amdur, M. O. (Eds) *Toxicology: The Basic Science of Poisons* (2nd edn), Macmillan, New York, pp. 84–138.

Williams, G. M. (1981) Liver carcinogenesis: the role for some chemicals of an epigenetic mechanism of liver-tumor promotion involving modification of the cell membrane. *Food Cosmet. Toxicol.* **19**, 577–583.

Williams, G. M. and Weisburger, J. H. (1983) New approaches to carcinogen bioassay. In: Holmberger, F. (Ed.) *Safety Evaluation and Regulation of Chemicals, Vol. 2*, S. Karger, Farmington, Connecticut, pp. 200–209.

Wilson, J. G. (1977) Current status of teratology. General principles and mechanisms derived from animal studies. In: Wilson, J. G. and Clarke Fraser, F. (Eds) *Handbook of Teratology. 1. General Principles and Etiology*, Plenum Press, New York.

WHO (World Health Organization) (1978) *Principles and Methods for Evaluating the Toxicity of Chemicals. Part I. Environmental Health Criteria 6*, World Health Organization, Geneva.

WHO (World Health Organization) (1987) *Principles for the Safety Assessment of Food Additives and Contaminants in Food, Environmental Health Criteria 70*, World Health Organization, Geneva.

WHO (World Health Organization) (1989) *Guidelines for Predicting Dietary Intake of Pesticide Residues*, World Health Organization, Geneva.

WHO (World Health Organization) (1990) Principles for the toxicological assessment of pesticide residues in food, *Environmental Health Criteria 104*, World Health Organization, Geneva.

Yamasaki, H. (1984) Modulation of cell differentiation by tumour promotors. In: Slaga, T. J. (Ed.) *Mechanisms in Tumour Promotion, Vol. IV*, CRC Press, Boca Raton, Florida, pp. 1–26.

12 Ecological Effects of Pesticides on Non-target Species in Terrestrial Ecosystems

DAVID PIMENTEL
Cornell University, New York, USA

12.1 INTRODUCTION

The quantity of pesticides applied in world agriculture annually is estimated to be about 2.5 million tonnes at a cost of about $16.3 billion (US) (Helsel, 1987). Despite the use of this 5 million tonnes of pesticides and all other controls, pests in the world are probably destroying about 35 per cent of all potential crops before harvest (Pimentel and Pimentel, 1979). These losses to pests are primarily due to insects, plant pathogens, and weeds. After the crops are harvested, an additional 20 per cent of the crops are probably destroyed by insects, microorganisms, rodents, and birds. Thus, nearly half of all potential food in the world is being destroyed annually by pests, despite all efforts to control pests with pesticides and other types of controls.

Although large quantities are applied to crops, only a small percentage of the applied pesticides reach the target pests—this is estimated to be less than 0.1 per cent (Pimentel and Levitan, 1986). Thus, more than 99 per cent of applied pesticides go off into the environment and affect non-target sectors of the ecosystem, including soil, water, atmosphere, and the non-target biota. Pesticides, however, are generally profitable to use in crop production. On average, pesticide use on crops returns about $4 (US) per $1 invested for pest control (Pimentel *et al.* 1991). These are direct benefits, and do not include the social and environmental costs of using pesticides (Pimentel *et al.*, 1980a).

Integrated pest management (IPM) is playing a role in slowing the use of pesticides in the world, but IPM practices that actually result in reducing pesticide use have been only gradually adopted (Pimentel, 1986). One important reason for the slowness is the problem of developing non-chemical controls to replace chemicals. Also, non-chemical controls are sophisticated, and this

Methods to Assess Adverse Effects of Pesticides on Non-target Organisms
Edited by R. G. Tardiff
©1992 SCOPE Published by John Wiley & Sons Ltd

contributes to the difficulty of farmers adopting the new approaches for pest control.

It is hoped that biotechnology and genetic engineering will help to develop new biological pest controls using microorganisms, and that these will be easy to use and effective (NRC, 1987; Pimentel, 1987). Although the new biotechniques for pest control will help reduce the use of pesticides, biotechnology and genetic engineering will probably create some serious environmental problems themselves (Pimentel, 1987; Pimentel et al., 1989).

The objective of this paper is to investigate the ecological effects of pesticides and genetically engineered pest control organisms on non-target species in terrestrial ecosystems. Particular attention will be given to methodology for conducting sound ecological investigations of the effects of pesticides and genetically engineered biocontrol organisms on the environment.

12.2 TROUBLESOME PESTICIDES AND BIOLOGICAL CONTROL AGENTS

There are nearly a thousand different types of pesticides in use (Metcalf et al., 1962; WHO, 1988). Clearly, it would be difficult to list all pesticides that are hazardous to the environment and the kinds of ecological effects each has on the environment. This is especially true when the environment includes 5–10 million species. The United Nations (WHO, 1988) completed a listing of the most hazardous pesticides to humans. This is a valuable list, but its limitation is that it is restricted to lethal dosages to humans based on rat and other laboratory animal studies.

In general, the toxicity and the hazard to the environment have a relationship. Insecticides generally are the most hazardous to the environment, followed by fungicides and herbicides. This is a generalized statement, because certain herbicides are highly toxic and present a greater hazard to the environment than some insecticides. Thus, one has to be specific about which pesticide (including its dosages and methods of application) is being investigated in an ecological study.

DDT and related chlorinated pesticides are noted for their deleterious impact on non-target species. An important reason for the serious ecological effects of the chlorinated pesticides is that these pesticides have a high lipid/water coefficient, and thus have a tendency to accumulate in organisms (Pimentel and Edwards, 1982). Most organisms contain lipids and, hence, are likely to take up lipophilic pesticides (such as many of the organochlorine insecticides) from the soil and water environments. In certain environments, organisms may bioconcentrate these fat-soluble pesticides at 10–1000 times the level found in the ambient environment (Pimentel, 1971). Pesticides that are water soluble may also be a serious hazard because of their movement in water in the terrestrial ecosystem. For example, pesticides such as aldicarb and several herbicides have a tendency to be washed from the treated crop area to other parts of the ecosystem, including the aquatic system (Pimentel and Edwards, 1982).

Another attribute that can make some pesticides hazardous is their relatively high activity at relatively low concentrations. Aldicarb and parathion are pesticides with these characteristics. This is why the UN (WHO, 1988) lists these materials as highly toxic and hazardous to use.

Persistence is another characteristic that makes pesticides hazardous to the environment (Pimentel and Edwards, 1982). Obviously, the longer a chemical remains in the environment, the greater the chance that it will have adverse effects, and the greater the likelihood that it will spread or be transported from the treated crop ecosystem to other ecosystems. Also, the pesticide may accumulate in the environment if the life of the chemical is greater than the frequency of application. Classic examples of pesticides that persist for years are many of the organochlorine insecticides like dieldrin (Pimentel, 1971) and the herbicide paraquat. Some pesticides that are readily adsorbed into organic matter or clay particles persist longer in the environment (Pimentel and Edwards, 1982). However, these polar compounds may be less biologically active than non-polar compounds. Conversely, non-polar compounds tend to persist for shorter periods, because they are not adsorbed and thus are readily available to living organisms.

Biotechnology has promised new biological controls to replace pesticides. Although these new biological pest controls will have some advantages over the use of pesticides, the new biotechnology and biological controls are not without risks themselves (Pimentel *et al.*, 1984, 1989). For example, five vertebrate species that were intentionally introduced for biological controls have all become pests themselves in the United States (Pimentel *et al.*, 1989). These biocontrol species include the Indian mongoose, the English sparrow, and the grass carp.

Such genetically engineered microbes as bacteria and viruses for biological control may reduce pesticide use but also may cause environmental problems (Pimentel *et al.*, 1989). Several microbes have already been engineered for biological control. One of these is *Pseudomonas syringae* (Ps), which was modified for the biological control of frost-causing types of Ps (Lindow, 1982). Spraying enormous numbers of the altered bacterium, known as the 'ice minus strain', on potatoes, tomatoes, strawberries, corn, and other crops allows the bacterium to outproduce and replace the wild form of *Pseudomonas*. This could extend the crops' growing seasons and increase yields.

Although preliminary tests suggest that this engineered organism may be relatively safe, Lindow reported that the naturally occurring Ps is an 'important plant pathogen' in 17 crops and will also infect at least 100 species of plants in nature (Lindow *et al.*, 1978). Clearly, under these circumstances, tests in contained environments were advisable to demonstrate that the modified strain was non-pathogenic in both crops and wild plants (Pimentel, 1987).

12.3 INJURIOUS EFFECTS ON ECOSYSTEMS

The injurious ecological effects of pesticides and biotechnology on terrestrial ecosystems are summarized based on currently available data.

12.3.1 STABILITY

Pesticides have been reported to influence populations of organisms and thus change the interactions and stability among species within ecosystems (Müller et al., 1981). The best documented cases of such ecological effects are from agroecosystems. When insecticides were first used on tropical cotton crops, for example, they controlled the two or three major pests of the crop and greatly increased yields. Within a few seasons, however, the chemicals reduced populations of parasites and predators, and a number of other arthropod species became serious pests (ICAITI, 1977).

Orchards are complex ecosystems that are easily perturbed by the extensive use of pesticides, and there are many instances of increased pest attacks in orchards after the use of pesticides (Pimentel, 1971). These include outbreaks of codling moth, leaf rollers, aphids, scales, and tetranychid mites because controlling parasite and predator populations had been drastically reduced (Brown, 1978; Tolstova and Atanov, 1982; Bostanian et al., 1984). Also, intensive use of herbicides, insecticides, and fungicides in orchards leads to reduced soil fauna and microflora and increased leaching of nutrients from the soil (Rusek and Kunc, 1983).

Pesticides can affect animal reproduction directly, as evidenced by the deleterious effect of the persistent organochlorine insecticides on reproduction in raptors and other birds. Eggshell thinning due to the uptake of organochlorine insecticides that affect calcium (Ca) metabolism has been observed in predacious birds (Keith et al., 1970; Newton et al., 1986; Wiemeyer et al., 1986; Opdam et al., 1987). Fish-eating birds are more severely affected than terrestrial predatory birds, because the fish-eating birds acquire more pesticides via their food chain than the other predators (Pimentel, 1971; Littrell, 1986).

Pesticides can also affect reproduction in the invertebrates; for example, sublethal doses of DDT, dieldrin, and parathion increased egg production by the Colorado potato beetle by 50, 33 and 65 per cent, respectively, after two weeks (Abdallah, 1968). The herbicide 2,4,5-T was found to reduce the reproduction of soil-inhabiting Collembola (Eijsackers, 1978). Populations of invertebrates with high rates of increase can recover stable populations much more rapidly than those of bird and mammal populations (Pimentel and Edwards, 1982).

In some cases, insect pests have altered their behaviour to avoid insecticides. For example, houseflies were found to avoid resting inside treated barns. Instead, the resistant flies rested most frequently on untreated vegetation outside the barns.

12.3.2 WASTE DISPOSAL AND NUTRIENT CYCLING

Most dead organic matter is broken down by the activities of the soil fauna and microflora, which together fragment and decompose the material (Pimentel and Warneke, 1989). These organisms assist in organic matter decomposition, incorporate the degraded material into the soil, and help to convert mineral elements into forms available for plant growth (Pimentel et al., 1980b). A large portion of the pesticides used ultimately reaches the soil, where it can affect soil organisms directly or indirectly (Fletcher, 1960; Edwards and Thompson, 1973; Broadbent and Tomlin, 1982; Prasse, 1985). Populations of earthworms, for example, which are among the most important decomposer organisms, are decreased drastically by some pesticides (particularly chlordane, endrin, parathion, phorate) and nematocides, fungicides, and carbamate pesticides (Edwards, 1980; Barker, 1982; Lofs-Holmin, 1982).

Soil microarthropod populations and rates of decomposition and mineralization have been reduced by insecticide treatments in agricultural and grassland ecosystems (Perfect et al., 1981; Pimentel and Warneke, 1989), forest areas (Weary and Merriam, 1978), and a desert ecosystem (Santos and Whitford, 1981). Such effects generally are transient, but they may result in a reduction in soil fertility and productivity (Perfect et al., 1979).

Most nutrients, especially carbon, nitrogen, phosphorus, potassium, and sulphur, are taken up by plants, which in turn may be eaten by animals. The amounts and forms of nutrients in soil and plants may be changed by pesticides affecting the dynamics of these elements in the ecosystem. For example, the herbicide simazine increased water and nitrate uptake in barley, rye, and oat seedlings, resulting in increased plant weight and total protein content of the plants (Ries and Wert, 1972).

12.3.3 DIVERSITY AND FOOD CHAINS

Pesticides are notorious for altering the interrelationships of species in ecosystems (Pimentel, 1971). Some species are sensitive to some or all pesticides and may be exterminated from an ecosystem so that species diversity (richness) is reduced (Pimentel and Edwards, 1982; Tolstova and Atanov, 1982; Prasse, 1985). For instance, the number of species of soil-inhabiting arthropods in a cereal crop were reduced considerably by a single recommended dose of DDT, and a greater reduction resulted from the use of aldrin (Edwards et al., 1967).

Parasites and predators frequently suffer greater mortality from insecticides than do their herbivorous hosts (Pimentel, 1971; Croft and Brown, 1975), either because of greater susceptibility to the chemical or because their food supply is drastically reduced after pesticide use. For example, treatment of cole (Brassica) crop plants with either DDT or parathion reduced the number of taxa of herbivores, but reduced the number of parasitic and predacious taxa even more (Pimentel, 1961a), with consequent effects on species diversity and the

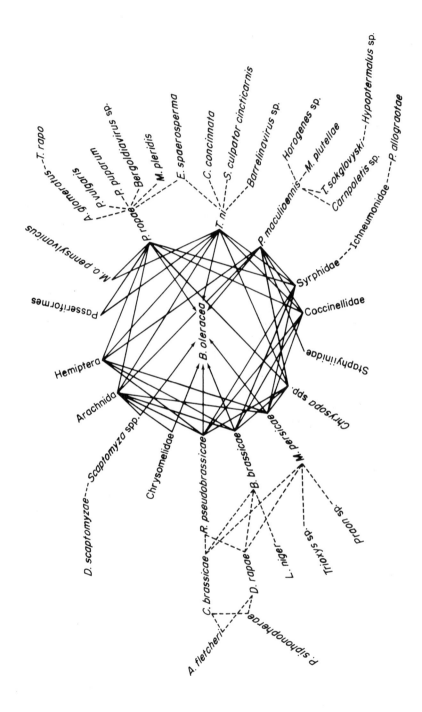

Figure 12.1. Relationships between the cole crop plant (*Brassica oleracea*), insect pests (——), and parasitic (----) and predacious (· · · ·) enemies of the pests (Pimentel, 1961a)

complex structure of this ecosystem (Figure 12.1). The selective application of some insecticides may, through the reduction of some predacious species, increase species diversity (Risch and Carroll, 1982).

In terrestrial ecosystems, herbicides can either increase or decrease plant diversity, depending on the initial floristics of the area and specificity of the chemicals used (Tomkins and Grant, 1977; Wakefield and Barrett, 1979). Where herbicides affect plant species composition, animal populations have been shown to respond in turn (Malone, 1969; Spencer and Barrett, 1980). For example, the large-scale application of herbicides in southern England suggests that the presence of these pesticides in cereals is leading to the elimination of insect-desirable plants. This has led to decreasing numbers of partridges, because there are fewer insects on which the young partridge chicks can feed (Potts, 1977).

12.3.4   ENERGY FLOW

Energy flow through ecosystems can be influenced by pesticides that alter primary production. The use of pesticides in agroecosystems usually increases primary production, and there is good evidence that primary production in grassland and forests is also increased (Shure, 1971). However, frequent use of pesticides does not always concomitantly increase crop and forest yields. For example, regular use of some insecticides on cotton and in orchards has created new insect and mite pests, thus sometimes reducing productivity (Edwards, 1973; ICAITI, 1977).

In orchards, the use of the fungicides benomyl or methyl thiophanate to control scab has sometimes led to increased outbreaks of the disease and reduced productivity (Edwards and Lofty, 1977; Lofs-Holmin, 1982). These chemicals are toxic to earthworms, which help to control apple scab by removing most of the infected apple leaves from the soil surface.

Organisms in ecosystems exist in complex interdependent associations, and the transfer of food energy dominates most interspecies relationships in ecosystems (Elton, 1927). In ecosystems, energy flows from producers through the lower trophic levels to higher levels in food chains. Clearly, if pesticides kill organisms lower in the trophic levels, less energy will be available for those species at the higher levels (Müller et al., 1981; Pimentel and Edwards, 1982). In the first years of herbicide application in orchards, an increased food supply (dead organic matter) and more favourable soil moisture led to a higher population density of Enchytraeidae and higher soil respiration activity in the soil (Rusek and Kunc, 1983).

12.3.5   POLLINATION

Cross-pollination is essential to reproduction in many plants. A total of 90 US crops, valued at more than $4 billion (US), are dependent upon insect pollination; and nine additional crops, valued at more than $4.5 billion (US) are significantly benefited by insect pollination (USDA *et al.*, 1969). In addition to the cultured plants, large numbers of wild plants require cross-pollination.

An estimated 20 000 species of US native flowering plants are dependent upon biotic cross-pollination mechanisms (Pimentel *et al.*, 1980c). Honey bees and wild bees carry out most of this pollination, and many of these species are highly susceptible to pesticides (Pimentel, 1971; Pimentel *et al.*, 1980a). In some circumstances, farmers have had to rent honey bees or by other means encourage the presence of bees on their farms.

12.3.6   RECOMBINANT-DNA BIOTECHNOLOGY

12.3.6.1   Ecological effects

The planned release of genetically engineered organisms (GEO) into terrestrial and aquatic environments raises concerns about potential short- and long-term effects that GEOs could have on processes and populations associated with many diverse ecosystems (Rissler, 1984; Milewski, 1985; Pimentel, 1987; Pimentel *et al.*, 1989). A list of research issues includes:

1. Determination of the effects of GEOs on various components of ecosystem structure and function
2. Delineation of geochemical and biological processes most useful for describing ecosystem structure and function
3. Microcosm and/or field studies (i.e., verification of laboratory-derived methodologies and results) that estimate ecosystem responses in potentially impacted areas or under GEO-use conditions
4. Verification of biological indicators developed in the laboratory on population, community, and ecosystem responses to GEO exposure
5. Development of model systems to predict resiliency (impact and recovery) of populations, communities, and ecosystems exposed to GEOs
6. Assessment of risks associated with release of GEOs by integration and interpretation of biological, chemical, and physical data on aquatic and terrestrial ecosystems (Crane and Moore, 1984; Lance and Gerba, 1984; Corapcioğlu and Haridas, 1985).

12.3.6.2   Adverse ecological effects

Although we are fortunate that no environmental disaster has resulted to date from genetic engineering, some environmental problems will probably result from the release of genetically engineered organisms for several reasons. First, none of the test protocols will allow us to predict with 100 per cent accuracy the impact of genetically engineered organisms on the environment (Pimentel *et al.*, 1989). There is no way in which sufficient tests can be run in the laboratory and in controlled microcosms to eliminate all possibilities of a disaster (Hagedorn and Lacy, 1988).

Historically, we have been unable to distinguish accurately all beneficial organisms from potential pests (Pimentel *et al.*, 1989). More than 128 species of crops and animals, for example, that were intentionally introduced as beneficial have become some of the most serious pests known in the United States. Farmers spend several billion dollars annually for their control. Johnsongrass, for instance, is the most serious weed pest in the southern United States (Williams and Hayes, 1984). Other potential adverse effects of biotechnology (Pimentel *et al.*, 1989) include the following.

1. Developing crop resistance to herbicides will encourage the use of a wider array of herbicides on a variety of crops and probably increase the use of herbicides, thus intensifying the ecological problems associated with these pesticides.

2. Developing microbial agents with recombinant-DNA (R-DNA) technology may help reduce pesticide use. The same agents, however, may harm or displace beneficial organisms.

3. Although genetically engineered microbes released to attack specific chemical pollutants have the potential to improve the environment, these microbes must be compound-specific and produce harmless by-products; otherwise, they could pose environmental hazards.

4. When unique genetic characters are released into the environment via microbes and other organisms, a few of these novel DNA sequences may be transferred to other microbes and other organisms.

5. Because most pest species are of native origin, using native organisms to genetically engineer new organisms is probably not any safer than selectively introducing foreign organisms.

6. Few ecological niches in the ecosystem are completely filled; therefore, natural communities are unlikely to resist invasion by foreign organisms, including genetically engineered organisms.

7. Although R-DNA technology has the potential to increase genetic diversity in agriculture and forestry, it is expected to reduce further genetic diversity in these systems.

8. Accuracy in predicting the adverse ecological effects of releasing a genetically engineered organism depends on the specific organism, the type of genetic information introduced, the particular environment into which it is released, and the availability of detailed ecological information.

12.3.6.3 Research approach

A lack of scientific understanding and a lack of appropriate methodologies exist for examining the effects of GEOs on ecosystem structure and function. Studies dealing with the effects of adding a GEO to a natural ecosystem will usually require more highly detailed microcosm simulations. Three principal research approaches that appear to be useful include:

1. Expanded use of microcosms as representations of various ecosystems including appropriate design features, characterization of the most critical parameters, calibration to the field, and standardization of the protocols;
2. Establishment of ecosystem baseline data for any particular habitat to permit confident analysis of ecological effects (and the degree of change required to detect a significant effect);
3. The generation of positive controls to ensure that test systems are appropriate for assessing ecosystem effects (Brezjnev et al., 1974; Hunter et al., 1986). However, Hagedorn and Lacy (1988) emphasize that, although these tests including microcosms are helpful, they are relatively poor in predicting ecological effects in nature.

With the wide diversity in ecosystem populations (especially microbial) and processes, it will be a major undertaking to attribute changes in any one ecosystem parameter to the presence or activities of a GEO. By using an appropriate modelling program, conducting experiments in a reasonable microcosm, and focusing on the most important processes, it may be possible to determine the potential that a GEO may have for causing environmental perturbations (Corapcioğlu and Haridas, 1984; Kook et al., 1987).

Research trends in examining ecosystem effects must include some element of experimental procedure that incorporates:

1. Designing a microcosm to simulate some important aspects of the proposed release area;
2. Evaluating the GEO by monitoring a set of parameters that are deemed 'most critical' for the particular microcosm;
3. Developing a descriptive model of the microcosm that can account for process rates, perturbations, and analyses (Minogue and Fry, 1983; Hicks and Newell, 1984; Thingstad and Pengerud, 1985; Pimentel et al., 1989). Lastly, numerical analysis of data assumes a uniquely important aspect in ecosystem studies because of the large variation inherent in the components of the system and the difficulty of establishing cause and effect relationships (Rouse, 1985). It will be necessary to attempt to define normal ranges of variability and function for specific ecological populations and/or processes and naturally occurring levels of change (Gladden and Ginzburg, 1982). Only then can perturbations be detected and the probability be determined that the alteration was associated with the presence and/or activities of a GEO.

12.4 METHODS FOR DETECTION AND QUANTIFICATION

The methods employed for detection of the adverse effects of pesticides and biotechnology agents on terrestrial ecosystems depend on whether the

Table 12.1. Measuring the adverse ecological effects of pesticides and biotechnology agents on terrestrial ecosystems. Various aspects of potential investigations are listed herein

Type of terrestrial ecosystem	Natural biota assessed	Ecosystem dynamics measured
Crop	Plants	Stability
Grassland	Mammals	Energy flows
Forest	Birds	Species diversity and food chain
Soil	Invertebrates	Waste decomposition and cycling
	Microorganisms	Pollination
		Productivity

system is a crop, grassland, forest, or soil terrestrial ecosystem (Table 12.1). Another important dimension of the experimental assessment is which species or groups of species will be assessed in the quantified investigation. In addition, the methods employed will depend on whether stability, species diversity, energy flows, waste decomposition (biogeochemical cycles), pollination, or a combination of these ecological factors will be assessed in the study (Table 12.1).

Since it is impossible to describe all experimental methods that might be employed for the detection and quantification of the adverse effects of pesticides and biotechniques on all the categories listed in Table 12.1, measuring the impact of pesticides on cole crops will be used as an example. In this model assessment, attention will be focused on the crop plants, invertebrates, and microorganisms both above ground and in the soil system. All aspects of the ecosystem dynamics are measured related to these species, except for pollination.

Often, the fauna and flora of crop ecosystems have fewer species than a natural forest and grassland; however, when all the species included in the soil ecosystem are taken into account, species richness is enormous (Odum, 1971).

For the proposed model study, *Brassica oleracea* or cole plants (broccoli, Brussels sprouts, cabbage, cauliflower, collards, and kale) are proposed to investigate the ecological effects of pesticides on the ecosystem for the following reasons:

1. Cole plants grow easily and rapidly;
2. Cole plants are attacked by an abundance of insect pests and plant pathogens (Walker and Larson, 1958; Pimentel, 1961a; Root, 1973; Kareiva, 1985);
3. Cole plants grow rapidly under favourable conditions and therefore can tolerate relatively heavy pest attack without the need of pesticides (control untreated) for survival (without pesticides, however, the crop is usually unmarketable);
4. A wide array of different insect pests (aphids, caterpillars, beetles, and plant bugs) and plant pathogens (fungi, bacteria, and viruses) offer potential for possible extrapolation of the results to other crops;
5. Cole crops are an important food crop in the world;

6. Cole plant ecosystems have a rich fauna and flora that make them similar to natural ecosystems.

Collards will be used as the representative crop plant species because of their morphological structure—open flat leaves that make insect and plant pathogen sampling relatively easy compared with other genotypes, like cabbage, of this species.

12.4.1 ABOVE-GROUND INSECT NUMBERS

The insect community associated with collards (*Brassica oleracea*) is ideal for study because the community is rich in numbers of both species and individuals (Pimentel, 1961b; Root, 1973). In addition, all animals occur on both natural and cultivated cruciferae in the northeastern US region; however, the arthropods are attracted to and prefer the cultivated *B. oleracea* species. Also important is the fact that the plant is a biennial and thus can be maintained in the field for an added season. Bimonthly, starting the first week in June, 15 plants per plot are measured and insect populations sampled for potential ecological effects of pesticides. To avoid bias in the choice of individual plants to be sampled, every fourth plant is selected for sampling. The starting plant is selected at random.

An estimate of the total surface area of the plant is made by placing a plastic sheet, which has been etched in centimetre squares, against the leaves and stem. Only one side of the leaf is included in the measurements. In making the visual counts of arthropods, only a single stage in the life history of each is used. The stages selected are those that give the best estimate of the density of the species and also its parasitism.

The bimonthly arthropod population samples detect a 10–50 per cent difference in abundance at the $P=0.05$ level, depending on the variability in the species population (Southwood, 1978). Simultaneously, the bimonthly population samples (throughout the summer) often will suggest important trends, even if these samples are not statistically different (Steel and Torrie, 1980). These consistent trends are extremely important in the analysis and interpretation of the data (Risch *et al.*, 1986).

12.4.2 SOIL AND LITTER INVERTEBRATE POPULATIONS

Litter and soil samples are taken during the summer at about one-month intervals during July and August. Sampling consists of taking 10 soil units (12 cm diameter × 8 cm deep). Before a soil sample is removed, any litter on the surface of the sample will be removed and placed in a ¼ in mesh screen cylinder (12 cm diameter × 8 cm) lined with tissue paper. The screen cylinder is used to keep the soil sample intact during handling and extraction. Both the cylinder and soil samples are then placed in a plastic bag and labelled.

A total of 10 litter and soil samples are selected at random locations within each test plot. Tullgren funnels are used to separate the invertebrates from the litter (Southwood, 1978). These funnels are 20 cm in diameter at the top. Hardware cloth (¼ in mesh) covers the funnel about 5 cm from the top, where the diameter is 16 cm. About 60 cm above the funnels, reflector floodlights of 75 W drive the invertebrates from the litter.

The litter samples are first sprinkled with water and then covered with a piece of wet cheesecloth. Glass jars containing 75 per cent ethyl alcohol placed below the funnels are used to collect the invertebrates. After 96 h, the alcohol is strengthened and the jars labelled and closed for counting the organisms later.

To estimate the numbers of surface-dwelling invertebrates (e.g., *Coleoptera*, *Diplopoda*), pitfall-traps are used (Dunger, 1983).

12.4.3 BIRD AND MAMMAL POPULATIONS

If pesticide effects on bird and mammal populations are to be measured, then extremely large ecosystems have to be treated. To locate dead birds and small mammals after death is in itself most difficult because of the rapid disappearance of carcasses. For example, Balcomb (1986) reported that about 80 per cent of the bird carcasses disappeared within 24 h after death. In addition, if the birds die in a grassland or forest, it becomes almost impossible to detect even one out of 100 deaths. Attaching tracking devices to birds and mammals will help to locate them, but the cost of making more than a few would be enormous.

12.4.4 PLANT PATHOGEN INFECTIONS

The incidence of plant pathogen infections in the experimental treatments is measured by two procedures. First, starting the first week in June, each plant in each plot is visually searched bimonthly for signs of disease that include wilting, yellowing, black spots, brown spots, white spots, and other suspicious symptoms of potential disease. The diseased plants are removed, roots and all, and placed into a plastic bag with an appropriate label. At the laboratory, the plants are carefully examined and a diagnosis made of the disease. Then the plants are measured for leaf-surface area using the methodology described earlier for insect measurements. The intensity of the infection is assessed by measuring the extent of area of infection. In addition, in the last two weeks of June and in early September, 15 plants are selected at random and totally removed from each plot in each treatment. These plants are also placed in plastic bags, labelled, and taken to the laboratory for examination. This procedure helps us to detect any potential infections that are not sufficiently severe to cause noticeable wilting and yellowing conditions in the plants in the experimental treatments.

The common diseases of cole plants include clubroot, yellows, black rot, black leg, rhizoctonia, bacterial soft rot, white blight, black leaf spot, ring spot, powdery mildew, downey mildew, white rust, mosaic, and damping off (Walker and Larsen, 1958).

12.4.5   PLANT PRODUCTIVITY

Net primary production is one of the most important parameters of plant quality and measure of stress effects. Plant production supplies the food to the insects and plant pathogens and, therefore, plays a major role in the dynamics of the system. Some of the pesticide treatments are expected to reduce plant productivity.

To measure plant productivity, 15 plants selected at random in each plot are measured bimonthly for total above-ground surface area. This is accomplished by placing a plastic measuring device (25 × 25 cm etched in centimetre squares) against each leaf and stem and estimating plant surface area. At the close of each experimental season, 10 plants in each plot are dug up and the roots washed clean of soil. These plants are then oven-dried and weighed to determine dry weight.

12.4.6   NUTRIENT AVAILABILITY TO THE PLANTS

Some pesticide treatments should influence leaching and availability of soil nutrients to the plants in the different treatments. The availability of these nutrients to the vegetation is assessed to associate net primary production and possible insect, herbivore, parasite, predator, and saprophyte and plant pathogen abundance with these nutrient changes. The nutrients selected for investigation in the experimental ecosystems are Al, As, B, Ca, Cd, Co, Cr, Cu, Fe, K, Mg, Mn, Mo, N, Na, Ni, P, Pb, S, Se, and Zn. These nutrients were selected because of their role in the biotic function of the experimental systems. Total nitrogen and KCl-extractable ammonium and nitrate in the soil receive particular attention because nitrogen is frequently a limiting nutrient, and the cycling dynamics of this element are largely determined by biologically mediated processes (e.g., ammonium mineralization, nitrification).

Ten 3 cm^2 soil cores (15 cm deep) are collected during May and September from each plot and these combined into one bulk sample for each plot. These are thoroughly mixed on a clean plastic surface. While in the field, 6 g subsamples of soil (approximate weights) are added to preweighed 120 ml polyethylene bottles containing 200 ml of $2 \text{ N KCl} + \text{PMA}$ (phenyl mercuric acetate: 0.5 p.p.m.). Precise sample weights are determined by reweighing the KCl bottles upon return to the laboratory. Moisture correction factors, ash content, and total nitrogen determinations are made on the remaining bulk samples. In addition, bulk samples collected prior to treatment and at the end of the growing season are analysed for cation exchange capacity (CEC), total phosphorus, Ca, K, Mg, and S.

Nutrient movement and availability measurements are made in the plots of each treatment to determine nitrogen and calcium leaching from the soil. These measurements include soil sampling at depths of 20 and 50 cm to determine movement and concentration of plant nutrients. Soil samples are taken weekly in June and then once per month in July, August, and September. For these purposes, soil sampling is a superior method to lysimeters, although the method is more laborious (personal communications from E. R. Watson, 1986, and T. W. Scott, 1987, Cornell University, Ithaca, New York).

During May and September, one leaf at the top and one at mid-height of 10 plants in each plot is sampled. These are combined on a 1 : 1 ratio, based on weight, into one sample for each plot. The leaves are analysed for the nutrients listed.

12.4.7 DECOMPOSITION

Decomposition of organic matter in the experimental systems is essential to normal nutrient cycling in these systems. Because pesticides may influence the rate of organic matter decomposition, we plan to assess this component (Edwards, 1980).

Standard litterbag methods are used to determine the effects of pesticide applications on litter decomposition (Edwards and Heath, 1963; Hagvar and Kjondal, 1981). Collards are used as standard organic matter. About 4 g (oven dry weight) of collards are placed in nylon mesh litterbags (approximately 15×15 cm of 1 mm mesh). The litterbags are placed in the field in May. Each bag is placed 5 cm below the soil surface. A total of 10 replicate bags are placed within each plot and these are collected in early October. Weight loss determinations for litterbag materials returned to the laboratory are made after drying at 60 °C. These samples are ground to pass through a #20-mesh screen, and sent to a soil-testing laboratory for an assessment of total nitrogen and nitrate.

12.5 SUMMARY AND CONCLUSIONS

About 2.5 million tonnes of pesticides are applied annually in the world at an estimated cost of $16.3 billion (US). Generally, these pesticides provide a significant benefit to agriculture and public health. At the same time, pesticide use is causing major problems:

1. Approximately 20 000 fatalities occur worldwide annually
2. Large amounts of food products are contaminated
3. Beneficial natural biota are destroyed
4. The injurious effects to terrestrial environments include reduced (a) stability, (b) energy flow, (c) species diversity, (d) pollination, and (e) waste decomposition and cycling.

Methods for the detection and quantification of the ecological effects of pesticides on terrestrial ecosystems are complex and costly, depending on what aspects and what combinations of pesticides are the target of the investigation. There is a clear need for a single accepted procedure for assessing the ecological effects of pesticides on non-target species in terrestrial ecosystems.

12.6 REFERENCES

Abdallah, M. D. (1968) The effect of sublethal dosages of DDT, parathion, and dieldrin on oviposition of the Colorado potato beetle (*Leptinotarsa decemlineata* Say) (*Coleoptera: Chrysomelidae*). *Bull. Entomol. Soc. Egypt Econ. Ser.* **2**, 211–217.

Balcombe, R. (1986) Songbird carcasses disappear rapidly from agricultural fields. *Auk* **103**, 817–820.

Barker, G. M. (1982) Short-term effects of methiocarb formulations on pasture earthworms (*Oligochaeta: Lumbricidae*). *N.Z. J. Exp. Agric.* **10**, 309–311.

Bostanian, N. J., Dondale, C. D., Binns, M. R. and Pitre, D. (1984) Effects of pesticide use on spiders (Arachneae) in Quebec apple orchards. *Can. Entomol.* **116**, 663–675.

Brezjnev, A. I., Ginzburg, L. R. and Poluektov, R. A. (1974) The structural optimization of exploited populations. *Econ. Math. Methods* **10**, 808–811 (in Russian).

Broadbent, A. B. and Tomlin, A. D. (1982) Comparison of two methods for assessing the effects of carbofuran on soil animal decomposers in corn fields. *Environ. Entomol.* **11**, 1036–1042.

Brown, A. W. A. (1978) *Ecology of Pesticides*. John Wiley, New York.

Corapcíoğlu, M. Y. and Haridas, A. (1985) Microbial transport in soils and groundwater: a numerical model. *Adv. Water Resour.* **8**, 188–200.

Crane, S. R. and Moore, J. A. (1984) Bacterial pollution of ground water, a review. *Water Air Soil Pollut.* **22**(1), 67–84.

Croft, B. A. and Brown, A. W. A (1975) Responses of arthropod natural enemies to insecticides. *Ann. Rev. Entomol.* **20**, 285–335.

Dunger, W. (1983) *Tiere im Boden. Die Neue Brehm-Bucherei*, Ziemser Verlag, Wittenberg, Lutherstadt, 380pp.

Edwards C. A. (Ed.) (1973) *Environmental Pollution by Pesticides*, Plenum, London.

Edwards, C. A. (1980) Interactions between agricultural practice and earthworms. In: Dindal, D. L. (Ed.) *Soil Biology as Related to Land Use Practices*, US Environmental Protection Agency, Office of Pesticides and Toxic Substances, Washington, DC, pp 3–11.

Edwards, C. A. and Heath, G. W. (1963) The role of soil animals in breakdown of leaf material. In: Doeksen, J. and van der Drift, J. (Eds) *Soil Organisms*, North Holland, Amsterdam, pp 76–84.

Edwards, C. A. and Thompson, A. R. (1973) Pesticides and the soil fauna. *Residue Rev.* **45**, 1–79.

Edwards, C. A. and Lofty, J. R. (1977) *The Biology of Earthworms 4*, Chapman and Hall, London.

Edwards, C. A., Dennis, E. B. and Empson, D. W. (1967) Pesticides and the soil fauna: effects of aldrin and DDT in an arable field. *Ann. Appl. Biol.* **60**, 11–22.

Eijsackers, H. (1978) Side effects of the herbicide 2,4,5-T on reproduction, food consumption, and moulting of the springtail *Onychiurus quadriocellatus* Gisin (Collembola). *Z. Angew. Entomol.* **85**, 341–360.

Elton, C. (1927) *Animal Ecology*, Macmillan, New York.

Fletcher, W. W. (1960) The effect of herbicides on soil microorganisms. In: Woodford, E. K. and Sagar, G. R. (Eds) *Herbicides and the Soil*, Blackwell, Oxford, pp 20–62.

Gladden, J. and Ginzburg, L. R. (1982) Variation and persistence in stochastic population models with differing age structures. *Bull. Ecol. Soc. Am.* **63**, 139.

Hagedorn, C. and Lacy, G. H. (1988) Methods of study of potential effects of biotechnology on integrated pest managment. Paper presented at SGOMSEC Workshop, Budejovice, Czechoslovakia, October 3–7, 1988.

Hagvar, S and Kjondal, B. R. (1981) Effects of artificial acid rain on the microarthropod fauna in decomposing birch leaves. *Pedobiologia* **22**, 409–422.

Helsel, Z. R. (1987) Pesticide use in world agriculture. In: Stout, B. A. (Ed.) *Energy in World Agriculture, Vol. 2*, Elsevier, New York, pp. 179–195.

Hicks, R. E. and Newell, S. Y. (1984) The growth of bacteria and the fungus *Phaeosphaeria-Typharum Eumycota Asomycotina* in salt march microcosms in the presence and absence of mercury. *J. Exp. Mar. Biol. Ecol.* **78**(1–2), 143–156.

Hunter, M., Stephenson, T., Kirk, P. W. W., Perry, R. and Lester, J. N. (1986) Effect of salinity gradients and heterotrophic microbial activity on biodegradation of nitrilotriacetic-acid in laboratory simulations of the estuarine environment. *Appl. Environ. Microbiol.* **51**(5), 919–925.

ICAITI (Instituto Centro Americano de Investigacion y Technología Industrial) (1977) *An Environmental and Economic Study of the Consequences of Pesticide Use in Central American Cotton Production: Final Report*, Central American Research Institute for Industry (Guatemala), United Nations Environment Programme, Nairobi, Kenya.

Kareiva, P. (1985) Finding and losing host plants by *Phyllotreta*: patch size and surrounding habitat. *Ecology* **66**, 1809–1816.

Keith, J. O., Woods, L. A. and Hunt, E. C. (1970) Reproductive failure in brown pelicans on the Pacific coast. *Transactions of the 35th North American Wildlife and Natural Resources Conference*, Wildlife Management Institute, Washington, DC, pp. 56–63.

Kool, J. B., Parker, J. C. and Van Genuchten, M. T. H. (1987) Parameter estimation for unsaturated flow and transport models—a review. *J. Hydrol.* **91**, 255–293.

Lance, J. C. and Gerba, C. P. (1984) Virus movement in soil during saturated and unsaturated flow. *Appl. Environ. Microbiol.* **47**(2), 335–337.

Lindow, S. E. (1982) Epiphytic ice nucleation-active bacteria. In: Mount, M. S. and Lacy, G. H. (Eds) *Phytopathogenic Prokaryotes, Vol. 1*, Academic Press, New York, pp. 335–362.

Lindow, S. E., Arny, D. C. and Upper, C. D. (1978) Distribution of ice nucleation-active bacteria on plants in nature. *Appl. Environ. Microbiol.* **36**, 831–838.

Littrell, E. E. (1986) Shell thickness and organochlorine pesticides in osprey eggs from Eagle Lake, California. *Calif. Fish Game* **72**, 182–185.

Lofs-Holmin, A. (1982) Measuring cocoon production of the earthworm *Allolobophora caliginosa* (Sav.) as a method of testing sublethal toxicity of pesticides. *Swed. J. Agric. Res.* **12**, 117–119.

Malone, C. R. (1969) Effects of diazinon contamination on an old-field ecosystem. *Am. Midland Naturalist* **82**, 1–27.

Metcalf, C. L., Flint, W. P. and Metcalf, R. L. (1962) *Destructive and Useful Insects— Their Habits and Control* (4th edn), McGraw Hill, New York, 1087pp.

Milewski, E. A. (1985) Field testing of microorganisms modified by recombinant techniques: applications, issues, and development of 'points to consider'. *Recomb. DNA Tech. Bull.* **8**, 102–108.

Minogue, K. P. and Fry, W. E. (1983) Models for the spread of disease: model description. *Phytopathology* **73**, 1168–1173.

Müller, P., Nagel, P. and Flacke, W. (1981) Ecological side effects of dieldrin application against tsetse flies in Adamaoua, Cameroon. *Oecologia* **50**, 187–194.

NRC (National Research Council) (1987) *Agricultural Biotechnology: Strategies for National Competitiveness*, National Academy Press, Washington, DC, 224pp.

Newton, I., Bogan, J. A. and Rothery, P. (1986) Trends and effects of organochlorine compounds in sparrowhawk eggs. *J. Appl. Ecol.* **23**, 461–478.

Odum, E. P. (1971) *Fundamentals of Ecology* (3rd edn), Saunders, Philadelphia.

Opdam, P., Burgers, J. and Müskens, G. (1987) Population trend, reproduction, and pesticides in Dutch sparrowhawks following the ban on DDT. *Ardea* **75**(2), 205–212.

Perfect, T. J., Cook, A. G., Critchley, B. R., Critchley, U., Davies, A. L., Swift, M. J., Russell-Smith, A. and Yeadon, R. (1979) The effect of DDT contamination on the productivity of a cultivated forest soil in the sub-humid tropics. *J. Appl. Ecol.* **16**, 705–719.

Perfect, T. J., Cook, A. G., Critchley, B. R. and Russell-Smith, A. (1981) The effect of crop protection with DDT on the microarthropod population of a cultivated forest soil in the sub-humid tropics. *Pedobiologia* **21**, 7–18.

Pimentel, D. (1961a) Competition and the species-per-genus structure of communities. *Ann. Entomol. Soc. Am.* **54**, 323–333.

Pimentel, D. (1961b) An ecological approach to the insecticide problem. *J. Econ. Entomol.* **54**, 108–114.

Pimentel, D. (1971) *Ecological Effects of Pesticides on Non-Target Species*, Executive Office of the President, Office of Science and Technology, Washington, DC, 220pp.

Pimentel, D. (Ed.) (1986) *Some Aspects of Integrated Pest Management*, Cornell University, Department of Entomology, Ithaca, New York, 368pp.

Pimentel, D. (1987) Down on the farm: genetic engineering meets technology. *Technol. Rev.* **90**, 24–30.

Pimentel, D. and Edwards, C. A. (1982) Pesticides and ecosystems. *BioScience* **32**, 595–600.

Pimentel, D. and Pimentel, M. (1979) *Food, Energy, and Society*, Edward Arnold Ltd, London, 165pp.

Pimentel, D. and Levitan, L. (1986) Pesticides: amounts applied and amounts reaching pests. *BioScience* **36**, 86–91.

Pimentel, D. and Warneke, A. (1989) Ecological effects of manure, sewage sludge, and other organic wastes on arthropod populations. *Agric. Zool. Rev.* **3**, 1–30.

Pimentel, D., McLaughlin, L., Zepp, A., Lakitan, B., Kraus, T., Kleinman, P., Vancini, F., Roach, W. J., Graap, E., Keeton, W. S. and Selig, G. (1991) Environmental and economic impacts of reducing US agricultural pesticide use. In: Pimentel, D. (Ed.) *Handbook of Pesticide Management in Agriculture, Volume 1, (2nd edn)*, Boca Raton, Florida: CRC Press, pp. 679–718.

Pimentel, D., Andow, D., Dyson-Hudson, R., Gallahan, D., Jacobson, S., Irish, M., Kroop, S., Moss, A., Schreiner, I., Shepard, M., Thompson, T. and Vinzant, B. (1980a) Environmental and social costs of pesticides: a preliminary assessment. *Oikos* **34**, 127–140.

Pimentel, D., Garnick, E., Berkowitz, A., Jacobson, S., Napolitano, S., Black, P., Valdes-Cogliano, S., Vinzant, B., Hudes, E. and Littman, S. (1980b) Environmental quality and natural biota. *BioScience* **30**, 750–755.

Pimentel, D., Andow, D., Dyson-Hudson, R., Gallahan, D., Jacobson, S., Irish, M., Kroop, S., Moss, A., Schreiner, I., Shepard, M., Thompson, T. and Vinzant, B. (1980c) Pesticides: environmental and social costs. In: Pimentel, D., and Perkins, J. H. (Eds) *Pest Control: Cultural and Environmental Aspects*, Westview Press, Boulder, Colorado, pp. 99–158.

Pimentel, D., Glenister, C., Fast, S. and Gallahan, D. (1984) Environmental risks of biological pest controls. *Oikos* **42**, 283–290.

Pimentel, D., Hunter, M. S., LaGro, J. A., Efroymson, R. A., Landers, J. C., Mervis, F. T., McCarthy, C. A. and Boyd, A. E. (1989) Benefits and risks of genetic engineering in agriculture. *BioScience* **39**, 606–614.

Potts, G. R. (1977) Population dynamics of the grey partridge: overall effects of herbicides and insecticides on chick survival rates. *Proc. Int. Congr. Game Biol.* **13**, 203–211.

Prasse, I. (1985) Indications of structural changes in the communities of microarthropods of the soil in an agroecosystem after applying herbicides. *Agric. Ecosyst. Environ.* **13**, 205–216.

Ries, S. K. and Wert, V. (1972) Simazine-induced nitrate absorption related to plant protein content. *Weed Sci.* **20**, 569–572.

Risch, S. J. and Carroll, C. R. (1982) Effect of a keystone predaceous ant, *Solenopsis geminata*, on arthropods in a tropical ecosystem. *Ecology* **63**, 1979–1983.

Risch, S. J., Pimentel, D. and Grover, H. D. (1986) Corn monoculture versus old fields: effects of low levels of insecticides. *Ecology* **67**, 505–515.

Rissler, J. (1984) Research needs for detecting environmental effects of genetically engineered microorganisms. *Recomb. DNA Tech. Bull.* **7**, 20–30.

Root, R. B. (1973) Organization of a plant-arthropod association in simple and diverse habitats: the fauna of collards *(B. oleracea)*. *Ecol. Monogr.* **43**, 95–124.

Rouse, D. I. (1985) Construction of temporal models: I. Disease progress of air-borne pathogens. *Adv. Plant Pathol.* **3**, 11–29.

Rusek, J. and Kunc, F. (1983) Impact of herbicides on edaphon and their decomposition in soil. Synthetics report, Institute of Landsc. Ecology and Institute of Microbiology, Czech. Academy of Sciences, Prague, 79pp. (in Czech, unpublished).

Santos, P. F. and Whitford, W. G. (1981) The effects of microarthropods on litter decomposition in a Chihuahuan desert ecosystem. *Ecology* **62**, 654–663.

Scott, T. W. (1987), unpublished work.

Shure, D. J. (1971) Insecticide effects on early succession in an old field ecosystem. *Ecology* **52**, 271–279.

Southwood, T. R. E. (1978) *Ecological Methods*, Halsted Press, London, 524pp.

Spencer, S. R. and Barrett, G. W. (1980) Meadow vole population response to vegetational changes resulting from 2,4-D application. *Am. Midl. Nat.* **103**, 32–46.

Steel, R. G. D. and Torrie, J. H. (1980) *Principles and Procedures of Statistics*, McGraw-Hill, New York, 633pp.

Thingstad, T. F. and Pengerud, B. (1985) Fate and effect of allochthonous organic material in aquatic microbial ecosystems: an analysis based on chemostat theory. *Mar. Ecol. Prog. Ser.* **21**(1–2), 47–62.

Tolstova, Y. S. and Atanov, N. M. (1982) Action of chemical substances for plant protection on the arthropod fauna of the orchard. I. Long-term action of pesticides in agrocoenoses. *Entomol. Rev.* **61**, 1–14.

Tomkins, D. J. and Grant, W. F. (1977) Effects of herbicides on species diversity of two plant communities. *Ecology* **58**, 398–406.

WHO (World Health Organization) (1988) *The WHO Recommended Classification of Pesticides by Hazard and Guidelines to Classification 1988–1989*, World Health Organization, Division of Vector Biology and Control, Geneva.

USDA and the State Universities and Land-Grant Colleges (1969) *A National Program of Research for Bees and Other Pollinating Insects Affecting Man*, US Department of Agriculture, Washington, DC.

Wakefield, N. G. and Barrett, G. W. (1979) Effects of positive and negative nitrogen perturbations on an old-field ecosystem. *Am. Midl. Nat.* **101**, 159–169.

Walker, J. C. and Larson, R. H. (1958) *Diseases of Cabbage and Related Plants*, USDA Agricultural Handbook No. 144, US Department of Agriculture, Washington, DC, 41pp.

Watson, E. R. (1986), MS thesis, Cornell University, USA.

Weary, G. C. and Merriam, H. G. (1978) Litter decomposition in a red maple woodlot under natural conditions and under insecticide treatment. *Ecology* **59**, 180–184.

Wiemeyer, S. N., Porter, R. D., Hensler, G. L. and Maestrelli, J. R. (1986) *DDE, DDT & Dieldrin: Residues in American Kestrels and Relations to Reproduction*, Fish and Wildlife Technical Report 6, US Department of the Interior, Fish and Wildlife Service.

Williams, C. S. and Hayes, R. M. (1984) Johnsongrass (*Sorghum halepense*) competition in soybeans (Glycine max). *Weed Sci.* **32**, 498–501.

13 Methods to Assess Toxicity to Aquatic Systems in Functional Ecosystems

V. LANDA and T. SOLDÁN
Czechoslovak Academy of Sciences, Institute of Entomology, Česke Budějovice, Czechoslovakia

13.1 INTRODUCTION

Many of the more than 1000 pesticides currently used in most of the countries of the world inadvertently reach the aquatic ecosystems. The several possibilities for pesticide penetration into water, substrates and aquatic biota include:

1. Surface runoff of pesticides used in agriculture and forestry—undoubtedly the most significant one;
2. Pesticides from rainfall, accidental spraying of water bodies, accidental spills, and continuous release from industrial wastewater;
3. Use of pesticides to control unwanted aquatic animals or plants, such as lampreys, some imported fishes, mosquitos, midges, black flies, pond weed, water milfoil, and water hyacinth.

The effects of pesticides on aquatic ecosystems are relatively well-known, because considerable attention has been paid to dose–response relationships resulting in both safe and economical levels of pesticide application (Muirhead-Thomson, 1971). However, unwanted side-effects of even strictly controlled uses of pesticides on non-target aquatic organisms are extremely difficult to avoid. Uptake and accumulation of a pesticide by aquatic organisms seem to be more likely a function of habitat, habits, life cycle, and exchange equilibria than of food uptake; but they are also affected by many other factors, such as size of organism, pharmacokinetics, and physical and chemical properties of the pesticide (Rosenberg, 1975). Transport routes and accumulation processes of pesticides communicated by substrates are much more complicated than often assumed. Global transport mechanisms brought some residues even into

Methods to Assess Adverse Effects of Pesticides on Non-target Organisms
Edited by R. G. Tardiff
©1992 SCOPE Published by John Wiley & Sons Ltd

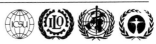

Antarctica (Tatton and Ruzicka, 1967). Moreover, our knowledge is restricted mostly to direct acute effects and mortality, while effects on the population and community level are practically unknown. Vertebrates (mostly fish) have been studied much more intensively than invertebrates.

The objective of this paper is to summarize the methods used to assess:

1. Pesticide toxicity and occurrence of pesticides in substrates of aquatic biotopes;
2. Acute and chronic effects in aquatic organisms;
3. Acute and chronic effects leading to population and community changes or changes in productivity of the ecosystem;
4. Research needs to improve the scientific bases for measurement of effects on the ecosystem.

13.2 PESTICIDES: TOXICITY TO AND OCCURRENCE IN AQUATIC SYSTEMS

To identify the major routes of pesticide exposure to aquatic systems and biota, the following parts of a global biocycle should be considered:

1. The water column, which usually first comes in contact with pesticides;
2. Organic substrates (algae, mosses, vascular hydrophytes, leaf litter, and branches);
3. Inorganic substrates, which include sedimentary material ranging from microscopic silts to coarse sand particles.

Naturally, pesticide content of interstitial water and sediments is usually much lower than that in the water column; and lithic biotopes are mostly less contaminated than standing waters. For instance, permethrin residues after application to a 640 ha forested block in Ontario attained peak concentrations of $147 \mu g/l$ in ponds, but only $2.5 \mu g/l$ in streams; while accumulation and persistence of pesticides in bottom sediment was negligible (Kingsbury and Kreutzweiser, 1980).

The determination of pesticide content in water, organic substrates, sediments (and animal tissues as well) is solely chemical. The solid materials or animal/plant tissues are usually homogenized, and 2–3 or less are extracted (e.g., with acetone/hexane), evaporated to a small volume, cleaned and dried, and analysed by a gas chromatographic procedure.

The effects, including acute toxicity, of pesticide-contaminated water on non-target organisms (NTOs) should be determined using biological methods. The concept of *in situ* bioassays is based on exposure of test animals at field sites without disturbing contaminated sediment, and the determination of percentage survival. The process of exposing fish to test the toxicity of water is relatively simple: cages containing fish are hung in the water column or anchored at the bottom, and mortality is measured after exposure for 96 h or longer.

The use of invertebrates to test undisturbed sediments, organic matter, or water presents additional problems such as predation and recovery of test animals. Only planktonic organisms (e.g., *Daphnia magna*) can be used to test water, since benthic organisms not exposed to the test substrate increase respiratory and metabolic rates by several fold, and results can be easily overestimated (Hynes, 1970). Nebecker *et al.* (1984) recommends testing sediments with a 9×20 cm cylindrical stainless steel screen (1.5 mm mesh) enclosed in petri dishes. Twenty adult *Hyalella*, juvenile *Gammarus*, or *Hexagenia* larvae (only 10 larger specimens) should be used in each case. One quarter of the cage is gently forced lengthwise into the sediment and anchored by stakes. Animals are exposed for 96 h using at least two replicate cages, then gently washed free of sediment and evaluated.

For an acute-lethal *in situ* mortality test, the crayfish (*Orconectes virilis*) can also be used at the same moult stage (Leonhard, 1974). A suitable cage size for six adult crayfish is $20 \times 15 \times 10$ cm. One cage is removed from each site at each sample period (e.g., 2, 4, 8, 16, 24 h exposure on day 1, and one sample per day for the following 30 days). The number of deaths is recorded; weights, lengths, and other characteristics are noted. Death is defined as complete immobility with no flexion of the abdomen upon forced extension. Animals are frozen for residue analysis to identify bioaccumulation at successive exposure intervals.

Some laboratory bioassays are unable to test pesticide-contaminated water or sediments. These include the liquid phase elutriate test and the solid phase sediment and water beaker test (Nebecker *et al.*, 1984). The solid phase sediment and water test can be modified according to Prater and Anderson (1977), who use a recirculating system containing both *Daphnia* (about 1 day old) and *Hexagenia* (20 and 5 per replicate, respectively). It seems to be more time-consuming to construct, calibrate, and use the beaker test; yet the results are comparable (Malueg *et al.*, 1983). By contrast, a similar device can be used for acute toxicity testing of pesticides on any invertebrates (see the tests for lampricide residues with *Hexagenia bilineata* in artificial substrates in Fremling (1975).

13.2.1 METHODS TO DETECT ACUTE AND DELAYED TOXICITY AMONG INDIVIDUALS

Of about a million species, only several invertebrate organisms have been selected to test adverse effect of toxicants: predominantly, the snail *Helisoma trivolvis*, the clams *Sphaerium*, *Corbicula*, and *Musculium*, the amphipods *Hyalella azteca*, *Gammarus lacustris* and *G. pulex fossarum*, the burrowing mayfly larvae *Hexagenia rigida* and *H. bilineata*, and larvae of the midge *Chironomus tentans*. Rarely, marine amphipods or freshwater benthic oligochaetes are used (Swartz *et al.*, 1982; Bailey and Liu, 1980).

The major criterion to select a test organism is the relative ease of mass rearing in the laboratory; others include small size, short life-span, maintenance and testing, and uniformity of organisms (Lawrence, 1981).

About 25 fish species are currently used to test waterborne pesticides. Among them, the common carp (*Cyprinus carpio*), the rainbow trout (*Salmo gairdneri*), the brown trout (*Salmo trutta*), the goldfish (*Carassius auratus*), the zebrafish (*Brachidanio rerio*), and the bluegill (*Lepomis macrochirus*) represent the most often used test vertebrate organisms. Nevertheless, any invertebrate animal or any fish can be used for chronic tests including those not necessarily advantageous for acute tests. For instance, the freshwater clam *Corbicula fluminea* has been found to be very useful for long-term field monitoring studies, but is of little or no value in acute studies, since it often closes its shell when exposed to high pulses of toxicants (Nebecker *et al.*, 1984).

Dose–response relationships are routinely examined in laboratory procedures for acute toxicity of aquatic invertebrates (Muirhead-Thomson, 1973). However, the substrate and other abiotic conditions should be similar to natural ones. Pelagic or planktonic organisms are simply tested in natural water. To test benthic organisms, the apparatus suggested by Prater and Anderson (1977) can be used; whereas, that of Rodrigues and Kaushik (1984) is helpful to test organisms living on substrates in the stream (e.g., black flies), and requires that the larvae of test invertebrates be fed and allowed to acclimate for a minimum of 16 h prior to treatment.

Acute toxicity results are usually expressed as $LC_{50}/48$ h and $LC_5/48$ h (Mayer and Ellersieck, 1986). In fish, the mechanism of toxic effect is the inhibition of some hydrolytic enzymes, mostly of acetylcholine hydrolase. Pesticides produce inhibition that varies from 40 per cent with fenitrothion to 78 per cent with dichlorvos. The major bioassays used to measure acute or delayed toxic effects of pesticides on aquatic organisms are as follows.

1. Egg test of the burrowing mayfly *Hexagenia*. Eggs are obtained from live females, placed in petri dishes (300 to 500 eggs for the standard size of 9 cm diameter), and tested at 20 °C for hatch rate (cumulative percentage hatch per treatment) and initiation of hatching. Eggs should be taken from numerous females to prevent use of unfertilized eggs. Eggs can be stored at 8 °C for up to 10 months and returned to 20 °C without considerably affecting hatch parameters (Friesen, 1979). With this test, the effects of methoxychlor ranged from partial suppression of hatching to a delay in hatching to total suppression of embryogenesis with the incipient LC_{50} estimated to be less than 0.06 mg/l.

2. *Chironomus* adults emergence test used to test for pesticides in sediments. A 2 or 3 cm deep layer of sediment is placed in 20 l containers overlaid with 15 cm of aerated water. The test starts with 10-day-old (20 °C) second instar larvae; the endpoint is the number of emerged adults collected in an erlenmayer flask trap. One hundred larvae fed on a mixture of 600 mg caerophyl and 100 mg tetralin are always used in replicate (Nebecker *et al.*, 1984).

3. *Daphnia magna* life-cycle test. This test exposes 5-day old *Daphnia* for 10 days through maturation and release of young (three broods), at which time adults and young specimens are counted. Experimental animals are fed at the rate of 2 mg/l of algae such as *Selenastrum* every other day. For water or sediment toxicity, total number of survivors are reported.

4. Measurement of mortality, growth, and fecundity of successive generations of the ramshorn snail, *Helisoma trivolvis*. Snail are cultured according to standard conditions and exposed to various concentrations (Flannagan, 1974). If mortality occurs during the egg-laying period, fecundity can be adjusted by multiplying the number of offspring produced by the standard number of days of egg laying divided by the actual number of days of egg laying (Flannagan and Cobb, 1979).

5. Sublethal crayfish *Orconectes virilis* test on intermolt phase and haemolymph calcium. This test is based on cyclical changes throughout the moult cycle, with normally higher levels of exoskeletal calcification present during premoult than during intermoult. Absence of elevation of calcium concentration in specimens exposed to pesticides in the laboratory defines failure to moult. Hemolymph samples are taken directly from the heart and analysed for calcium spectrophotometrically (Leonhard, 1974).

6. Testing embroyonic and larval life stages of fish. Acute-lethal tests are based on direct mortality; however, the most common effects of pesticides are changes in rates of respiration, fin and body movements, heartbeat, and response to light or touch. Chronic sublethal responses can be monitored in long-term toxicity tests. Rates of development, growth, yolk utilization, chorion strength, the occurrence of abnormalities, the timing and duration of hatch, and the initiation of larval feeding behaviour are all indicators of toxicity. For instance, triazine pesticides cause accumulation of an exudate in the body cavity and sometimes even ruptures of the body wall. The most common test is performed in petri dishes using eggs of rainbow trout; eggs and larvae of *Pimephales promelas*, *Salvelinus fontinalis*, *Schizostedion vitreium*, and *Brachydanio rerio* can be used as well (McKim, 1977; McDonald, 1979).

7. Residual oxygen test to estimate acute-lethal toxicity in fish. Using *Salmo gairdneri*, a 2–5 g trout contained in a 300 ml vessel is tested with five replicated pesticide concentrations at 10–15 °C. The time to death and the residual oxygen concentration at death are recorded. Residual oxygen concentrations, as mg O_2/l, are plotted against the logarithm of pesticide concentration, and the relationships are examined for a well-defined inflection point (Giles and Klaprat, 1979).

8. Test on cardiovascular and respiratory functions in fish. A surgical procedure is used to implant a buccal or opercular catheter to measure cough frequency, ventilation rate, and changes in pressure. Generally, an anaesthetized fish weighing from 0.3–2.0 kg is used. For electrocardiogram data, needle electrodes are inserted under the skin slightly anterior to the pectoral fins (recording electrode) and midventrally to the pelvic fins (reference electrode). An

alternative method has also been suggested (Majewski and Klaverkamp, 1975). Other 'physiological or ethological' tests include optomotor response or responsiveness to overhead light stimulation.

9. Fish serum and brain cholinesterase bioassays. Dissected brain or samples of serum are analysed by laboratory procedures using acetylcholine as the substrate. The supernatant of brain extract from $10\,\mu l$ of serum is examined for absorbance changes at 406 nm against air every 30 s for 3 min. The enzyme activity is related to the slope of the absorbance change. Other changes may occur in serum glucose, serum protein, or total serum lipid (Lockhart et al., 1951). Since most organophosphate pesticides are known to inhibit cholinesterase, this method seems to be most efficient. It was applied to monitor field applications of the organophosphates fenitrothion and malathion and the carbamate propoxur.

Tests with fish for chronic toxicity and bioaccumulation are somewhat difficult, because of the relatively long life cycles (e.g., 2–3 years in the carp). A possible exception is the zebrafish (*Brachydanio rerio*) because this small, egg-laying, tropical cyprinid has a life cycle of approximately 75 days. The fish are placed in chambers that allow the eggs to drop to the bottom, and eliminates their predation. The eggs are collected by scraping a slanted divider and siphoning them out (Lillie et al., 1979).

Morphological and pathological effects caused by pesticides are known to be non-specific. They are practically unknown in invertebrates, where generally only the nervous system shows morphological changes. For instance, treatment of mayfly larvae with nematocides at various concentrations led to a brownish precipitate in numerous cells of the sub-oesophageal ganglion. The deposit was intensely concentrated in a well-localized connective tissue, and sporadically it was found in the adjoining commissures and ganglia (Gysels, 1975).

Histopathological effects of pesticides in fishes have been studied intensively. Pathological changes occur mainly in the liver, blood vessels, kidneys, and gills. Liver cells exhibit cytoplasmic granularity, partial loss of liver plate radial orientation, and shrinkage of some liver cell mass. Glomeruli in the posterior kidney show pycnotic changes of cell nuclei, vocalization of cytoplasm, and atrophy of some cells. Gill filaments and lamellae show the precipitated masses that have plugged the central capillaries. The pathological changes of large blood vessels caused by methoxychlor are described in bluegill by Kennedy et al. (1970). Also changes in haematocrit levels and in morphology and quantity of blood cells have been found in various fish species. Boyd (1964) found that sublethal amounts of several chlorine insecticides induced abortions. The highest levels of DDT (2.0 mg/kg per week for 156 days) produced more mature ova than the untreated fish; also mortality among sac-fry was higher when one of the gametes came from a treated parent than when both gametes came from untreated fish. The reproduction of some other species (e.g, cutthroat goldfish) seems to be unaffected by DDT treatment (Allison et al., 1964).

13.3 BIOCONCENTRATION AND BIOINDICATION OF PESTICIDES

The bioconcentration tests are of principal importance, second only to those for determining chronic toxicity in the environment. A large number of bioconcentration assays have been described.

The *Chironomus* larval survival and growth test follows the same procedure used for the adult emergence test, except that exposure is for 15 days. The larvae are then placed in water overnight to clear the gut; then they are killed with warm water, dried, weighed, measured, and frozen for later tissue analysis. Other tests include the *Hyalella* partial life cycle test (for 28 days) with *Gammarus* or *Hexagenia* (Arthur, 1980; Fremling and Mauck, 1980). In larger animals, limited numbers of tissues are used. For example, at the conclusion of the *Orconectes virilis* sublethal test, only the following tissues are extracted: gills, liver, stomach, intestine, gonad, heart, tail muscle, haemolymph, and carapace (Leonhard, 1974).

Kinetics (i.e., rates of accumulation and elimination) of pesticides are determined using ^{14}C-labelled insecticides, followed by depuration of radioactivity after transfer to clean water for 96 h. A two-component curve consisting of a rapid initial uptake rate during the first 2 h followed by a reduced linear rate for the remainder of the 24 h exposure is characteristic for 20 plant and animal species in the case of the lampricide uptake (Figure 13.1). Rates

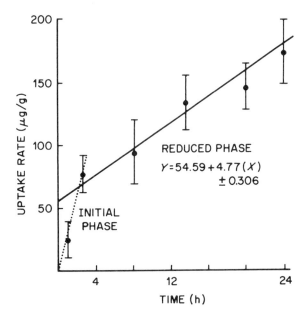

Figure 13.1. Rate of uptake of ^{14}C-labelled lampricide by the amphipod *Gammarus pseudolimnaeus* during 24 hour exposure to 9 mg/l (Maki and Johnson, 1977)

of uptake ranged from 0.36 μg/g/h for the crayfish *Orconectes propinquus* to 17.9 μg/g/h for the caddis fly larvae *Brachycentrus americanus* (Maki and Johnson, 1977). Rates of loss (Figure 13.2) and half-life figures varied from 7.2 h for the crayfish to 5295 for annelid worms. Continued accumulation of labelled residues from the organic matter is suggested for some pool species in the case of fenitrothion. Although the level of an initial 64 μg/l had declined to traces of 0.1 μg/l in water a few hours after treatment, it peaked in the whole crayfish *Orconectes virilis* at 1.37 μg/g at 19 days after application, and persisted at lower levels for 30 days (Leonhard, 1974).

The bioconcentration factor (BCF) is defined by solving the uptake equation for total body residue after 24 h exposure, and dividing this value by the mean initial pesticide water concentration (Maki and Johnson, 1977; Muir *et al.*, 1975). For instance, the BCF of some synthetic pyrethroids ranged in invertebrates from 135 for *trans*-permethrin to 316 for δ-methrin, but they were two- or four-fold less than those observed in oysters (Schimmel *et al.*, 1983) or carp (Ohkawa *et al.*, 1980).

In contrast to that for organophosphates and pyrethroids, the bioaccumulation of DDT and PCBs is a very aggressive and long-term process. Detritus-feeder organisms especially are exposed to a pronounced pesticide stress. For instance, mayfly larvae (*Ephemera danica*) accumulate DDT and PCB (Figure 13.3) to a steady state of 310 μg/g and 130 μg/g, respectively, according to a first-order kinetic equation (Södergren and Svensson, 1973). The same species showed DDE/DDT accumulation greater than that of detritus, Plecoptera, *Ancylus*,

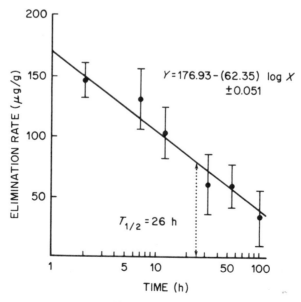

Figure 13.2. Rate of elimination of ^{14}C-labelled lampricide by the amphipod *Gammarus pseudolimnaeus* following 24 hour exposure to 0.9 mg/l (Maki and Johnson, 1977)

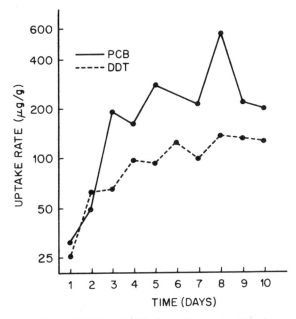

Figure 13.3. Accumulation of DDT and PCBs by sediment-dwelling larvae of the mayfly *Ephemera danica* (Sodergren and Swenson, 1973)

Gammarus, Trichoptera, *Tipula*, *Baetis*, or *Salmo* (Södergren *et al.*, 1972). The bioaccumulation and magnification of pesticides are very efficient, especially in the food chain of detritivore invertebrate fish. The bioconcentration factor in fish may even reach levels of 10^4 (Macek and Korn, 1970). Tolerances for DDT and PCBs in food range in most countries from 0.2 p.p.m. in baby food to 5.0 p.p.m. in fish. In the past, at the time of large-scale use of DDT, these tolerances were exceeded (Mauck and Olson, 1977).

The study of distribution of pesticides in different aquatic biotopes is urgently needed. Invertebrates as primary consumers and relatively short-lived organisms seem to be more useful than top consumers (fish), which accumulate pesticide for a long time. For instance, Södergren *et al.* (1972) successfully used an amphipod, *Gammarus pulex*, to indicate the levels of DDT and PCB in southern Swedish streams. Residue levels (less than 5 p.p.m. of lipid weight) were generally low in February, when streams were fed by underground water and the ground was frozen and snow-covered. They were very high (more than 35 p.p.m. of lipid weight) in April, associated with peak flow volumes caused by melting snow sweeping organic and inorganic material into streams.

When evaluating bioindicators of pesticide levels in the environment, one might keep in mind the reduced resistance and different accumulation rates of young and smaller specimens (Freeden, 1972; Eidt, 1975) and those with higher metabolic rates (Jensen and Gaufin, 1964) compared to others. Food selection and microhabitat may influence the susceptibility to soluble and insoluble pesticides (e.g., methoxychlor and its derivatives); filter-feeding organisms (unwanted blackflies and caddis flies) showed that a large number of non-target, scrapper, and collector feeding category species (Cummins, 1973) were heavily influenced (Flannagan et al., 1980). The populations of animals that live on the upper surface of stones and pelagic organism (most fish) as well as those entering aquatic habitats occasionally are more likely to be exposed to a pesticide during short to moderate exposure than those that dwell deeper in a substrate (Wiederholm, 1984). Moreover, a short pulse of pesticide at high concentration usually exerts a more pronounced effect than a long exposure to that pesticide at low concentration, even though the product of the concentration times the period of exspoure may be identical (Muirhead-Thomson, 1973).

13.4 EFFECTS OF PESTICIDES ON NON-TARGET COMMUNITIES

The successive physiological disturbances induced by pesticides (including hyperactivity, loss of equilibrium, tremors and convulsions) are capable of producing an avoidance mechanism, causing population movements. This mechanism in vertebrates (fish) has been reported frequently (Alabaster and Lloyd, 1980; Baier et al., 1985; Murty, 1986), but is much less known than the drift of aquatic invertebrates. Some species, such as rainbow trout (*Salmo gairdneri*), tend to remain motionless for several minutes; others, such as whitefish (*Coregonus clupeaformis*), show consistent swimming patterns. The apparatus to test for avoidance behaviour has been described in detail by Scherer and Nowak (1973). The avoidance of fenitrothion by goldfish provides an immediate read-out of time spent in places with concentration variations as great as 50 per cent (Scherer, 1975). Avoidance chamber responses of invertebrates and fry of rainbow trout to some herbicides (copper sulphate, acrolein, xylene emulsion, Dalapon, and Roundup) have been described by Folmar (1978).

Pesticide-induced downstream drift of invertebrates can be easily sampled with drifting nets (usually 1×1 m or smaller, mesh size about 0.14–0.30 mm). Pesticides may often induce invertebrate drift of catastrophic proportions. Numbers of drifting specimens increase at least several times during the 2–4 h after application, as in the case of large-scale treatment of forest with Actellic and Ambush in Czechoslovakia (Tonner et al., 1983; Figure 13.4). For instance, Flannagan et al. (1980) found that 50 000 specimens entered a 15 cm diameter sampler during a 4 h period after treatment of the Athabasca River with methoxychlor. An estimated 2.5 billion animals drifted past a particular site during that period of time. Dead specimens reached more than 50 per cent (Figure 13.5; Tonner et al., 1983). Gibbs et al. (1984) described the effects of carbaryl application in Maine. Invertebrate drift increased up to 170 times two days after treatment, and virtually all organisms in the samples were dead. Surface benthic communities (mainly Ephemeroptera, Trichoptera, and Plecoptera) can be eliminated (Wallace and Hynes, 1975).

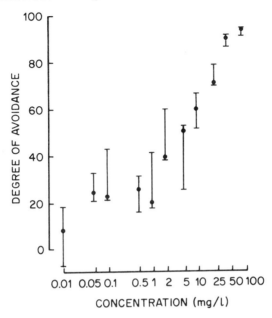

Figure 13.4. Avoidance of fenitrothion by goldfish *Carassius auratus*; values are median response, and bars are standard errors (Scherer, 1975)

Benthos recovery is usually accomplished within several months. For fenitrothion applied at 73 μg/l, benthos recovered after its total elimination at about 350 m downstream (23 μg/l) 50 days after treatment (Eidt, 1981). Organophosphates and carbamates rarely penetrate the sediments deeply, and substrate-dwelling animals remain mostly unaffected (e.g., oligochaetes and Chironomidae). On the other hand, penetration by DDT and PCB is more pronounced, and recovery of benthic invertebrates required at least 4 years in New Brunswick (Ide, 1960).

Toxic effects of pesticides also influence more tolerant species of aquatic communities, in that their qualitative presentation and types of competitors, predators, and prey-organisms may expand or contract as niche space is vacated or eliminated. Changing densities are detected by quantitative sampling—usually electrofishing or Surber benthometry of invertebrates. The effects are summarized as follows:

1. Top predator elimination usually results in a several-fold increase in density of benthic insects. For example, elimination of fish from a Wisconsin lake by toxaphene was followed by a 200-fold increase in the *Chironomus* population, which declined again when fish were restocked (Hilsenhoff, 1965).

2. Reduction of invertebrate predators showed similar effects; for example, the number of blackflies (filtrators) increased greatly following the treatment of streams with DDT and the subsequent reduction of predatory Plecoptera and Trichoptera (Hurlbert, 1975).

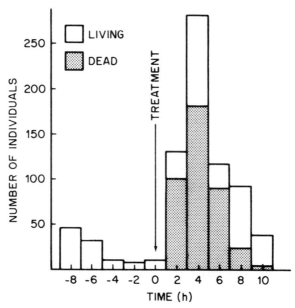

Figure 13.5. Drifting specimens of the stonefly *Protonemura auberti* during application of pirifosmethyl (Actelic) and decamethrin (Ambush) (Tonner *et al.*, 1983)

3. Similarly, massive increases in attached algae in streams have been attributed to the elimination of grazers by pesticides (Yasuno *et al.*, 1982). However, increased densities of benthic invertebrates following some herbicide treatment presumably resulted from the changes in oxygen levels associated with decaying plants; this may also give rise to higher phytoplankton production before the macrophytes begin to reappear. Species closely associated with macrophytes (e.g., some Ephemeroptera, Plecoptera, or Chironomidae) can be reduced greatly when substrate availability and complexity are reduced (Brooker and Edwards, 1975).

4. The removal of competitors causes expansion of species with similar niche requirements. For example, in a malaria eradication programme, pesticide-resistant populations of *Anopheles* mosquitoes have benefited from the pesticide-caused mortality of species that compete for their preferred prey (Hurlbert, 1975).

5. Non-target species populations can be eliminated as a consequence of effects on some abiotic factors, as in the case of herbicide treatment. The decay of large amounts of plant material can reduce the amount of dissolved oxygen and alter pH conditions, thus affecting many organisms (especially fish).

Data on pesticide effects at the aquatic ecosystem level are very scarce. Thus far, measurements have been made of only the quantity of nutrients and levels of energy. Both primary and secondary production have been measured by hydrobiological methods, mostly in conjunction with methoxychlor or lampricide treatment of running waters. While methoxychlor caused reduction of densities and biomass to less than 10 per cent, the following parameters were unaffected: counts of fungal hyphae, respiration rates of conditioned leaf discs, and adenosine triphosphatase (ATP) content of coarse organic matter. However, ATP levels of fine particulate organic matter were significantly higher in a treated stream representing potentially increased food quality and generation of subsequent transport to downstream reaches (Cuffney et al., 1984). Generally, both secondary production of benthic organisms and the turnover ratio (production + biomass) are decreased by any toxic quantity of a pesticide, mostly as a consequence of density reduction. The production quotient between primary and secondary consumers seem to be very suitable for assessing the effects of pesticides on running water biocenoses. The production quotient is approximately 15 in undisturbed biocenosis and increases with greater disturbances (Frutiger, 1985).

13.5 REFERENCES

Alabaster, J. S. and Lloyd, R. (1980) *Water Quality Criteria for Fresh-Water Fish*, Butterworths, London, pp. 297–298.

Allison, D., Kallman, B. J., Cope, O. B. and Van Valin, C. C. (1964) *Some Chronic Effects of DDT on Cutthroat Trout*, Research Report 64, US Department of Interior, Bureau of Sport Fisheries and Wildlife, Washington, DC, 30pp.

Arthur, J. W. (1980) Review of freshwater bioassay procedures for selected amphipods. In: Buikema, A. L. and Cairns, J. (Eds) *Aquatic Invertebrate Bioassays*, ASTM Special Technical Publication 715, American Society for Testing and Materials, Philadelphia, Pennsylvania, pp. 98–108.

Baier, Ch., Hurle, K. and Kirchhoff, J. (1985) *Datensammlung zur Abschatzung des Gefahrdungspotentials von Pflanzenschutzmiettel—Wirkstoffen fur Gewasser*, Paul Parey, Verlag.

Bailey, H. C. and Liu, D. H. E. (1980) *Lumbriculus veriegatus*, a benthic oligochaete, as a bioassay organism. In: Eaton, J. C., Parrish, P. R. and Hendrick, A. C. (Eds) *Aquatic Toxicology*, ASTM Special Technical Publication 707, American Society for Testing and Materials, Philadelphia, Pennsylvania, pp. 205–215.

Boyd, C. E. (1964) Insecticides cause mosquitofish to abort. *Prog. Fish-Cult.* **26**, 138.

Brooker, M. P. and Edwards, R. W. (1975) Review paper: aquatic herbicides and the control of water weeds. *Water Res.* **9**, 1–15.

Cuffney, T. F., Wallace, J. B. and Webster, J. R. (1984) Pesticide manipulation of a headwater stream: invertebrate response and their significance for ecosystem processes. *Freshwater Invertebr. Biol.* **3**, 153–171.

Cummins, K. W. (1973) Tropic relations of aquatic insects. *Ann. Rev. Entomol.* **18**, 183–206.

Eidt, D. C. (1975) The effect of fenitrothion from large-scale forest spraying on benthos in New Brunswick headwater streams. *Can. Entomol.* **107**, 743–760.

Eidt, D. C. (1981) Recovery of aquatic arthropod populations in a woodland stream after depletion by fenitrothion treatment. *Can. Entomol.* **113**, 303–313.

Flannagan, J. F. (1974) Influence of trisodium nitrilotriacetate on the mortality, growth and fecundity of the freshwater snail (*Helisoma trivolvis*). *Fish. Res. Board Can.* **31**, 155–161.

Flannagan, J. F. and Cobb, D. G. (1979) The use of the snail *Helisoma trivolvis* in a multingeneration mortality, growth and fecundity test. In: Scherer, E. (Ed.) *Toxicity Tests for Freshwater Organisms*, Can. Spec. Publ. Fish. Aquat. Sci. **44**, 19–26.

Flannagan, J. F., Townsend, B. E. and de March, B. G. E. (1980) Acute and long-term effects of methoxychlor larviciding on the aquatic invertebrates of the Athabasca River, Alberta. In: Haufe, W. O. and Croome, G. C. R. (Eds) *Control of Black Flies in the Athabasca River*, technical report, Alberta Environment, Edmonton, pp. 151–158.

Folmar, L. C. (1978) Avoidance chamber responses of mayfly nymphs exposed to eight herbicides. *Bull. Environ. Contam. Toxicol.* **17**, 312–318.

Freeden, F. J. H. (1972) Reactions of the larvae of three rheophilic species of *Trichoptera* to selected insecticides. *Can. Entomol.* **104**, 944–953.

Fremling, C. R. (1975) Acute toxicity of the lampricide 3-trifluoro-methyl-4-nitrophenyl (TFM) to nymphs of mayflies (*Hexagenis* sp.). *Invest. Fish Control* **58**, 1–6.

Fremling, C. R. and Mauck, W. L. (1980) Methods for using nymphs of burrowing mayflies (Ephemeroptera, *Hexagenia*) as toxicity test organisms. In: Buikema, A. L. and Cairns, J. (Eds) *Aquatic Invertebrate Bioassays*, ASTM Special Technical Publication 715, American Society for Testing and Materials, Philadelphia, pp. 81–97.

Friesen, M. K. (1979) Toxicity testing using eggs of the burrowing mayfly *Hexagenia rigida* (Ephemeroptera, Ephemeridae), with methoxychlor as toxicant. *Proceedings of the Fifth Annual Aquatics Workshop*, Report 862, pp. 266–277.

Frutiger, A. (1985) The production quotient PQ: a new approach for quality determination of slightly to moderately polluted running waters. *Arch. Hydrobiol.* **104**, 513–526.

Gibbs, K. E., Mingo, T. M. and Courtemanch, D. L. (1984) Persistence of carbaryl (Sevin-4-oil) in woodland ponds and its effects on pond macro invertebrates following forest spraying. *Can. Entomol.* **116**, 203–204.

Giles, M. A. and Klaprat, D. (1979) The residual oxygen test: a rapid method for estimating the acute-lethal toxicity of aquatic contaminants. In: Scherer, E. (Ed.) *Toxicity Tests for Freshwater Organisms*, Can. Spec. Publ. Fish. Aquat. Sci. **44**, pp. 37–45.

Gysels, H. (1975) Electrophoretical and histochemical investigations on some noxious *Lepidoptera* and on the impact of pesticide upon *Ephemera danica*, a water-dwelling, innocuous mayfly. *Acta Zool. Pathol. Antverp.* **62**, 127–141.

Hilsenhoff, W. L. (1965) The effect of toxaphene on the benthos in a thermally-stratified lake. *Trans. Am. Fish. Soc.* **94**, 210–213.

Hurlbert, S. H. (1975) Secondary effects of pesticides on aquatic ecosystems. *Res. Rev.* **57**, 81–148.

Hynes, H. B. N. (1970) *The Ecology of Running Waters*, University Press, Toronto, 555pp.

Ide, F. P. (1960) Effects of forest spraying with DDT on aquatic insects, food of salmon and trout, in New Brunswick. *Proc. Entomol. Soc. Ontario* **91**, 39–40.

Jensen, L. A. and Gaufin, A. R. (1964) Long-term effects of organic insecticides on two species of stonefly naiads. *Trans. Am. Fish. Soc.* **93**, 357–363.

Kennedy, H. D., Eller, L. L. and Walsh, D. F. (1970) *Chronic Effects of Methoxychlor on Bluegills and Aquatic Invertebrates*, Tech. Pap. Bureau Fish. Wildl. 53, pp. 3–18.

Kingsbury, P. D. and Kreutzweiser, D. P. (1980) *Environmental Impact Assessment of a Semi-Operational Permethrin Application*, Forestry Service Report FPM-X-30, Environment Canada, Ottawa, pp. 1–47.

Lawrence, S. G. (Ed.) (1981) *Manual for the Culture of Selected Freshwater Invertebrates*, Can. Spec. Publ. Fish. Aquat. Sci. 54, 169.

Leonhard, S. L. (1974) Uptake of fenitrothion by caged crayfish *Orconectes virilis* in Pine Creek, Manitoba. *Manitoba Entomol.* **8**, 16–18.

Lillie, W. R., Harrison, S. E., Macdonald, W. A. and Klaverkamp, J. F. (1979) The use of the zebrafish (*Brachydanio rerio*) in whole-life-cycle tests. In: Scherer, E. (Ed.) *Toxicity Tests for Freshwater Organisms*, Can. Spec. Publ. Fish. Aquat. Sci. 44, pp. 104–111.

Lockhart, W. L., Rosenbrough, N. J., Farr, A. L. and Randall, R. J. (1951) Protein measurement with folin phenol reagent. *J. Biol. Chem.* **193**, 267–275.

Macdonald, W. A. (1979) Testing embryonic and larval life stages of fish. In: Scherer, E. (Ed.) *Toxicity Tests for Freshwater Organisms*, Can. Spec. Publ. Fish. Aquat. Sci. 44, pp. 131–138.

Macek, K. J. and Korn, S. (1970) Significance of the food chain in DDT accumulation by fish. *J. Fish. Res. Board Can.* **27**, 1496–1498.

Majewski, H. S. and Klaverkamp, J. F. (1975) An acute bioassay for cardiovascular and respiratory functions in rainbow trout. In: Craig, G. R. (Ed.) *Proceedings of the Second Annual Aquatic Toxicity Workshop, 1975, Toronto, Ontario*, Ontario Ministry of the Environment, Ottawa, pp. 165–178.

Maki, A. W. and Johnson, H. E. (1977) Kinetics of lampricide (TFM, 3-trifluoromethyl-4-nitrophenol) residues in model stream communities. *J. Fish. Res. Board Can.* **34**, 276–281.

Malueg, K. W., Schuytema, G. S., Gakstatter, J. H. and Krawczyk, D. F. (1983) Effects of *Hexagenia* on *Daphnia* response in sediment toxicity tests. *Environ. Toxicol. Chem.* **2**, 73–82.

Mayer, F. L. and Ellersieck, M. R. (1986) *Manual of Acute Toxicity: Interpretation and Data Base for 410 Chemicals and 66 Species of Freshwater Animals*, US Department of Interior, Fish and Wildlife Service, Washington, DC, 582pp.

Mauck, W. L. and Olson, K. E. (1977) Polychlorinated biphenyls in adult mayflies (*Hexagenia bilineata*) from the upper Mississippi River. *Bull. Environ. Contam. Toxicol.* **17**, 387–390.

McKim, J. M. (1977) Evaluation of test with early life stages of fish for predicting long-term toxicity. *J. Fish. Res. Board Can.* **34**, 1148–1154.

Muir, D. C. G., Rawn, G. P., Townsend, B. E., Lockhart, W. L. and Greenhalgh, R. (1975) Bioconcentration of cypermethrin, deltamethrin, fenvalerate and permethrin by *Chironomous tentans* larvae in sediment and water. *Environ. Toxicol. Chem.* **4**, 51–61.

Muirhead-Thomson, R. C. (1971) *Pesticides and Freshwater Fauna*, Academic Press, London, New York, 248pp.

Muirhead-Thomson, R. C. (1973) Laboratory evaluation of pesticide impact on stream invertebrates. *Freshwater Biol.* **3**, 479–498.

Murty, A. S. (1986) *Toxicity of Pesticides to Fish*, CRC Press, Boca Raton, Florida, 143pp.

Nebecker, A. V., Cairns, M. A., Gakstatter, J. H., Malueg, K. W., Schuytema, G. S. and Krawczyk, D. F. (1984) Biological methods for determining toxicity of contaminated freshwater sediments to invertebrates. *Environ. Toxicol. Chem.* **3**, 617–630.

Ohkawa, H., Kikuchi, R. and Miyamoto, J. (1980) Bioaccumulation and biodegradation of the (S)-acid isomer of fenvalerate (Sumicidin) in an aquatic model ecosystem. *J. Pest. Sci.* **5**, 11–22.

Prater, B. L. and Anderson, M. A. (1977) A 96-hour bioassay of Duluth and Superior harbor basins (Minnesota) using *Hexagenia limbata*, *Asellus communis*, *Daphnia magna*, and *Pimephales promelas* as test organisms. *Bull. Environ. Contam. Toxicol. Chem.* **2**, 73–82.

Rodrigues, C. S. and Kaushik, N. K. (1984) A bioassay apparatus for the evaluation of black fly (*Diptera simuliidae*) larvicides. *Can. Entomol.* **116**, 75–78.

Rosenberg, D. M. (1975). Food chain concentration of chlorinated hydrocarbon pesticides in invertebrate communities: a re-evaluation. *Quest. Entomol.* **11**, 97–110.

Scherer, E. (1975) Avoidance of fenitrothion by goldfish. *Bull. Environ. Contam. Toxicol.* **13**, 492–496.

Scherer, E. and Nowak, S. (1973) Apparatus for recording avoidance movements of fish. *J. Fish Res. Board Can.* **30**, 1594–1596.

Schimmel, S. C., Garnas, R. L., Patrik, J. M. and Moore, J. C. (1983) Acute toxicity, bioconcentration and persistence of AC222, 705, benthiocarb, chloropyrifos, fenvalerate, methyl parathion and permethrin in the estuarine environment. *J. Agric. Food Chem.* **31**, 104–113.

Södergren, A. and Svensson, B. (1973) Uptake and accumulation of DDT and PCB by *Ephemera danica* (Ephemeroptera) in continuous-flow systems. *Bull. Environ. Contam. Toxicol.* **9**, 345–350.

Södergren, A., Svensson, B. and Ulfstrand, S. (1972) DDT and PCB in south Swedish streams. *Environ. Pollut.* **3**, 25–36.

Swartz, R. C., DeBeb, W. A., Sercu, K. A. and Lamberson, J. O. (1982) Sediment toxicity and the distribution of amphipods in Commencement Bay, Washington, USA. *Pollut. Bull.* **13**, 359–364.

Tatton, J. O'. G. and Ruzicka, J. H. A. (1967) Organochlorine pesticides in Antarctica. *Nature (Lond.)* **215**, 346–348.

Tonner, M., Vavra, N., Syrovatka, O. and Soldan, T. (1983) Einfluss der Luftbespritzung gegen grauen Larchenwickler (*Zeiraphera diniana*) auf die Entomofauna des Rhithrons in Krkonose (Riesengebirge). *Vest. Cesk. Spol. Zool.* **47**, 293–303.

Wallace, R. R. and Hynes, H. B. N. (1975) The catastrophic drift of stream insects after treatments with methoxychlor (1,1,1-trichloro-2,2-*bis*-[o-methoxyphenyl] ethane). *Environ. Pollut.* **8**, 255–268.

Wiederholm, T. (1984) Responses of aquatic insects to environmental pollution. In: Resh, V. S. and Rosenberg, D. M. (Eds) *The Ecology of Aquatic Insects*, Praeger, New York, pp. 508–557.

Yasuno, M., Ohkita, J. and Hatakeyma, S. (1982) Effects of temephos on macrobenthos in a stream of Mt Tsukuba. *Jpn. J. Ecol.* **32**, 29–38.

14 Methods to Assess Adverse Effects on Plants

J. VELEMINSKY and T. GICHNER

Institute of Experimental Botany, Czechoslovak Academy of Sciences, Prague, Czechoslovakia

14.1 INTRODUCTION

Plants are the main recipients of pesticides, regardless of whether they themselves represent the target organism (e.g., weed) or whether the targets are pests, pathogenic fungi, etc. They are exposed to pesticides from direct application, through the uptake from soil and water, and from atmospheric drift. It has been shown (Ware *et al.*, 1970) that about half of pesticides applied by aircraft land outside the target cropland or forest and fall out either on adjoining ecosystems or drift into distant ecosystems.

Pesticides tend to be very reactive, mostly electrophilic, compounds that can react with various nucleophilic centres of cellular biomolecules, including DNA (Crosby, 1982), or form even more reactive electrophilic products that either modify cellular components or are metabolized to more or less stable products. Ideally, pesticides should affect only the target organism; however, this ideal is rarely attained because of similarities in the basic life processes of both target and non-target plants. Toxicity, including mutagenicity, is the consequence; it is mediated by various changes in the metabolism of plants, including formation of metabolic pathways of pesticide degradation.

Differential sensitivity of plant species to toxic and genotoxic effects of pesticides has been shown to cause overall changes in species ratios, both among weeds in a crop field and in natural plant communities, due to the reduced abundance of susceptible species with concurrent increases in naturally tolerant species. This may have further consequences for the entire ecosystem (Pimentel and Edwards, 1982). An important factor in this situation is the occurrence of herbicide-resistant forms within susceptible plant species. Here, pesticides can play roles as agents favouring the selection of pre-existing resistant mutants and as potential inducers of genetic changes (Grant, 1972, 1982a; Brown, this

Methods to Assess Adverse Effects of Pesticides on Non-target Organisms
Edited by R. G. Tardiff
©1992 SCOPE Published by John Wiley & Sons Ltd

volume). Genotoxic pesticides are potentially able to increase mutations in DNA, controlling the expression of various qualitative and quantitative traits that could cause genetic instabilities of natural plant populations and in crop varieties (Crosby, 1982).

Another important consideration is the possible formation of stable metabolites and their accumulation in plants to such an extent that they can become harmful to both human and animal populations via their respective food chains. Attention must be given to this problem despite the observation that bound residues incorporated into lignin, hemicellulose, and other carbohydrate components of the cell wall of plants are generally considered to be less toxic to the biosphere than corresponding adducts produced in animal cells (Lamoureux and Rusness, 1986).

Pesticides have also produced changes in plant metabolism and in nutritional patterns that may have secondary effects on the ecology. Even when applied at recommended dosages, some herbicides have been found to increase unwanted insects and plant pathogens (Pimentel, 1971; Oka and Pimentel, 1974). For example, when corn was treated with 2,4-dichlorophenoxyacetate (2,4-D) at the recommended dosage of 1 kg/ha, the numbers of corn leaf aphids increased by threefold; corn borers were 26 per cent more abundant and were also 33 per cent larger than the same insects on untreated corn (Oka and Pimentel, 1974). The larger size corn borers produced one third more eggs, and thus contributed to the overall build-up of corn borers in corn fields.

The insecticides monocrotophos and phosphamidon likewise increased concentrations of nitrogen and phosphorus in rice plants; these changes were thought to contribute to a resurgence in numbers of the rice blue leafhopper (Mani and Jayraj, 1976). In addition to the increased number of plant insect pests, herbicides can also increase plant pathogen attack. For instance, when corn was treated with a recommended dosage of 2,4-D (1 kg/ha), black corn smut grew fivefold larger than on untreated corn (Oka and Pimentel, 1974). Also, corn treated with 2,4-D and resistant to southern corn leaf-blight lost its resistance to the blight.

Increasing insect pest and plant pathogen attacks on crops due to the use of some herbicides may in turn increase the application of more pesticides, such as insecticides and fungicides. Thus, the environmental problem in using herbicides may be amplified beyond that of the herbicide itself.

Most nutrients, especially C, K, N, P, and S, are taken up by plants, which in turn may be eaten by animals. These nutrients are eventually returned to the soil or atmosphere via decomposition of decaying organisms. The amounts and forms of nutrients in soil and plants may be changed by pesticides affecting the dynamics of these animal in the ecosystem.

Pesticides can alter the chemical composition of plants. The changes that occur appear to be specific for both the plant and the pesticides involved. For example, certain organochlorine insecticides have increased the amounts of some macro- and micro-element constituents (Al, B, Ca, Cu, Fe, K, Mg, Mn, N, P, Sr, and Zn) of corn and beans, and decreased the amounts of others (Cole *et al.*, 1968). In another study, DDT, aldrin, endrin, and lindane were found to stimulate synthesis of the important amino acids arginine, histidine, leucine, lysine, proline, and tyrosine in corn, but decreased the content of tryptophane (Thakre and Saxena, 1972). The herbicide simazine increased water and nitrate uptake in barley, rye, and oat seedlings, resulting in increased plant weight and total protein content (Ries and Wert, 1972). Soil treatment of carrot with insecticides Nexion, Birlane, and Dyfonate increased the concentration of free sugars in roots, whereas an opposite effect was observed after the action of the herbicide Dosanex (Rouchaud *et al.*, 1983).

In this chapter attention is paid mostly to the methods and experimental approaches suitable for detection of immediate and delayed toxicity of pesticides, their harmful metabolites and residues on plants. The chapter does not describe all methods used to measure pesticide metabolites and residues, changes in the plant metabolism, or nutritional requirements caused by pesticides.

14.2 MEASURING PESTICIDE-INDUCED TOXICITY IN PLANTS

The toxic effects of pesticides accumulated in soil or water can be measured on intact plants grown in the natural communities or in the field, on intact plants cultivated in the greenhouse or growth chambers, or on plant cell cultures *in vitro*.

14.2.1 PLANTS IN THE FIELD AND IN NATURAL COMMUNITIES

Several endpoints are available to measure an immediate toxic effect of pesticides on crop plants in the field. Standardized procedures in field trials simulating the conditions of agricultural utilization exist, and are recommended by authorities for evaluation of toxic effects of pesticides, especially herbicides, on crops. They measure toxicity to the target organism and to crops by using endpoints such as plant emergence or seed germination, crop stand or survival, growth rate, various types of injury during plant growth (e.g., chlorosis), seed setting fresh or dry weight of plants at harvest, and crop yield. Data from these trials may serve to decide suitable doses of pesticides in fields to avoid harmful effects on crop species or varieties under specific climatic conditions (Frans *et al.*, 1988).

Similar experimental protocols can be followed for studies dealing with quantitative and qualitative changes caused by herbicides among weed species in crop fields and among those in natural plant communities on roadsides, grasslands, and forests (Way and Chancellor, 1976). The experimental territory is to be divided into standard plots exposed to a test herbicide or a mixture of herbicides and to untreated plots as controls. In each plot, individual species and the number of individuals within each species are determined before the application of pesticides and at various times during and after pesticide application. Finally, plants are harvested; various endpoints are measured separately according to species and plots. Survival to harvest, dry or wet weight of plants or their parts, and seed setting or seed weight can be measured and statistically analysed using principal-component analysis or linear regression modelling (Tomkins and Grant, 1974, 1976; Campbell *et al.*, 1981)

In general, herbicides in experiments lasting even several years do not eradicate susceptible species, but rather reduce their abundance. With reductions in susceptible species, a concurrent increase in species naturally tolerant to the tested compound(s) is typical. This situation results in an overall change in species ratios, but with no change in the number of species present (Chancellor, 1979). For instance, in plots sprayed annually with 2,4-D for 36 years, no new major species has become established (Hume, 1987).

14.2.2   PLANTS IN GREENHOUSES AND GROWTH CHAMBERS

Greenhouse and growth-chamber conditions are especially suitable for determining the importance of individual external factors like temperature, light intensity and quality, day length, water stress, nutrition, and air humidity on the uptake, absorption, transport, translocation, metabolism, persistence, disappearance and overall toxicity of pesticides in the whole plants (Cole, 1983; Lamoureux and Rusness, 1986).

Greenhouse or growth-chamber toxicity tests on individual plant species are often used as bioassays to detect pesticides residues in soil or to assay herbicide toxicity on crop plants, but these tests can be applied to all other studies of pesticide–plant interactions. The tests are simple, rapid, and highly standardized with regard to number of plants per dose of pesticide, stage of plant development, dose range and number of repetitions, conditions of plant cultivation, positive and negative controls, and handling of data.

Principally, they follow techniques of classical growth analysis (Evans, 1972; Cartwright, 1976), but various protocols are available for different testing purposes (Hance and McKone, 1976; Horowitz, 1976; Banki, 1978; Nyffeler *et al.*, 1982). Pesticides are applied to soil or sprayed on seedlings, and their effects are measured mostly by the wet or dry weight of either the whole plant or separate shoots, roots, and leaves. Toxic effects are usually expressed by constants like LD_{50} or ED_{50} that correspond to the pesticide concentration causing 50 per cent plant death or 50 per cent reduction in plant growth or weight compared to untreated controls (Hance and McKone, 1976).

14.2.3   PLANT TISSUE CULTURES

Plant tissue cultures are used increasingly in pesticide studies to screen new compounds, understand the mechanism(s) of pesticide action, bioassay metabolites, ensure experiments without microbial contamination, and save time and reduce costs. Cells in cultures rapidly absorb chemicals with which they come into contact, can be maintained for a long time, and have a high rate of metabolite formation; experiments can be standardized to a greater extent with cultures than with intact plants; and metabolic products are easily isolated and separated. By contrast, plant tissue culture techniques in pesticide research are useless in evaluating contributions of plant-associated microorganisms or cuticular or vascular transport-mediated phytotoxicity or in testing for the phytotoxicity of herbicides acting as photosynthetic inhibitors, unless they produce additional toxic effects independent of the main pathway. Sufficient pieces of evidence are available indicating both similarities and differences in the response of plant tissue cultures and intact plants to pesticides (Mumma and Davidonis, 1983; Swisher, 1987; Gressel, 1987). Consequently, *in vitro* test results must be validated in whole plants.

Phytotoxicity of pesticides is measured either on calluses grown on agar solidified medium or on cell suspension cultures dispersed in liquid media. The suspension cultures are more capable of being standardized and tend to produce substantial reproducibility. Various simple and standard procedures can be recommended (Mumma and Davidonis, 1983; Swisher, 1987; Langebartels and Harms, 1986). The toxicity of pesticides is estimated according to the depression of growth and vitality of cells or calluses. The simplest way is to measure the wet weight of calluses, packed volume of cell suspensions (determined after centrifugation in graduated tubes), or their settled volume (in nephelometric flasks). Commonly used methods include the determination of dry weight of cell suspension, measurement of cell number, optical density in sonicated cell suspension, electrical conductivity, permeability of fluorescein, reduction of triphenyltetrazolium chloride, and incorporation of ^{14}C-leucine into proteins (Langebartels and Harms, 1986; Gressel, 1987; Swisher, 1987).

14.3 DETECTING GENOTOXIC EFFECTS OF PESTICIDES IN PLANTS

Genetic changes induced by pesticides, their metabolites, and residues are expressed by various endpoints, which include:

1. Structural changes in chromosomes and chromatids, called chromosomal aberrations (breaks, deletions, inversions, gaps, translocations, rings) and other disturbances (stickiness, clumping, erosion)
2. Disturbances in the mitotic or meiotic division, like spindle inactivation, causing so-called c-mitosis, non-disjunction, and other irregularities in the chromosome distribution during anaphase, resulting in polyploid or aneuploid cells
3. Recombinational events like somatic crossing over and sister chromatid exchanges

4. Sterility and embryonic lethality
5. Mutations in somatic tissues expressed as sectors on leaves and flowers
6. Mutation in generative cells expressed either on pollen grains (in haplophase) or in sexual progeny.

To determine these endpoints, a number of plant assays have been developed, based mostly on laboratory application with test compounds, followed by cultivation of plants or their parts (roots) in the laboratory, greenhouse or field. Only a few of them are suitable or have been adapted for testing genetic effects of pesticides *in situ*, under conditions of their utilization in agriculture, horticulture and forestry, or to assess exposures in natural plant communities (Grant, 1982a; Plewa, 1985; Ma and Harris, 1985). In addition, several plant assay systems frequently used for monitoring genotoxic substance in the air and water as a part of assessing risks to humans (Grant and Zura, 1982; Constantin, 1982) have been employed occasionally to test pesticides. As pointed out by Grant (1982a), over 230 plant species have been used in various studies on mutagenesis; however, only a limited number of plant assays are available for routine screening for genotoxicity of pesticides.

14.3.1 CYTOGENETIC ASSAYS

Assays for detection of chromosome aberrations in plants are some of the oldest, simplest, most reliable, and least expensive methods in the field of environmental mutagenesis. Cytogenetic abnormalities can be detected in mitotic and meiotic divisions. Analyses of somatic chromosome aberrations are carried out in cells of growing root tips, stem apexes, or in pollen tubes, whereas studies of meiosis are carried out with pollen mother cells (PMC). Most advantageous for cytogenetic analysis are the species having small numbers of morphologically distinguishable chromosomes that can be viewed microscopically by staining and preparation of squashed slides from soft meristematic tissues. These conditions are met in root tips of the broad bean *Vicia faba* (Kihlman and Anderson, 1984), onion *Allium cepa* (Grant, 1982b), hawks beard *Crepis capillaris, pea* Pisum sativum, in root tips and PMC of barley *Hordeum vulgare*, corn *Zea mays*, and spiderwort *Tradescantia* (Grant *et al.*, 1981; Ma, 1982). This is the reason why these organisms have been used to test for clastogenicity of environmental mutagens, including pesticides. Techniques for staining and slide preparation are so universally known and relatively simple that many other species, including crop and wild plants, may be screened for cytogenetic changes induced by pesticides *in situ* or under laboratory conditions.

Two groups of cytogenetic tests are used in plants:

1. Laboratory assays. These are characterized by a short-term (1-24 h) application of test pesticides on seeds or root tips, often at higher doses than used in agriculture, horticulture, or forestry. The evaluation of

chromosomal structural changes is performed during the first cell cycle after pesticide application. Mostly *Vicia faba*, *Allium cepa*, and barley root tips or seeds are used for this assay.

2. *In situ* assays. They enable application of pesticides under conditions and stage of plant development similar to that in agricultural practice. Experiments of this type can be carried out under field conditions using plants of a single species (mostly barley, corn, *Vicia faba*) or multiple species forming the components of natural plant communities.

Experiments of this type have been carried out by Tomkins and Grant (1974, 1976; Grant and Zura, 1982), who analysed 12 different species among 50 detected in experimental plots on roadsides close to agricultural fields. Plants in these plots were sprayed with selected herbicides (picloram, simazine, and diurone) at doses used in agriculture, and their cytogenetic effects were determined in somatic and meiotic cells of flower buds collected at different sampling periods. The researchers observed a significant but differential increase in the frequency of aberrant cells in various species, the highest being in the mid-season of spraying (June and July) and the lowest in the off-season.

Two other types of rapid and efficient assays in plants do not detect the cytogenetic damage itself, but rather its consequences: formation of micronuclei, and pollen abortion of sterility and lowered seed setting.

The micronucleus test in *Tradescantia* is based on the fact that this organism's chromosomes in early meiotic prophase are extremely prone to breakage; and, subsequently, acentric fragments lead to formation of micronuclei in the tetrade stage of pollen development. Ma (1982) has developed a sensitive assay for scoring micronuclei in flower bud cells after exposition of inflorescences to gaseous or liquid forms of environmental pollutants. The assay is very rapid, because the number of micronuclei can be determined 24–30 h after the action of the tested compound. A special vegetatively propagated clone of *Tradescantia paludosa*, recommended for the assay, can be transferred to the exposed area either as cuttings or as plants in pots. This assay has been applied also for fumigants and several pesticides in the liquid form (Ma *et al.*, 1984).

Reduced pollen fertility and seed setting are assumed to be consequences of chromosome aberrations induced in the meiotic stage. Indeed, pesticides that induce chromosome aberrations in meiosis also reduce pollen viability (Grant, 1982a).

The pollen sterility assay can be explored for studies in natural plant communities. This kind of research may follow the protocol described by Kurinnyj (1983), based on random sampling of flowers of various species in areas exposed to pesticides and detection of pollen viability by acetocarmine squash technique or by fluorescence techniques.

Several test systems in plants are suitable for detection of gene mutations either in many (multiple loci systems) or in one or two specific gene markers (specific locus systems). Mutations are expressed as hereditary changes in the phenotypes observed in haplophase (pollen grains), in somatic tissues of the exposed plants or in the sexual progeny of exposed plants (where mutations of a recessive character are induced in the germ cells of self-pollinated plants).

14.3.2   ASSAYS FOR DETECTION OF GENE MUTATIONS

Multiple-loci system tests are very sensitive, because a variety of genetic events in a large number of loci are measured. In the most frequently used systems (i.e., in barley and *Arabidopsis thaliana*), based on determination of chlorophyll and/or embryonic recessive lethals, 700–800 loci are involved (Nilan, 1978). The multilocus system tests in plants are comparable to the *Drosophila* mutation assay, and are considered to be more relevant than specific-locus system tests for prediction of mutagenic response in people. Both in barley and in *Arabidopsis thaliana*, test compounds are usually applied in liquid form on seeds, and the mutations are evaluated after self-pollination and formation of seeds in plants grown in the greenhouse or in the field. Whereas in barley chlorophyll-deficient mutants are recognized at seedling stage in *Arabidopsis* they can be detected on unripe seeds in the siliquae (Grant *et al.*, 1981; Redei *et al.*, 1984). The *Arabidopsis* assay is much less time- and space-consuming, and cheaper than the barley assay. In both systems, a large number of mutagenic compounds, including pesticides, have been screened (Grant, 1982a; Redei, 1982); but seldom *in situ*. A similar protocol to the barley assay is used principally to detect chlorophyll-deficient mutants in wheat, rice, oats, pea, and tomato (Nilan, 1978).

Much more experience in the *in situ* monitoring of pesticides is available with the waxy specific locus system in corn (Plewa, 1985). The assay is based on the detection of mutations in the 'waxy' character of pollen grains. In brief, the starch of pollen grains having the dominant wild-type allele *Wx* consists of a mixture of amylose and amylopectine, and it stains bluish-black with iodine. Mutation from dominant to recessive (*wx*) allele leads to the loss of amylose, and the pollen grain stains red. Since over 10^6 pollen grains per treatment group can be scored by a rather simple technique in a short time, this genetic analysis has a statistical power comparable to that obtained in the microbial mutagenesis assays. In the *in situ* experiments, Plewa *et al.* (1984) evaluated the genotoxic activity of pesticides in field plots (2×0.5 m or 10×3 m) situated randomly within the corn field. Insecticides and herbicides were applied in their field grade formulation at doses similar to that recommended for the control of pests and weed (Grant *et al.*, 1981; Plewa, 1985). The waxy system is not specific to corn only, and similar assays have been explored in barley and other species (Nilan *et al.*, 1981).

Mutations in haploid pollen grains can be explored for the estimation of induced changes in the gene Adh^+ coding for alcohol dehydrogenase. Grains of corn having Adh^- mutations stain yellow, whereas Adh^+ stains blue (Schwartz, 1981).

Another group of specific locus mutation assays in plants, used occasionally to test the genotoxicity of pesticides, is based on specially constructed tester strains, or clones, that are heterozygotic in one or two loci. This enables the manifestation of somatic mutations shortly after the application of a test compound. Somatic mutations are expressed as sectors of differently coloured tissues on leaves (soybean, tobacco, clover, corn) or on flower petals and stamen hairs (*Tradescantia*). The stamen hair assay in *Tradescantia* interspecific hybrids is one of the most sensitive laboratory tests; it has also been used for *in situ* monitoring of gaseous air pollutants, giving the results 2–3 weeks after the exposure of flower buds (Schairer et al., 1981). The test has been explored also for fumigants (e.g., 1,2-dibromoethane) and pesticides in liquid form (e.g., maleic hydrazide) (Gichner et al., 1982; Veleminsky and Gichner, 1988). The tobacco assay, based on the detection of green and white sectors on yellow-green leaves, seems to be very suitable for testing pesticides (e.g., maleic hydrazide) in the soil (Briza et al., 1984). This assay, as well as the soybean assay (Vig, 1975), detects not only reversion or forward mutations, but also somatic recombinations. A tester strain of perennial white clover, with the leaf-colour marker gene, could be a good indicator for long-term monitoring *in situ* (Nilan, 1978), but has never been used for this purpose.

14.3.3 DETECTION OF GENOTOXIC METABOLITES FORMED IN PLANTS FROM PESTICIDES

Formation of mutagenic metabolites from xenobiotics is a well-known phenomenon in animals (Bartsch et al., 1982). Such a mechanism was not considered in plants until it was found to occur in corn sprayed with atrazine and in barley treated with sodium azide. Stable metabolites were isolated, and they caused mutations in microbial tester strains (Plewa and Gentile, 1976; Owais and Kleinhofs, 1988). These observations stimulated research to find suitable and efficient methods to detect mutagenic metabolites in plants formed from environmental compounds including pesticides. Recently, the state of the art in this field has been summarized by Plewa et al. (1988).

There are at least three ways to detect the metabolic activation of pesticides into mutagenic products in plants (Gentile et al., 1986; Veleminsky and Gichner, 1988):

1. Exposure of plants or plant-cell cultures to pesticides and testing for mutagenic activity of plant extracts in any mutagenicity assay like *Salmonella*, yeast, or human and rodent cell assay. If extracts from pesticide-treated plants increase the mutagenicity and extracts from unexposed plants are non-mutagenic, the plant genotoxic product can be further purified and characterized. For atrazine's mutagenic metabolite in corn, this can be done by centrifugal

fractionation, gel permeation on Sephadex, and HPCL chromatography (Means *et al.*, 1988), whereas for azidoalanin (a mutagenic product of sodium azide in barley), purification and identification are performed by other procedures (Owais and Kleinhofs, 1988).

2. Preparation of extracts from untreated plants that retain enzyme activities and their co-incubation with pesticides of interest and with an indicator organism (e.g., bacteria, yeasts, or animals cells). The activation of the pesticide to the mutagenic product mediated by plant enzymes is scored according to the frequency of mutations in the indicator organism. This system has been used successfully by numerous laboratories for pesticide studies to detect the formation of mutagenic metabolites from captan, diquat, maleic hydrazide, triallate, and ziram (Rasquinha *et al.*, 1988).

3. Co-incubation of cultured plant cells (instead of plant extract) with the pesticide and with the indicator strain for mutagenicity. This system overcomes many differences associated with the preparation of plant extracts and maintenance of their enzymatic activity (Plewa *et al.*, 1988).

14.4   CONCLUSIONS

This chapter deals mostly with the biological assays that are, or might be, used for detection of toxic, principally genotoxic, effects of pesticides in plants. Compared to chemical and biochemical methods, these assays are simple, inexpensive, less laborious, and able to detect toxicity without the researcher's knowing or understanding the steps that produce the ultimate effect(s). This observation does not imply that chemical and biochemical methods are less important or less used than bioassays. Attempts have been made to detect metabolites that may be formed, and residues and impurities that may remain or that may accumulate in plants used either as human food or as animal feed and forage. In general, experimental strategies and chemical or biochemical methods of extraction, clean-up, and quantitative and qualitative determinations are the same for plants as for animals. Radioactively labelled pesticides, combined with thin-layer and high-performance liquid chromatography or gas chromatogaphy have contributed substantially to great progress in the residue and metabolite analysis in plants (Klein and Scheunert, 1982; Lord, 1982; Shimabukuro *et al.*, 1978; Mumma and Davidonis, 1983; Lamoureux and Rusness, 1986).

Crops and wild plants are some of the most frequent recipients of pesticides among biota. Different species and forms (varieties, cultivars) respond differently to different pesticides in terms of their uptake, translocation, degradation or activation, and accumulation of residues and metabolites, the consequence of which is differential toxicity, including genotoxicity. Nevertheless, such data on plants are generally not taken into account in the assessment of the environmental hazard of pesticides (Hardy, 1982; Costa *et al.*, 1987).

14.5 REFERENCES

Banki, L. (1978) *Bioassay of Pesticides in the Laboratory*, Akademiai Kiado, Budapest.

Bartsch, H., Kuroki, T., Roberfroid, M. and Malaveille, C. (1982) Metabolic activation systems *in vitro* for carcinogen/mutagen screening tests. In: DeSerres, F. J. and Hollaender, A. (Eds) *Chemical Mutagens*, Plenum Press, New York, London, pp. 95–161.

Briza, J., Gichner, T. and Veleminsky, J. (1984) Somatic mutations in tobacco plants after chronic exposure to maleic hydrazide and its diethanolamine and potassium salts. *Mutat. Res.* **139**, 25–28.

Brown, T. (1992) Chapter 15 in this volume.

Campbell, T. A., Gentner, W. A. and Danielson, L. L. (1981) Evaluation of herbicide interactions using linear regression modeling. *Weed Sci* **29**, 378–381.

Cartwright, P. M. (1976) General growth responses of plants. In: Audus, L. J. (Ed.) *Herbicides, Physiology, Biochemistry, Ecology, Vol. 1*, Academic Press, London, New York, San Francisco, pp. 55–82.

Chancellor, R. J. (1979) The long-term effects of herbicides on weed populations. *Ann. Appl. Biol.* **91**, 125–146.

Cole, D. J. (1983) The effects of environmental factors on the metabolism of herbicides in plants. *Aspects Appl. Biol.* **4**, 245–252.

Cole, H., Mackenzie, D., Smith, C. B. and Bergman, E. L. (1968) Influence of various persistent chlorinated insecticides on the macro and micro element constituents of *Zea mays* and *Phaseolus vulgaris* growing in soil containing various amounts of these materials. *Bull. Environ. Contam. Toxicol.* **3**, 141–153.

Constantin, M. J. (1982) Plant genetic systems with potential for the detection of atmospheric mutagens. In: Tice, R. R., Costa, D. L. and Schaich, K. M. (Eds) *Genotoxic Effects of Airborne Agents*, Plenum Press, New York, London, pp. 159–177.

Costa, L. G., Galli, C. L. and Murphy, S. D. (Eds) (1987) *Toxicology of Pesticides: Experimental, Clinical and Regulatory Perspectives*, NATO ASI Series Vol. H 13, Springer-Verlag, Berlin, Heidelberg, 320pp.

Crosby, D. G. (1982) Pesticides as environmental mutagens. In: Fleck, R. A. and Hollaender, A. (Eds) *Genetic Toxicology: An Agricultural Perspective*, Plenum Press, New York, London, pp. 201–218.

Evans, G. C. (1972) *The Quantitative Analysis of Plant Growth*, Blackwell Scientific Studies in Ecology, University of California Press, Berkeley, 734pp.

Frans, R., Corbin, B., Johnson, D. and McClelland, M. (1988) *Herbicide Field Evaluation Trials on Field Crops, 1987*, Arkansas Agricultural Experiment Station Res. Series Report No. 365, University of Arkansas, Little Rock, 80pp.

Gentile, S. M., Gentile, G. J. and Plewa, M. J. (1986) *In vitro* activation of chemicals by plants: a comparison of techniques. *Mutat. Res.* **164**, 53–58.

Gichner, T., Veleminsky, J. and Pokorny, V. (1982) Somatic mutations induced by maleic hydrazide and its potassium and diethanolamine salts in the *Tradescantia* mutation assay. *Mutat. Res.* **103**, 289–293.

Grant, W. F. (1972) Pesticides—subtle promoters of evolution. IV Symposium Biol. Hung. **12**, 43–50. Hungarian Academy of Sciences, Budapest.

Grant, W. F. (1982a) Cytogenetic studies of agricultural chemicals in plants. In: Fleck, R. A. and Hollaender, E. (Eds) *Genetic Toxicology. An Agricultural Perspective*, Plenum Press, New York, London, pp. 353–378.

Grant, W. F. (1982b) Chromosome aberrations assays in *Allium*. *Mutat. Res.* **99**, 273–291.

Grant, W. F., Zinoveva-Stahevitch, A. E. and Zura, K. D. (1981) Plant genetic test systems for the detection of chemical mutagens. In: Stich, H. F. and San, R. H. C.

(Eds) *Short-Term Tests for Chemical Carcinogens*, Springer-Verlag, New York, Heidelberg, Berlin, pp. 200–216.

Grant, W. F. and Zura, K. D. (1982) Plants as sensitive *in situ* detectors of atmospheric mutagens. In: Heddle, J. A. (Ed.) *Mutagenicity: New Horizons in Genetic Toxicology*, Academic Press, New York, pp. 407–434.

Gressel, J. (1987) *In vitro* plant cultures for herbicide prescreening. In: LeBaron, H. M., Mumma, R. O., Honeycutt, R. C. and Duesing, J. H. (Eds) *Biotechnology in Agricultural Chemistry*, American Chemistry Society, Washington DC, pp. 41–52.

Hance, R. J. and McKone, C. E. (1976) The determination of herbicides. In: Audus, L. J. (Ed.) *Herbicides, Physiology, Biochemistry, Ecology. Vol. 2*, Academic Press, London, New York, San Francisco, pp. 393–446.

Hardy, A. R. (1982) Ecotoxicology of pesticides: the laboratory and field evaluation of the environmental hazard presented by new pesticides. In: Costa, L. G., Galli, C. L. and Murphy, S. D. (Eds) *Toxicology of Pesticides: Experimental, Clinical and Regulatory Perspectives*, NATO ASI Series Vol. H 13, Springer-Verlag, Berlin, Heidelberg, pp. 185–196.

Horowitz, M. (1976) Application of bioassay techniques to herbicide investigations. *Weed Res.* **16**, 209–215.

Hume, L. (1987) Long-term effects of 2,4-D application on plants. I. Effects on the weed community in a wheat crop. *Can. J. Bot.* **65**, 2530–2536.

Kihlman, B. A. and Anderson, H. C. (1984) Root tips of *Vicia faba* for the study of the induction of chromosomal aberrations and sister chromatid exchanges. In: Kilbey, B. J., Legator, M., Nichols, W. and Ramel, C. (Eds) *Handbook of Mutagenicity Test Procedures*, Elsevier, Amsterdam, New York, Oxford, pp. 531–554.

Klein, W. and Scheunert, I. (1982) Bound pesticide residues in soil, plants and foot with particular emphasis on the application of nuclear techniques. In: *Agrochemicals: Fate in Food and the Environment*, IAEA Proceedings Series, International Atomic Energy Agency, Vienna, pp. 177–205.

Kurinnyj, A. I. (1983) Indication of environmental pollution by mutagenic pesticides according to their gametocidic action on plants. *Tsitol. Genet.* **4**, 32–35 (in Russian).

Lamoureux, G. L. and Rusness, D. G. (1986) Xenobiotic conjugation in higher plants. In; Paulson, G. D., Caldwell, J., Hutson, D. H. and Menn, J. J. (Eds) *Xenobiotic Conjugation Chemistry*, ACS Symposium, Vol. 299, American Chemical Society, Washington DC, pp. 62–107.

Langebartels, C. and Harms, H. (1986) Plant cell suspension cultures as test system for an ecological evaluation of chemicals. Growth inhibition effects and comparison with the metabolic fate in intact plants. *Angew. Botanik* **60**, 113–123.

Lord, K. A. (1982) Metabolism of pesticides in plants. In: *Agrochemicals: Fate in Food and the Environment*, IAEA Symposium Series, International Atomic Energy Agency, Vienna, pp. 213–222.

Ma, T. H. (1982) *Tradescantia* cytogenetic tests (root-tip mitosis, pollen mitosis, pollen mother cell meiosis): a report of the US Environmental Protection Agency Gene-Tox Program. *Mutat. Res.* **99**, 293–302.

Ma, T. H. and Harris, M. M. (1985) *In situ* monitoring of environmental mutagens. In: Saxena, J. (Ed.) *Hazard Assessment of Chemicals. Vol. 4*, Academic Press, New York, pp. 77–106.

Ma, T. H., Harris, M. M., Anderson, V. A., Ahmed, I., Mohammad, K., Bare, J. L. and Lin, H. (1984) *Tradescantia* micronucleus (Trad-MCN) tests on 140 health-related agents. *Mutat. Res.* **138**, 157–167.

Mani, M. and Jayraj, S. (1976) Biochemical investigations on the resurgence of rice blue leaf hopper *Zygina maculifrons* (Motch.). *Indian J. Exp. Biol.* **14**, 636–637.

Means, J. C., Plewa, M. J. and Gentile, J. M. (1988) Assessment of the mutagenicity of fractions from s-triazine-treated *Zea mays*. *Mutat. Res.* **197**, 325–336.

Mumma, R. O. and Davidonis, G. H. (1983) Plant tissue culture and pesticide metabolism. In: Hutson, D. H. and Roberts, T. R. (Eds) *Progress in Pesticide Biochemistry and Toxicology*, Wiley, Chichester, pp. 255–278.

Nilan, R. A. (1978) Potential of plant genetic systems for monitoring and screening mutagens. *Environ. Health Perspect.* **27**, 181–196.

Nilan, R. A., Rosichan, J. L., Arenaz, P., Hodgdon, A. L. and Kleinhofs, A. (1981) Pollen genetic markers for detection of mutagens in the environment. *Environ. Health Perspect.* **37**, 19–25.

Nyffeler, A., Gerber, H. R., Hurle, K., Testermer, W. and Schmidt, R. R. (1982) Collaborative studies of dose–response curves obtained with different bioassay methods for soil-applied herbicides. *Weed Res.* **22**, 213–222.

Oka, I. N. and Pimentel, D. (1974) Corn susceptibility to corn leaf aphids and common corn smut after herbicide treatment. *Environ. Entomol.* **2**(6), 911–915.

Owais, W. M. and Kleinhofs, A. (1988) Metabolic activation of the mutagen azide in biological systems. *Mutat. Res.* **197**, 313–323.

Pimentel, D. (1971) *Ecological Effects of Pesticides on Non-Target Species*, Executive Office of the President, Office of Science and Technology, Washington DC, 220pp.

Pimentel, D. and Edwards, C. A. (1982) Pesticides and ecosystems. *BioScience* **32**, 595–600.

Plewa, M. J. (1985). Plant genetic assays and their use in studies on environmental mutagenesis in developing countries. In: Muhammed, A. and Von Borstel, R. C. (Eds) *Basic and Applied Mutagenesis*, Plenum, New York, London, pp. 249–268.

Plewa, M. J. and Gentile, J. M. (1976) Mutagenicity of atrazine: A maize-microbe bioassay. *Mutat. Res.* **38**, 287–292.

Plewa, M. J., Wagner, E. D., Gentile, J. J. and Gentile, J. M. (1984) An evaluation of the genotoxic properties of herbicides following plant and animal activation. *Mutat. Res.* **136**, 223–245.

Plewa, M. J., Wagner, E. D. and Gentile, J. M. (1988) The plant cell/microbe coincubation assay for the analysis of plant-activated promutagens. *Mutat. Res.* **197**, 207–219.

Rasquinha, I. A., Woldeman, A. G. and Nazar, R. M. (1988) Studies on the use of plant extracts in assessing the effects of plant metabolism on the mutagenicity and toxicity of pesticides. *Mutat. Res.* **197**, 261–272.

Redei, G. P. (1982). Mutagen assay with *Arabidopsis*: a report of the US Environmental Protection Agency Gene-Tox Program. *Mutat. Res.* **99**, 243–255.

Redei, G. P., Acedo, G. N. and Sandhu, S. S. (1984) Mutation induction and detection in *Arabidopsis*. In: Chu, E. H. Y. and Generoso, W. M. (Eds) *Mutation, Cancer, and Malformation*, Plenum Press, New York, London, pp. 285–314.

Ries, S. K. and Wert, V. (1972) Simazine-induced nitrate absorption related to plant protein content. *Weed Sci.* **20**, 569–572.

Rouchaud, J., Moons, C. and Meyer, J. A. (1983) Effects of selected insecticides and herbicides on free sugar contents of carrots. *J. Agric. Food Chem.* **31**, 206–210.

Schairer, L. A., Santkulis, R. C. and Tempel, N. R. (1981) Monitoring ambient air for mutagenicity using the higher plant *Tradescantia*. In: Tice, R. C., Costa, D. L., and Scheich, K. M. (Eds) *Genotoxic Effects of Airborne Agents*, Plenum Press, New York, pp. 123–140.

Schwartz, D. (1981) *Adh* locus in maize for detection of mutagens in the environment. *Environ. Health Perspect.* **37**, 75–77.

Shimabukuro, R. H., Lamoureux, G. L. and Frear, D. S. (1978) Glutathione conjugation: a mechanism for herbicide detoxication and selectivity in plants. In: Pallos, F. M.

and Casida, J. E. (Eds) *Chemistry and Action of Herbicide Antidotes*, Academic Press, New York, pp. 133–149.

Swisher, B. A. (1987) Use of plant cell cultures in pesticide metabolism studies. In: LeBaron, H. M., Mumma, R. O., Honeycutt, R. C. and Duesing, J. H. (Eds) *Biotechnology in Agricultural Chemistry*, American Chemical Society, Washington DC, pp. 18–40.

Thakre, S. K. and Saxena, S. N. (1972) Effect of soil application of chlorinated insecticides on amino acid composition of maize (*Zea mays*). *Plant Soil* **37**, 415–418.

Tomkins, D. J. and Grant, W. F. (1974). Differential response of 14 weed species to seven herbicides in two plant communities. *Can. J. Bot.* **52**, 525–533.

Tomkins, D. J. and Grant, W. F. (1976) Monitoring natural vegetation for herbicide-induced chromosomal aberration. *Mutat. Res.* **36**, 73–84.

Veleminsky, J. and Gichner, T. (1988) Mutagenic activity of promutagens in plants: indirect evidence of their activation. *Mutat. Res.* **197**, 221–242.

Vig, B. K. (1975) Soybean (*Glycine max.*): a new test system for study of genetic parameters as effected by environmental mutagens. *Mutat. Res.* **31**, 49–56.

Ware, G. W., Cahill, W. P., Gerhardt, P. D. and Witt, J. M. (1970) Pesticides drift IV: on-target deposits from aerial application of insecticides. *J. Econ. Entomol.* **63**, 1982–1983.

Way, J. M., and Chancellor, R. J. (Ed.) (1976) *Herbicides, Physiology, Biochemistry, Ecology, Vol. 2*, Academic Press, London, New York, San Francisco, pp. 345–372.

15 Methods to Evaluate Adverse Consequences of Genetic Changes Caused by Pesticides

T. BROWN

Clemson University, Department of Entomology, South Carolina, USA

15.1 INTRODUCTION

What are the genetic changes that result from the use of pesticides? In populations of many pests and some non-target organisms exposed to lethal doses of insecticides, resistance has developed, so that rare genes conferring decreased susceptibility to a pesticide become common genes in the population, due to selection. In many cases, susceptibility becomes very rare after many years of selection against it, so that even in the absence of the pesticides, resistance often remains in the population for many generations. This phenomenon is genetic change on the population level. Although certain pesticides are known to be mutagenic, it is unknown whether the rare alleles for resistance in the field have been produced through mutation caused by any pesticide.

Resistance in pests is generally an adverse consequence of pesticide use, and it has resulted in the loss of many formerly efficacious pesticides; however, in some cases resistance can be viewed as having benefit. In non-target organisms, resistance can be beneficial, as in resistant predatory mites, which have been exploited for their biological control ability in the presence of pesticides in orchards. Herbicide resistance genes found in weeds can be genetically engineered into crops that were formerly intolerant, so that the range of crops for which a particular herbicide is useful can be expanded. Resistance is a major factor reducing DDT use, which has been beneficial to certain species of wildlife. The recognition and anticipation of resistance serves as a stimulation for the discovery of more diverse pesticide chemicals.

The serious threat is that the development of new pesticide chemicals and the discovery of new targets in the pests might not keep pace with the evolution

Methods to Assess Adverse Effects of Pesticides on Non-target Organisms
Edited by R. G. Tardiff
©1992 SCOPE Published by John Wiley & Sons Ltd

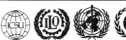

of resistance. While there are approximately 2000 active pesticide ingredients, they act upon only about 25 physiological target sites, most of which have been relied upon for many years. Uncontrollable pests will be of great consequence in agriculture and in public health. The objectives of this chapter are to review the status of resistance, to discuss the ways in which it develops, and to consider methods for assessing the hazards of resistance in the laboratory and in the field.

Certain pesticides are mutagenic (Klopman *et al.*, 1985); therefore, they could possibly cause change to the genetic code directly without lethality or population selection. These mutagenic changes may be heritable under certain circumstances, and they may be very difficult to detect. Mutagenicity of pesticides is of great concern, since the widespread use of pesticides in agriculture, in household pest control, and in public health leads to human and animal exposures on several levels, including residual amounts on agricultural products (for which legal tolerances have been established). The mutagenetic risk of pesticides is difficult to estimate, since mutagenic effects are often observed in the laboratory at concentrations much greater than those to which the public is exposed. The emphasis of this chapter is on resistance as a consequence of pesticide use. Mutagenicity is considered herein only as it relates to understanding the genesis of resistance genes.

15.2 STATUS OF PESTICIDE RESISTANCE

Resistance to pesticides has been established as a capability of a wide variety of pest species (Georghiou and Saito, 1983; Georghiou, 1986). Resistance has had the greatest impact on insecticides and acaricides (Brattsten *et al.*, 1986), but it is gaining in importance as more critical situations are detected for fungicides (Georgopoulos, 1986; Köller and Scheinpflug, 1987), herbicides (LeBaron and Gressel 1982; LeBaron and McFarland, 1990) and rodenticides (MacNicoll, 1986).

15.2.1 INSECTICIDES AND ACARICIDES

Resistance in arthropods is already a serious practical problem with major impact on public health and agricultural pest control. Over 490 species of arthropods are resistant (Georghiou, 1986), and this includes most of the major pests of agriculture and public health. In the last decade, there has been an alarming increase in resistance to organophosphorus, carbamate, and pyrethroid insecticides, so that many pests have developed resistance to multiple major classes of insecticides. The registration and use of insecticides of greater intrinsic toxicity has been a consequence of, and not a solution to, this problem. Approximately 50 species have resistance to photostable pyrethroid insecticides, which were marketed just 10 years ago (Brown, 1982; Georghiou, 1986). The

Table 15.1. Arthropod pests in which resistance has led to serious difficulty in control in many areas (adapted from Voss, 1987)

Order	Species	Common name
Acarina	*Amblyomma* spp.	Ticks
	Boophilus spp.	Cattle ticks
	Panonychus citri	Citrus red mite
	Panonychus ulmi	European red mite
	Rhipicephalus spp.	Ticks
	Tetranychus spp.	Spider mites
Anoplura	*Pediculus capitis*	Head louse
Coleoptera	*Leptinotarsa decemlineata*	Colorado potato beetle*
	Oryzaephilus surinamensis	Saw-toothed grain beetle
	Sitophilus oryzae	Rice weevil
	Tribolium castaneum	Red flour beetle
Diptera	*Aedes aegypti*	Yellowfever mosquito
	Anopheles spp.	Malaria mosquitoes
	Culex quinquefasciatus	Southern house mosquito
	Haemotobia irritans	Horn fly*
	Lucilia cuprina	Sheep blow fly
	Musca domestica	House fly*
	Simulium damnosum	Black fly
	Stomoxys calcitrans	Stable fly
Homoptera	*Aonidiella aurantii*	California red scale
	Bemisia tabaci	Sweetpotato whitefly
	Myzus persicae	Peach-potato aphid*
	Nephotettix cincticeps	Green leafhopper
	Nilaparvata lugens	Brown planthopper
	Psylla pyricola	Pear psylla*
	Trialeurodes vaporariorum	Greenhouse whitefly*
Lepidoptera	*Heliothis armigera*	Cotton bollworm*
	Liriomyza spp.	Serpentine leafminers*
	Plutella xylostella	Diamondback moth*
	Sitotroga cerealella	Angoumois grain moth
	Spodoptera exigua	Beet armyworm
Orthoptera	*Blattella germanica*	German cockroach

*Has developed resistance to pyrethroid insecticides

first practical problem in the field with full documentation and surveillance data was the devlopment of fenvalerate resistance in the diamondback moth on cole crops near Taipei (Liu *et al.*, 1981, 1984).

In 1987, the pesticide manufacturing industry noted that approximately 40 species of arthropods had developed resistance that caused serious practical difficulty for their control in many areas (Table 15.1). These were referred to as Category 1 species in regard to the seriousness of resistance; it was recommended that they be studied intensively (Voss, 1987). Additionally,

Table 15.2. Resistance to 12 types of herbicides in 64 species of weeds (LeBaron and McFarland, 1990)

Weed (number of species)	Herbicide(s)
Abutilon theophrastis	Triazines
Alopecurus myosuroides	Chlortoluron, triazines
Amaranthus spp. (8)	Triazines
Ambrosia artemisiifolia	Triazines
Arctotheca calendula	Paraquat
Arenaria serpyltifolia	Triazines
Atriplex patula	Triazines
Avena fatua	Diclofopmethyl
Bidens tripartita	Triazines
Brachypodium distachyon	Triazines
Brassica campestris	Triazines
Bromus tectorum	Triazines
Chenopodium spp. (6)	Pyrazon, triazines
Daucus carota	2,4-D
Digitaria sanguinalis	Triazines
Echinochloa crusgalli	Triazines
Eleusine indica	Trifluralin
Epilobium spp. (4)	Paraquat, triazines
Erigeron spp. (3)	Paraquat, triazines
Galinsoga ciliata	Triazines
Hordeum glaucum	Paraquat
Ixophorus unisetus	Imidazolinones
Kochia scoparia	Sulphonylureas, triazines
Lactuca serriola	Sulphonylureas
Lolium spp. (3)	Diclofopmethyl, paraquat, sulphonylureas, triazines
Lophochloa phleoides	Triazines
Matricaria matricarioides	Triazines
Panicum capillare	Triazines
Phalaris paradoxa	Triazines
Physalis longifolia	Triazines
Poa annua	Aminotriazole, paraquat, triazines
Polygonum spp. (5)	Triazines
Senecio vulgaris	Triazines
Setaria spp. (3)	Triazines, trifluralin
Sicyos angulatus	Triazines
Sinapis arvensis	Triazines
Solanum nigrum	Triazines
Sphenoclea zeylanica	2,4-D
Stellaria spp. (2)	Mecoprop, triazines
Xanthium strumarium	MSMA, DSMA

33 species were listed as Category 2 species—those in which resistance is of practical consequence in some, but not many, areas; careful monitoring of them was recommended, since the potential for more serious resistance exists. It is clear that only rapid advances in pesticide resistance management will prevent the increasingly serious impact of resistance in arthropods.

15.2.2 HERBICIDES

Herbicide resistance has been observed in the field and confirmed in 64 species of weeds (Table 15.2). Although the initial cases of herbicide resistance were considered as rather isolated curiosities, the problem is intensifying in that certain species are spreading, acquiring multiple resistances, and threatening major crops (LeBaron and McFarland, 1990). Triazine resistance has evolved in 53 species of weeds; however, it is clear that other classes of herbicides are inducing resistance at an increasing rate. Trifluralin resistance in cotton-field goosegrass (*Eleusine indica*), has spread in the US from South Carolina (Mudge *et al.*, 1984) to several neighbouring states, and has shown cross-resistance to oryzalin and phosphoric amide herbicides (Vaughn *et al.*, 1987). In Australia, the annual ryegrass *Lolium rigidum* has developed resistance to dinitroaniline, sulphonylurea, and aryloxyphenoxyproprionate herbicides, so that there are no herbicides registered that control multiple resistant populations of this type in wheat (Heap and Knight, 1982, 1986; Powles, *et al.*, 1990). Black-grass (*Alopecurus myosuroides*) has shown resistance to chlortoluron, diclofopmethyl and other herbicides in the United Kingdom (Kemp *et al.*, 1990).

15.2.3 FUNGICIDES AND BACTERICIDES

Fungicide resistance has been reported in at least 90 species of pathogens (Table 15.3). There are 59 species with benomyl resistance and 22 with resistance to other benzimidazole fungicides. Resistance to other single-site inhibitors is less common, and resistance to sterol biosynthesis inhibitors of the C-14 demethylation step has been slow to develop (Locke, 1986; Köller and Scheinpflug, 1987).

Benzimidazole resistance is of practical importance; however, it is fortunate that substitute chemicals are available for the majority of cases so that the problem is not as serious as the Category 1 arthropod resistance to insecticides. Multiple resistances may be of most immediate consequence in grey mould from *Botrytis cinerea*, powdery mildews caused by *Erysiphe cichoracearum*, *E. graminis*, or *Sphaerotheca fuligenea*, peach brown rot from *Monilinia fructicola*, and apple scab due to *Venturia inaequalis*. Resistance to copper was widespread in recent surveys for plasmid-borne resistance genes in certain strains of plant pathogenic bacteria (Cooksey, 1990).

15.2.4 RODENTICIDES

Rodenticide resistance has been limited to anticoagulants, mainly warfarin. Warfarin resistance in *Rattus norvegicus* is widespread in Europe and North America (Jackson and Ashton, 1986). Warfarin resistance is also common in the house mouse (*Mus musculus*) and to a lesser extent in the roof rat (*Rattus rattus*) in the US. Fortunately, second-generation halogenated anticoagulants,

Table 15.3. Pathogens having resistance to fungicides or bactericides applied in practice (Ogawa *et al.*, 1983; Cooksey, 1990)

Pathogen	Fungicide or bactericide
Alternaria spp. (2)	Polyoxin B
Aspergillus nidulans	Benomyl, calcium succinate
Botrytis spp. (2)	Benomyl, carbendazim, dichloran, iprodione, polyoxin B, quinomethionate, quintozene, tecnazene, thiophanate methyl
Ceratocystis ulmi	Benomyl
Cercospora spp. (4)	Benomyl, fentin acetate, fentin hydroxide
Cercosporella herpotrichoides	Benomyl, carbendazim
Cercosporidium personatum	Benomyl
Cladosporium spp. (2)	Benomyl
Cochiobolus carbonum	Cadmium succinate, thiram
Colletotrichum spp. (3)	Benomyl, carbendazim, thiabendazole, thiophanate methyl
Didymella ligulicola	Benomyl
Diplodia spp.	Diphenyl
Erwinia amylovora	Streptomycin
Erysiphe spp. (2)	Benomyl, ethirimol, thiophanate methyl, hydroxypyrimidine, SBI
Erythronium spp.	Benomyl
Fulvia fulva	Benomyl
Fusarium spp. (6)	Benomyl, tecnazene, thiabendazole, thiophanate methyl, thiram
Fusicalidium effusum	Benomyl
Gilbertelia persicaria	Dichloran
Hypomyces solani	Quintozene
Monilinia spp. (3)	Benomyl, iprodione, polyram
Mycospharella fragaries	Benomyl
Neurospara crassa	Benomyl
Oidiopsis taurica	Benomyl
Oidium begoniae	Benomyl
Penicillium spp. (6)	2-Aminobutane, anilazine, benomyl, diphenyl, 2-phenylphenol, thiabendazole, thiophanate methyl
Phytophthora infestans	Metalaxyl
Plasmopara viticola	Phenylamides
Pseudocercosporella herpotrichoides	Benomyl
Pseudomonas spp. (4)	Copper, streptomycin
Pseudoperonospora cubensis	Metalaxyl
Puccinia spp. (2)	Dichlone, oxycarboxin
Pyrenophora spp. (2)	Methoxyethylmercury, organomercury
Pyricularia oryzae	S-Benzyl-O,O-diisopropyl phosphorothioate, blasticidin-S, cadmium succinate, edifenphos, isoprothiolane, kasugamycin
Rhizoctonia solani	Benomyl, quintozene, thiram
Rhizopus stolonifer	Dichloran
Sclerotinia spp. (2)	Anilazine, benomyl, cadmium, succinate, thiram

(continued)

Table 15.3. *(continued)*

Pathogen	Fungicide or bactericide
Sclerotium spp. (2)	Benomyl, dichloran, quintozene
Septoria spp. (4)	Benomyl, carbendazim, edifenphos, thiophanate methyl
Sphaerotheca spp. (3)	Benomyl, dimethirimol, dinocap, pyrazophos, quinomethionate, thiophanate methyl
Sporobolomyces roseus	Carbendazim
Tilletia foetida	Hexachlorobenzene
Uncinula necator	Benomyl
Ustilago spp. (2)	Benomyl, carboxamide
Venturia spp. (3)	Benomyl, dodine, thiophanate methyl
Verticillium spp. (4)	Benomyl
Xanthomonas spp. (3)	Copper, streptomycin

such as brodifacoum, are not subject to cross-resistance to warfarin. Cases of resistance to the newer halogenated derivatives have been reported; should this become as widespread as warfarin resistance, then rodent control would depend on a very limited supply of viable replacement chemicals.

Thus, it appears that resistance to insecticides and acaricides is the most urgent problem; but this same status could apply to herbicides, fungicides, and rodenticides in the next decade. The greatest threat is the growing number of pest species with multiple resistances, whereas the number of new chemicals appears very limited. The challenge is to find practical ways to manage pesticides so that resistance is prevented before many more species become even more difficult to control.

15.3 DEVELOPMENT OF RESISTANT POPULATIONS

Resistance is a practical problem in population genetics. It is usually considered to be a consequence of rapid Darwinian selection brought about by the lethality of the pesticide to the normal susceptible organism, resulting in the concentration of rare, innately tolerant individuals, which then pass on to their progeny the genes responsible for a resistant population. Its consequences can be found on many levels, from the loss of a farm crop to resistant fungi, weeds, or arthropods, to the environmental hazard due to increased use of pesticides to gain some control of a resistant pest, to the decline of human health due to resistant vectors of disease or resistant rodents.

The potential hazard for resistance to a pesticide is difficult to predict from experimental evidence, due to the complex array of operational factors that can influence the degree of selection in the field, and the general lack of knowledge of pest genetics; however, several general principles have been learned through experience. Resistance generally develops most rapidly against those pesticides that are persistent in the field, so that one application exerts selection pressure on an entire generation or several consecutive generations of the pest. Examples of this phenomenon are the organochlorine insecticides, such as DDT and dieldrin, to which resistance had become widespread within ten years of their introduction.

Pesticides that are ephemeral due to photolability or reactivity are slower to induce resistance. Photolabile natural pyrethrins have produced only a few cases of low-level resistance due to their use alone (Brown, 1982). Organophosphorus and carbamate pesticides, most of which are reactive with nucleophiles and only moderately persistent, were used in enormous quantities for thirty years before resistance began seriously to diminish their effectiveness (Georghiou and Saito, 1983). Resistance is more likely to develop against pesticides with a specific mode of action (i.e., a single target), and less likely against general poisons with multiple targets and actions in the pest (Köller and Scheinpflug, 1987). Resistance generally develops in proportion to the intensity of selection pressure against the pest population. The resistance problem is aggravated by reliance upon broad-spectrum pesticides, which, when sprayed to control one problem pest, also apply selection pressure for resistance in other species that are present at levels not requiring concurrent control. This type of mismanagement was recognized as a major factor in multiple antibiotic resistance, so that an important countermeasure was replacement, whenever possible, of broad-spectrum antibiotics (Skurray *et al.*, 1988).

Resistance develops as a response of the target population to the selection to which it is subjected by pesticide. It requires that one or more gene alleles that confer reduced pesticide susceptibility be present in the population at some low level, or that such an allele arise through spontaneous or induced mutation. For plant pathogens, three general cases are recognized: unavailability of appropriate mutant; one-step pattern of development due to one major gene; and multistep pattern due to accumulation of several genes (Georgopoulos and Skylakakis, 1986).

In the presence of the pesticide, the rarer resistant genotype has a tremendous fitness advantage, because the susceptible genotype will be killed. When the pesticide is removed, this artificial fitness advantage is usually lost, but few resistance genes have been systematically studied to determine whether they inflict any fitness deficit in the absence of the pesticide that would contribute to reversion to susceptibility in the population. This gap is crucial to an understanding of the development of resistance and must be considered to design counter-strategies (Keiding, 1986; Roush and McKenzie, 1987).

It is also possible, but not proven or generally considered, that pesticides that are mutagenic in the target pest might induce resistance through the mutation of a normal gene into one that confers resistance, assuming the individual in which the mutation occurs is not killed by exposure to the pesticide. In one experiment in *Drosophila*, a chemical mutagen was used to produce a resistance gene, which was then subjected to selection pressure using a non-mutagenic pesticide, methoprene (Wilson and Fabian, 1986).

It is more likely that resistance in the field begins with the genetic diversity that is often present in pests; it has also been the basis of their evolution and survival of the many natural toxicants to which they have been exposed through the ages. In this regard, mutation leading to genetic diversity becomes an advantage. The mutagenicity of a variety of naturally occurring substances has recently been reviewed (Ames, 1983; Ames et al., 1987). Whereas genetic diversity and selection have led to an evolved natural resistance to toxicants in some species, the contribution of mutation induced by natural substances to observed genetic diversity is unclear. Mutagenicity is an individual consequence of exposure to certain pesticides, but it may or may not result in heritable change; resistance is a consequence of the selection of a rare allele in a population group, and it may or may not be due to an induced mutation.

Once resistance arises in one location, it can spread outward fastest if the surrounding areas remain treated, since resistant progeny will replace the susceptible ones at the interface of the genotypes. In the US, cyclodiene resistance in corn rootworm spread from one county in Nebraska to all the surrounding states over several years (Brown, 1971). Cypermethrin resistance in the tobacco budworm was detected in 1987 in Texas, and its spread will be closely monitored through a network of surveillance (Simonet et al., 1988). DDT and organophosphorus resistances in *Heliothis* spp. were also found first in the Midsouth (Sparks, 1981).

Resistance alleles can spread through mating, through natural migration of the pest, or even through the assistance of man, as in the case of resistant strains of stored-grain beetles which apparently escape fumigation efforts in commercial grain shipping and are often detected first at seaports of entry. Resistance to benomyl fungicide was spread across Michigan golf-course greens on the spikes of golf shoes as golfers moved from one course to another. Triazine herbicide resistance apparently spread most rapidly along railroad rights of way.

A much better understanding of the dynamics of resistance in the field is needed. This effect can be achieved only by observing the population genetics of resistance. The lack of techniques for estimating frequencies of expression of individual alleles has been the limiting factor in studying this phenomenon.

Compounds exist that can produce pest resistance to other pesticides within the same chemical class and to other classes of pesticides. This response is due to the breadth of action of the selected resistance mechanism in the pest, such as development of a less sensitive target or production of an enzyme catalysing the same form for detoxication of several compounds. Pyrethroids and DDT are common victims of reduced target sensitivity, probably in the sodium ion channel of nerve (Lund and Narahashi, 1983), and can be in the same cross-resistance group when the insect of interest has this mechanism, as noted in cattle ticks (Nolan et al., 1977), house flies (Plapp and Hoyer, 1968; DeVries and Georghiou, 1980), horn flies (Byford et al., 1985), tobacco budworms (Payne, 1982) and three mosquito species (Chadwick et al., 1984; Omer et al., 1980; Priester and Georghiou, 1980). It must be recognized that the unnecessary choice of a relatively dispensable compound might jeopardize a very valuable, economical, biodegradable, or selective compound by inducing cross-resistance. An example of this mismanagement is the use of persistent pyrethroid insecticides in situations where natural pyrethrins belonging to the same resistance group are more desirable, and would otherwise have practically no chance of falling to resistance (Keiding, 1986).

Cross-resistance has been distinguished from multiple resistance, in which a pest accumulates several mechanisms each giving resistance to one or more compounds (Metcalf, 1971). Certain species have accumulated multiple resistance to each of the pesticides used against them (Table 15.1). Some species seem to have an array of mechanisms to meet any challenge. Chemical control of certain populations of many of these pests cannot be achieved at the level of previous standards. On the other hand, a few important species, such as the boll weevil and the European corn borer, seemed to lack certain resistance mechanisms, so that they retained susceptibility to azinphosmethyl and DDT, respectively (Brown, 1971).

15.4   MECHANISMS OF RESISTANCE

15.4.1   BEHAVIOURAL AND PHYSIOLOGICAL MECHANISMS

Resistance usually results from genetically controlled biochemical or physiological changes from the normal type that alter pesticide pharmacokinetics or pharmacodynamics (Oppenoorth and Welling, 1976; Plapp, 1976; Soderlund and Bloomquist, 1990). Documented cases of behavioural avoidance of the pesticide are less common, but they can lead to serious consequences (Lockwood et al., 1984). Several cases of behavioural resistance selection are known, and they include both stimulus-independent phenomena, such as exophily of mosquitoes, and stimulus-dependent cases, generally known as increased irritability. The genetic bases of behavioural resistance have not been described.

Less methoprene uptake was the result of behavioural change selection in Culex pipiens (Brown and Brown, 1980). These larvae became quiesent when disturbed and exhibited significantly reduced movement and feeding behaviour for 3 h after disturbance. This selected behaviour was independent of methoprene stimulation. Lack of feeding behaviour was shown to reduce uptake by about 25 per cent, so that this mechanism alone did not confer all of the 100-fold increase in methoprene resistance in this strain. These larvae also produced 11 per cent more of an oxidative metabolite (Brown and Hooper, 1979); however, considering the wide range of juvenile hormone mimic chemistry to which there was full cross-resistance in this otherwise highly insecticide-susceptible strain (Brown et al., 1978), it is likely that behaviour and metabolism were combined with reduced sensitivity of an undefined molecular target to produce such a high level of resistance. Pyrethroid-resistant horn flies likewise displayed the behavioural mechanism combined with target insensitivity (Sparks et al., 1985).

Horn flies with an 85-fold increase in pyrethroid resistance were highly irritated by cypermethrin and delta-methrin (but not by DDT), and they were 50 times more cross-resistant to directly applied DDT. This latter effect may have been due to nerve insensitivity combined with low level metabolic resistance indicated by synergistic activity.

Physiological mechanisms can provide resistance without behavioural avoidance of the pesticide. A pesticide must penetrate the pest and reach the target, where a molecular lesion is initiated, leading to death. Pesticide pharmacokinetics include the processes of penetration, distribution and biotransformation of the pesticide; pesticide pharmacodynamics, by contrast, describe the interactions with the target site. Resistance has been associated with pharmacokinetics, pharmacodynamics, and combinations of these sets of processes.

One of the pharmacokinetic changes possible is pesticide detoxication, often increased in resistant strains due to increased amounts or increased efficiency of detoxication enzymes: less pesticide reaches the target site. There are many types of detoxicative reactions, so that one species might have several different mechanisms of detoxication resistance.

Targets of toxicity (often enzymes, receptor proteins, or ion channels) can be altered qualitatively (e.g., to have less affinity for the pesticide), so that a greater concentration must reach the target to cause death.

Resistance can be conferred by a single mechanism, as has been observed for many genes in mosquitoes and house flies (Brown, 1971; Tsukamoto, 1983). Clear segregation of resistance was demonstrated in progeny of appropriate backcrosses. In these cases, it is easy to determine the degree of dominance of the resistance gene allele and to identify doses that discriminate among genotypes; however, it would be a gross simplification to consider resistance as usually monofactorial.

In some strains combinations of mechanisms are present, as in the Learn, New York, strain of house flies having pyrethroid resistance conferred by genes on three chromosomes (Scott and Georghiou, 1986). Development of strains in which single mechanisms are combined has demonstrated that multiple mechanisms can interact synergistically as demonstrated by the addition of the *des* detoxication gene and *pen* permeability gene in diazinon-resistant house flies (Sawicki, 1970). This condition was confirmed in other strains of house flies, in which the permeability gene was named *tin* because it gave resistance to organotin compounds (Hoyer and Plapp, 1968).

Using genetic markers and the natural recombination that occurs in backcrosses, the relative importance of the various genes can be estimated. However, for most major agricultural pests, practically nothing is known of genetic linkage, which makes such evaluation nearly impossible. Even when one factor is strong enough that segregation of resistance can be observed, there may be secondary factors involved that complicate the interpretation of results (Payne *et al.*, 1988).

Changes in protein quality or quantity that cause resistance are inherited as alleles that vary from the normal type. Although few cases of resistance have been studied at the molecular genetic level, conferral of resistance through mutation of a single codon in a structural gene has been shown to result in an insensitive target protein, which is changed by only one amino acid substitution (Hirschberg and McIntosh, 1983). For the vast majority of resistance cases, very little is known of the inheritance of the trait. For many insecticides, the trait of resistance has been mapped genetically in the house fly and in several mosquitoes; however the structural and regulatory genes for the proteins likely to be involved as biochemical mechanisms have not been mapped. Work in this area has often been complicated by the multiplicity of isozymes occurring for the various detoxifying enzymes (Agosin, 1982; Motoyama *et al.*, 1983).

15.4.2 PROTEIN PRODUCTS INVOLVED IN RESISTANCE

Enzymes catalysing pesticide biotransformation have been implicated in pesticide resistance. Detoxication of many insecticides is catalysed by monooxygenase, glutathione *S*-transferase, or carboxylester hydrolase. Detoxication is a common mechanism for resistance in insects and plants, but it is very rarely a factor in resistance to fungicides. Decreased activation has been detected as a possible mechanism of resistance to the fungicides pyrazophos (De Waard and van Nistelrooy, 1980) and triadimenol (Kalamarkis *et al.*, 1986) and to the insecticide methyl parathion (Konno *et al.*, 1989).

Target proteins with reduced sensitivity to pesticides include β-tubulin in fungi resistant to benzimidazole fungicides, leaf plastid thylakoids in weeds resistant to triazine herbicides, and acetylcholinesterase in insects resistant to organophosphate and carbamate insecticides.

Detailed biochemical analysis of proteins from resistant and susceptible strains has been accomplished rarely. In the case of a carboxylester hydrolase, E4, from the aphid *Myzus persicae*, it was found that resistance was due to a much greater quantity of a protein with the same biochemical characteristics as that found in the susceptible strain (Devonshire and Moores, 1982). This protein has carboxylester hydrolase activity; however, its action is largely due to its very high titre and the noncatalytic reaction with, or the sequestering of, organophosphorus, carbamate, and pyrethroid insecticides. It is unusual that this appears to be the only resistance mechanism available to this aphid, while most insects have many possible mechanisms.

15.4.3 GENETIC MECHANISMS CONFERRING RESISTANCE

Increased detoxication enzyme activity can be the result of genetic changes at any of several levels. The quantity of protein with unchanged structure can be increased by: gene duplication or amplification, in which a pest acquires multiple copies of the same gene; increased gene transcription, which may result from a mutation of a regulatory sequence; or increased translation due to mutation in the processing rate of mRNA. Altered quality of protein (e.g., changed catalytic centre activity) can result either from changes in the structural gene coding protein sequence or from processing or regulatory gene changes. Similar alterations are possible for target proteins, which might have their affinity for the pesticide or their number reduced to provide a lower sensitivity.

Amplification of the carboxylester hydrolase gene responsible for 250 times the normal number of gene copies has been found to be a genetic mechanism of resistance to organophosphurus insecticides in mosquitoes (Mouches et al., 1986). Biochemically, this protein appears to resemble the E4 sequestering protein with carboxylester hydrolase activity in aphids which is also increased through gene amplification (Field et al., 1988); however, in mosquitoes, other mechanisms are also present, such as target insensitivity (Raymond et al., 1985).

The genetic basis has not been identified for a large number of species that have devloped increased detoxication rates through distinctly catalytic processes, such as those mediated by the microsomal monooxygenases. A report of the first cloning of the cytochrome P_{450} gene from an insect species suggest that resistant house flies have more constitutive transcription of this monooxygenase than their susceptible counterparts (Feyereisen et al., 1989). The sequence of the gene has been reported only for the resistant strain. The gene sequence for coding the haeme binding site of the house fly is similar to that of known, primarily mammalian, genetic codes; however, the overall sequence is sufficiently dissimilar from that of other species to be designated a new gene family for this species.

Resistance to the herbicide glyphosate can be genetically engineered into crops either by a gene for increased detoxication or by a gene for target site insensitivity. Experimental resistance to sulphonylurea herbicides is easily conferred by many nucleotide substitutions for several bases in the gene for the target enzyme acetolactate synthase (Yadav et al., 1986).

Perhaps the best studied gene encodes the target protein for triazine herbicides. In this case, a single amino acid substitution in the active site produces resistance that is maternally inherited, since the gene is a constituent of the chloroplast DNA and not the nuclear genome (Hirschberg and McIntosh, 1983).

Fungicide resistance to benzamidazoles has recently been studied at the level of the gene sequence for the target protein, which in this case is β-tubulin (Fujimura et al., 1990). In Neurospora crassa, as occurs in strain F914, benomyl resistance can be accompanied by hypersusceptibility to the N-phenylcarbamate fungicide, diethylfencarb. It was hypothesized that this negatively correlated cross-resistance would always result from benomyl selection, so that benomyl susceptibility would be restored by subsequent selection with diethylfencarb; however, that hypothesis is less likely to be correct, since other strains such as B511 are resistant to benomyl but are no more susceptible to diethylfencarb than wild-type strains. Single amino acid substitutions in β-tubulin that serve as a basis of these resistances are as follows: amino acid 198 is changed from glutamic acid to glycine in strain F914, making this strain benomyl-resistant but simultaneously very susceptible to diethylfencarb; if, instead, there is substitution of tyrosine for phenylalanine at position 167, then benomyl resistance is produced without the increased susceptibility to diethylfencarb.

15.5 METHODS TO ASSESS THE PROBABILITY OF RESISTANCE

Experimental selection for resistance in the laboratory provides some knowledge of the potential development of resistance to a given pesticide by a pest (Brown and Payne, 1988). The rapid and high-level development of resistance may indicate the presence of genes for resistance in this species; however, because of the genetically limited sample available in the laboratory, failure to develop resistance cannot be interpreted as a lack of its potential for expression. Many laboratory experiments on numerous compounds have demonstrated resistance, a phenomenon later observed in the wild (Brown and Payne, 1988). Since the mechanisms of resistance found in experimental laboratory strains are not known to be identical to those found in the field, the full significance of experiments remains unclear.

Another approach is selection of strains that are also exposed to mutagen. This exposure produces resistant strains whose mechanism(s) of resistance can be examined. However, the possibility of false-negative results exists and is complicated by the fact that induced mutations might not have occurred otherwise.

A refinement of this approach is to produce specific mutant genes through molecular site-directed mutagenesis and then to insert these genes into the organism of interest to determine whether resistance can be conferred. In the genetic engineering of crops, researchers have been successful with this approach by inserting the acetolactase synthase gene in the gene target of sulphonylurea herbicides (Falco et al., 1985). Resistance expressed in plants engineered in the laboratory, while not as yet observed elsewhere, suggests that it might be inducible in the field also.

Although this approach appears to be a very powerful and scientifically defined method of experimentally inducing resistance by anticipated mechanisms, it is less capable of uncovering unforeseen mechanisms than the cruder methods of experimental selection of the organism discussed previously.

15.5.1 CONVENTIONAL PESTICIDES

Resistance to DDT and its analogues, to cyclodiene, and to organophosphate, carbamate, and pyrethroid insecticides has been induced in over 143 experiments, in which insects were exposed to doses killing from 50 to 90 per cent of the colony for each of 10–60 generations (Brown and Payne, 1988). DDT, dieldrin, and permethrin generally induced resistance rapidly and to very high levels, while organophosphorus and carbamite insecticides produced a slower response to less intense resistance. In the broadest sense, this relationship was the same as that observed in the field, where DDT resistance was actually found prior to most laboratory studies, and organophosphate resistance had only limited occurrence for nearly 20 years.

15.5.2   JUVENILE HORMONE MIMICRY, *Bacillus thuringiensis* TOXIN, AND OTHER NOVEL PESTICIDES

Mimicry of juvenile hormone is not an exception to the phenomenon of resistance, as demonstrated in a completely susceptible wild strain of the northern house mosquito, *Culex pipiens*, which increased methoprene resistance 100-fold in 34 generations of selection and developed lesser levels of resistance to triprene and the chitin synthesis inhibitor diflubenzuron (Brown *et al.*, 1978). In a confirmatory selection of a new collection of larvae from the same site two years later, high methoprene resistance was developed in just nine generations. Hydroprene produced selective resistance in the confused flour beetle, *Tribolium confusum*, whereas the milkweed bug, *Oncopeltus fasciatus*, developed a fourfold increase in tolerance to kinoprene (Brown *et al.*, 1978). Methoprene resistance has also been developed in *Drosophila melanogaster* by selection following mutagen treatment of males (Wilson and Fabian, 1986). While there are no reports of resistance in agriculture to this class of novel insecticides, they are not used as extensively as conventional pesticides.

Bacillus thuringiensis toxin added to larval diet produced a 14-fold increase in resistance in 27 generations of selection of house fly larvae (Harvey and Howell, 1965). From that point, resistance was not increased in 23 additional generations of selection, but it was relatively stable in the absence of selection for 20 generations. This toxin has attracted renewed interest with successful expression of its recombinant gene in plants (Vaeck *et al.*, 1987). Protection of crop plants from lepidopterous and coleopterous pests is the primary goal of this research. Recently, two lepidopterous pests of stored products responded to selection with this toxin mixed into a wheat-based larval diet. The Indianmeal moth, *Plodia interpunctella*, developed a 310-fold increase in resistance in 35 generations, while the almond moth, *Cadra cautella*, exhibited a 7.8-fold increase in resistance in 23 generations (McGaughey and Beeman, 1988). Resistance was generated very rapidly in several Indianmeal moth colonies, even though the selecting dose was adjusted only once per experiment, and many generations were selected at less than the median lethal dose. No reports exist on the selection of insect pests with the genetically engineered toxin in plants or soil microbes.

When novel pesticides are employed in selection experiments, the results can be very dependent on the methods of application and timing of the dose because of the greater lability of many of these compounds in relation to conventional pesticides, and because dose effects differ according to the stage of physiological development of the pest. This situation could result in very uneven selection within a generation so that some individuals are not actually selected. High doses timed to correspond to the most susceptible stage(s) or the use of slow-release formulations may overcome this technical problem (Brown and Payne, 1988). Similarly, consistency in the expression of toxin dose should be determined in the design of selection experiments in genetically engineered plants.

15.6 MOLECULAR TECHNIQUES TO DETECT RESISTANCE

The new prospect for studying resistance before use requires advances in finding DNA cloning vectors for pests. To be fully exploited, the basic genetics of pest species should be studied by several approaches, including the development of genetic linkage maps. New technology of restriction fragment-length polymorphism mapping recently applied to the human genome can be used to make rapid progress in many pest species for which genetic information is usually absent.

Understanding of population genetics in resistance development is fragmented and incomplete. The major problem is that surveillance data are generally obtained for susceptibility of the population by measuring mortality due to the pesticide; from these data, the proportion of resistance is estimated. Since there are often several genetically distinct mechanisms of resistance to one pesticide, direct detection of individual mechanisms becomes necessary. From the perspective of the population geneticist, the allele frequency must be determined (Roush and McKenzie, 1987). This requires that both homozygous and heterozygous individuals be detected with substantial accuracy and that tests be capable of discriminating between multiple resistance mechanisms in an individual. Breakthroughs in this form of surveillance have been achieved with the aphid *Myzus persicae*, in which an immunosorbent assay for an active enzyme has been used, and in several mosquito species, in which exposure to the insecticide was followed by multiple assays for several mechanisms in aliquots from each individual.

In Haiti, microtitre plate assays for carboxylester hydrolase were found to be very sensitive in detecting resistant individuals of *Anopheles albimanus*, so that the initial development of fenitrothion resistance was documented in the field and diagnosed as this mechanism (Brogdon *et al.*, 1988). In Guatemala, the additional, independent mechanism of less sensitive target acetylcholinesterase was also found when both mechanisms were assayed in each of 1100 mosquitoes (Brogdon *et al.*, 1988). These studies demonstrate the potential for determining the frequencies of several different resistance genes in field populations with economical and practical field kits.

15.7 ECOLOGICAL CONSEQUENCES OF RESISTANCE

A major consequence of resistance is that it often leads to increased frequency of pesticide application. This increased application rate can be damaging to biological control and integrated pest management strategies.

In some situations, mixtures that are synergistic in the resistant pest have been marketed, so that some control is regained; however, the environmental consequences of these mixtures is usually unknown. Indeed, even the basic toxicology of such mixtures has seldom been investigated.

Genetic engineering of resistance in beneficial species of insects, or even in domestic animals, may be the logical extension of accomplishments with crops when adequate cloning vectors are identified. Inserting resistance genes uncommon in pests into beneficial species may pose a great risk; for instance, a resistance gene engineered through a transposon vector into a parasitic insect could lead to the unintended movement of that gene into the pest.

Genes for hydrolases that cause enhanced degradation of pesticides have been isolated and cloned for soil-inhabiting microorganisms. A catalytic hydrolase mechanism (in contrast to a sequestering type) is very rare for organophosphorothioate and carbamate insecticides in resistant insects; in fact, the lack of hydrolysis is probably a major factor in the insecticidal activity of these major insecticidal classes. The accidental introduction of this mechanism could lead to serious resistance problems in pests and must be avoided.

Progress at improving beneficial organisms will depend on an improved understanding of the biochemistry of herbivory versus predation. It appears that herbivores are more powerful in monooxygenase-catalysed detoxication of xenobiotics than are predatory arthropods (Mullin *et al.*, 1982). Generalist herbivores have at least seven times more *trans*-epoxide hydrolase than *cis*-epoxide hydrolase, which is useful for the detoxication of epoxides sometimes generated through oxidation reactions. specialized herbivores and predators have much lower ratios (Mullin and Croft, 1984).

15.8 MUTAGENICITY OF PESTICIDES

Certain pesticides are known mutagens in bacteria and yeast assays (Klopman *et al.*, 1985). In addition, it is known that certain pesticides are promutagens which are metabolized to mutagens (Casida and Ruzo, 1986). Since insects and plants are capable of activating promutagens (Zijlstra *et al.*, 1987; Veleminsky and Gichner, 1988), it is possible that both mutagenic and promutagenic pesticides could produce mutations for resistance in alleles.

15.9 REFERENCES

Agosin, M. (1982) Multiple forms of insect cytochrome P-450: role in insecticide resistance. In: Hietanen, E., Laitinen, M. and Hanniner, O. (Eds) *Cytochrome P-450, Biochemistry, Biophysics, and Environmental Implications*, Elsevier, Amsterdam, pp. 661–669.

Ames, B. N. (1983) Dietary carcinogens and anticarcinogens. *Science* **221**, 1256–1264.

Ames, B. N., Magaw, R. and Gold, L. S. (1987) Ranking possible carcinogenic hazards. *Science* **236**, 271–280.

Brattsten, L. B., Holyoke, C. W. Jr, Leeper, J. R. and Raffa, K. F. (1986) Insecticide resistance: challenge to pest mangement and basic research. *Science* **231**, 1255–1260.

Brogdon, W. G., Beach, R. F., Stewart, J. M. and Castanaza, L. (1988) Microplate assay analysis of organophosphate and carbamate resistance distribution. *Bull. WHO* **66**, 339–346.

Brown, A. W. A. (1971) Pest resistance to pesticides. In: White-Stevens, R. (Ed.) *Pesticides in the Environment, Part II, Vol. 1*, Marcel Dekker, New York, pp. 457–552.

Brown, T. M. (1982) Prevention of pest resistance to synthetic pyrethroid insecticides. *Chem. Times Trends* **5**, 33–35.

Brown, T. M. and Brown, A. W. A. (1980) Accumulation and distribution of methoprene in resistant *Culex pipiens* larvae. *Ent. Exp. Appl.* **27**, 11–22.

Brown, T. M. and Hooper, G. H. S. (1979) Metabolic detoxication as a mechanism of methoprene resistance in *Culex pipiens*. *Pest. Biochem. Physiol.* **12**, 79–86.

Brown, T. M. and Payne, G. T. (1988) Experimental selection for insecticide resistance. *J. Econ. Entomol.* **81**, 49–56.

Brown, T. M., DeVries, D. H. and Brown, A. W. A. (1978) Induction of resistance to insect growth regulators. *J. Econ. Entomol.* **71**, 223–229.

Byford, R. L., Quisenberry, S. S., Sparks, T. C. and Lockwood, J. A. (1985) Spectrum of insecticide cross-resistance in pyrethroid-resistant populations of *Haematobia irritans (Diptera: Muscidae)*. *J. Econ. Entomol.* **78**, 768–773.

Casida, J. E. and Ruzo, L. O. (1986) Reactive intermediates in pesticide metabolism: peracid oxidations as possible biomimetic models. *Xenobiotica* **16**, 1003–1015.

Chadwick, P. R., Slatter, R. and Bowron, M. J. (1984) Cross-resistance to pyrethroids and other insecticides in *Aedes aegypti*. *Pestic. Sci.* **15**, 112–120.

Cooksey, D. A. (1990) Genetics of bactericide resistance in plant pathogenic bacteria. *Annu. Rev. Phytopathol.* **28**, 201–219.

Devonshire, A. L. and Moores, G. D. (1982) A carboxylesterase with broad substrate specificity caused organophosphorus, carbamate, and pyrethroid resistance in peach-potato aphids (*Myzus persicae*). *Pestic. Biochem. Physiol.* **18**, 235–246.

DeVries, D. H. and Georghiou, G. P. (1980) A wide spectrum of resistance to pyrethroid insecticides in *Musca domestica*. *Experentia* **36**, 226–227.

DeWaard, M. A. and van Nistelrooy, J. G. M. (1980) Mechanism of resistance to pyrazophos in *Pyricularia oryzae*. *Neth. J. Plant Pathol.* **86**, 251–528.

Falco, S. C., Chaleff, R. S., Dumas, K. S., LaRossa, R. A., Leto, K. J., Mauvais, C. J., Mazur, B. J., Ray, T. B., Schloss, J. V. and Yadav, N. S. (1985) Molecular biology of sulfonylurea herbicide activity. In: Zaitlin, M., Day, P., Hollaender, A. and Wilson, C. M. (Eds) *Biotechnology in Plant Science: Relevance to Agriculture in the Eighties*, Academic Press, Orlando, Florida, pp. 313–328.

Feyereisen, R., Koener, J. F., Farnsworth, D. E. and Nebert, D. W. (1989) Isolation and sequence of cDNA encoding a cytochrome P-450 from an insecticide-resistant strain of the house fly, *Musca domestica*. *Proc. Natl. Acad. Sci. USA* **86**, 1465–1469.

Field, L. M., Devonshire, A. L. and Forde, B. G. (1988) Molecular evidence that insecticide resistance in peach-potato aphids (*Myzus persicae* Sulz.) results form amplification of esterase gene. *Biochem. J.* **251**, 309–312.

Fujimura, M., Oeda, K., Inoue, H. and Kato, T. (1990) Mechanism of Action *N*-phenylcarbamates in benzimidazole-resistant neurospora strains. In: Green, M. B., LeBaron, H. M. and Moberg, W. K. (Eds) *Managing Resistance to Agrochemicals: From Fundamental Research to Practical Strategies*, ACS Symposium Series No. 421, American Chemical Society, Washington DC.

Georghiou, G. P. (1986) The magnitude of the resistance problem. In: National Research Council, *Pesticide Resistance: Strategies and Tactics for Management*, National Academy Press, Washington DC, pp. 14–43.

Georghiou, G. P. and Saito, T. (Eds) (1983) *Pest Resistance to Pesticides*, Plenum, New York.

Georgopoulos, S. G. (1986) Plant pathogens. In: National Research Council, *Pesticide Resistance: Strategies and Tactics for Management*, National Academy Press, Washington DC, pp. 100–101.

Georgopoulos, S. G. and Skylakakis, G. (1986) Genetic variability in the fungi and the problem of fungicide resistance. *Crop Protection* **5**, 299–305.

Harvey, T. L. and Howell, D. E. (1965) Resistance of the house fly to *Bacillus thuringiensis*. *J. Invert. Pathol.* **7**, 92–100.

Heap, I. and Knight, R. (1982) A population of ryegrass tolerant to the herbicide diclofop-methyl *Lolium rigidum*, genotypes, South Australia. *J. Aust. Inst. Agric. Sci.* **48**, 156–157.

Heap, I. and Knight, R. (1986) The occurrence of herbicide cross-resistance in a population of annual ryegrass, *Lolium rigidum*, resistant to diclofop-methyl. *Aust. J. Agric. Res.* **37**, 149–156.

Hirschberg, J. and McIntosh, L. (1983) Molecular basis of herbicide resistance in *Amaranthus hybridus*. *Science* **222**, 1346–1349.

Hoyer, R. F. and Plapp, F. W. Jr (1968) Insecticide resistance in the house fly: effect of a modifier gene in combination with major genes which confer resistance. *J. Econ. Entomol.* **64**, 1051–1055.

Jackson, W. B. and Ashton, A. D. (1986) Case histories of anticoagulant resistance. In: National Research Council, *Pesticide Resistance: Strategies and Tactics for Management*, National Academy Press, Washington DC, pp. 355–369.

Kalamarkis, A. E., Ziogas, B. N. and Georgopoulos, S. G. (1986) Resistance to ergosterol biosynthesis inhibitors in *Nectria haematococca* var. *cucurbitae*. In: Greenhalgh, R. and Roberts, T. R. (Eds) *Pesticide Science and Biotechnology. Proceedings of the Sixth International IUPAC Congress of Pesticide Chemistry*, Ottawa, Canada, 10–15 August, 1986, International Union of Pure and Applied Chemistry, Blackwell Scientific, Oxford, Boston.

Keiding, J. (1986) Prediction or resistance risk assessment. In: National Research Council, *Pesticide Resistance: Strategies and Tactics for Management*, National Academy Press, Washington DC, pp. 279–297.

Kemp, M. S., Moss, S. R. and Thomas, T. H. (1990) Herbicide resistance in *Alopecurus myosuroides*. In: Green, M. B., LeBaron, H. M. and Moberg, W. K. (Eds) *Managing Resistance to Agrochemicals: From Fundamental Research to Practical Strategies*, ACS Symposium Series No. 421, American Chemical Society, Washington DC.

Klopman, G., Contreras, R., Rosenkranz, H. S. and Waters, M. D. (1985) Structure–genotoxic activity relationships of pesticides: comparison of the results from several short-term assays. *Mutation Res.* **147**, 343–356.

Köller, W. and Scheinpflug, H. (1987) Fungal resistance to sterol biosynthesis inhibitors: a new challenge. *Plant Disease* **71**, 1066–1074.

Konno, T., Hodgson, E. and Dauterman, W. C. (1989) Studies on methyl parathion resistance in *Heliothis virescens*. *Pestic. Biochem. Physiol.* **33**, 189–199.

LeBaron, H. M. and McFarland, J. (1990) Herbicide resistance in weeds and crops. In: Green, M. B., LeBaron, H. M. and Moberg, W. K. (Eds) *Managing Resistance to Agrochemicals: From Fundamental Research to Practical Strategies*, ACS Symposium Series No. 421, American Chemical Society, Washington DC.

LeBaron, H. M. and Gressel, J. (Eds) (1982) *Herbicide Resistance in Plants*, John Wiley and Sons, New York.

Liu, M. Y., Chen, J. S. and Sun, C. N. (1984) Synergism of pyrethroids by several compounds in larvae of the diamondback moth (Lepidoptera: *Plutellidae*). *J. Econ. Entomol.* **77**, 851–856.

Liu, M., Tzeng, Y. and Sun, C. (1981) Diamondback moth resistance to several synthetic pyrethroids. *J. Econ. Entomol.* **74**, 393–396.

Locke, T. (1986) Current incidence in the United Kingdom of fungicide resistance in pathogens of cereals. *Proceedings of the British Crop Protection Conference: Pests and Diseases—1986*, Vol. 2, BCPC Publications, Surrey, UK, pp. 781–786.

Lockwood, J. A., Sparks, T. C. and Story, R. N. (1984) Evolution of insect resistance to insecticides: a reevaluation of the roles of physiology and behavior. *Bull. Entomol. Soc. Am.* **30**, 41–51.

Lund, A. E. and Narahashi, T. (1983) Kinetics of sodium channel modification as the basis for the variation in nerve membrane effects of pyrethroids and DDT analogs. *Pestic. Biochem. Physiol.* **20**, 203–216.

MacNicoll, A. D. (1986) Resistance to 4-hydroxycoumarin anticoagulants in rodents. In: National Research Council, *Pesticide Resistance: Strategies and Tactics for Management*, National Academy Press, Washington DC, pp. 87–99.

McGaughey, W. H. and Beeman, R. W. (1988) Resistance to *Bacillus thuringiensis* in colonies of Indianmeal moth and almond moth (*Lepidoptera: Pyralidae*). *J. Econ. Entomol.* **81**, 28–33.

Metcalf, R. L. (1971) The chemistry and biology of pesticides. In: White-Stevens, R. (Ed.) *Pesticides in the Environment, Part II*, Vol. 1, Marcel Dekker, New York, pp. 1–144.

Motoyama, N., Hayashi, M. A. and Dauterman, W. C. (1983) The presence of two forms of glutathione S-transferases with distinct substrate specificity in OP (organophosphorylation)-resistant and -susceptible housefly strains (*Musca domestica*). In: Miyamoto, J. and Kearney, P. C. (Eds) *Pesticide Chemistry: Human Welfare and the Environment. Proceedings of the 5th International Congress of Pesticide Chemistry*, Kyoto, Japan, 29 August–4 September 1982, Pergamon Press, Oxford, pp. 197–202.

Mouches, C., Pasteur, N., Berge, J. B., Hyrien, O., Raymond, M., de Saint Vincent, B. R., de Silvestri, M. and Georghiou, G. P. (1986) Amplification of an esterase gene is responsible for insecticide resistance in a California Culex mosquito. *Science* **233**, 778–780.

Mudge, L. C., Gossett, B. J. and Murphy, T. R. (1984) Resistance of goosegrass (*Eleusine indica*) to dinitro-aniline herbicides. *Weed Sci.* **32**, 591–594.

Mullin, C. A. and Croft, B. A. (1984) Trans-epoxide hydrolase: a key indicator enzyme for herbivory in arthropods. *Experientia* **40**, 176–178.

Mullin, C. A., Croft, B. A., Stricker, K., Matsumura, F. and Miller, J. R. (1982) Detoxication enzyme differences between a herbivorous and predatory mite. *Science* **217**, 1270–1272.

Nolan, J., Raulston, W. J. and Wharton, R. H. (1977) Resistance to synthetic pyrethroids in a DDT-resistant strain of *Boophilus microplus*. *Pestic. Sci.* **8**, 484–486.

Ogawa, J. M., Manji, B. T., Heaton, C. R., Petrie, J. and Sonoda, R. M. (1983) Methods for detecting and monitoring the resistance of plant pathogens to chemicals. In: Georghiou, G. P. and Saito, T. (Eds) *Pest Resistance to Pesticides*, Plenum Press, New York, pp. 71–98.

Omer, S. M., Georghiou, G. P. and Irving, S. N. (1980) DDT/pyrethroid resistance inter-relationships in *Anopheles stephensi*. *Mosq. News* **40**, 200–209.

Oppenoorth, F. J. and Welling, W. (1976) Biochemistry and physiology of resistance. In: Wilkinson, C. F. (Ed.) *Insecticide Biochemistry and Physiology*, Plenum Press, New York, pp. 507–551.

Payne, G. T. (1982) Mechanisms of resistance to methyl parathion in the tobacco budworm, *Heliothis virescens* (*Lepidoptera: Noctuidae*). MS thesis, Clemson University, Clemson, South Carolina, 80pp.

Payne, G. T., Blenk, R. G. and Brown, T. M. (1988) Inheritance of permethrin resistance in the tobacco budworm (*Leipidoptera: Noctuidae*). *J. Econ. Entomol.* **81**, 65–73.

Plapp, F. W. Jr (1976) Biochemical genetics of insecticide resistance. *Ann. Rev. Entomol.* **21**, 179–198.

Plapp, F. W. Jr and Hoyer, R. F. (1968) Possible pleiotropism of a gene conferring resistance to DDT, DDT analogs, and pyrethrins in housefly and *Culex tarsalis*. *J. Econ. Entomol.* **61**, 761–765.

Powles, S. B., Holtum, J. A. M., Matthews, J. M. and Liljegren, D. (1990) Herbicide cross-resistance in annual ryegrass (*Lolium rigidum* Gaud). In: Green, M. B., LeBaron, H. M. and Moberg, W. K. (Eds) *Managing Resistance to Agrochemicals: From Fundamental Research to Practical Strategies*, ACS Symposium Series No. 421, American Chemical Society, Washington DC.

Priester, T. M. and Georghiou, G. P. (1980) Cross-resistance spectrum in pyrethroid-resistant *Culex quinquefasciatus*. *Pestic. Sci.* **11**, 617–624.

Raymond, M., Pasteur, N., Fournier, D., Cuany, A., Berge, J. and Magnin, M. (1985) Genetics of a propoxur insensitive acetylcholinesterase responsible for resistance in *Culex pipiens* L. *Comp. Rend. Acad. Sci. Paris* **300**, 509–512 (in French).

Roush, R. T. and McKenzie, J. A. (1987) Ecological genetics of insecticide and acaricide resistance. *Ann. Rev. Entomol.* **32**, 361–380.

Sawicki, R. M. (1970) Interaction between the factor delaying penetration of insecticides and desethylation mechanisms of resistance in organophosphorus-resistant house flies. *Pestic. Sci.* **1**, 84–87.

Scott, J. G. and Georghiou, G. P. (1986) Mechanisms responsible for high levels of permethrin resistance in the house fly. *Pestic. Sci.* **17**, 195–206.

Simonet, D. E., Riley, S. L., Watkinson, I. A. and Whitehead, J. R. (1988) PEG-US monitoring program: adult vial tests. In: Brown, J. M. (Ed.) *Proceedings of the Beltwide Cotton Production Research Conferences, New Orleans, Louisiana, January 3–8, 1988: Insects*, National Cotton Council, Memphis, Tennessee, pp. 334–336.

Skurray, R. A., Rouch, D. A., Lyon, B. R., Gillespie, M. T., Tennent, J. M., Byrne, M. E., Messerotti, L. J. and May, J. W. (1988) Multiresistant *Staphylococcus aureus*: genetics and evolution of epidemic Australian strains. *J. Antimicrob. Chemother.* **21**(Suppl. C), 19–39.

Soderlund, D. M. and Bloomquist, J. R. (1990) Molecular mechanisms of insecticide resistance. In: Roush, R. T. and Tabashnik, B. E. (Eds) *Pesticide Resistance in Arthropods*, Routledge, Chapman & Hall, New York, London.

Sparks, T. C. (1981) Development of insecticide resistance in *Heliothis virescens* in North America. *Bull. Entomol. Soc. Am.* **27**, 186–192.

Sparks, C., Quisenberry, S. S., Lockwood, J. A., Byford, R. L. and Roush, R. T. (1985) Insecticide resistance in the horn fly, *Haematobia irritans*. *J. Agric. Entomol.* **2**, 217–233.

Tsukamoto, M. (1983) Methods of genetic analysis of insecticide resistance. In: Georghiou, G. P. and Saito, T. (Eds) *Pest Resistance to Pesticides*, Plenum Press, New York, pp. 71–98.

Vaeck, M., Reynaerts, A., Hofte, H., Jansens, S., de Beuckeleer, M., Dean, C., Zabeau, M., van Montagu, M. and Leemans, J. (1987) Transgenic plants protected from insect attack. *Nature* **328**, 33–37.

Vaughn, K. C., Marks, M. D. and Weeks, D. P. (1987) A dinitroaniline-resistant mutant of Eleusine indica exhibits cross-resistance and supersensitivity to antimicrotubule herbicides and drugs. *Plant Physiol.* **83**, 956–964.

Veleminsky, J. and Gichner, T. (1988) Mutagenic activity of promutagens in plants: indirect evidence of their activation. *Mutation Res.* **197**, 221–242.

Voss, G. (1987) *Insecticide/Acaricide Resistance: Survey and Recommendations by Industry*, GIFAP Insecticide Resistance Action Committee, International Group of National Associations of Agrochemical Manufacturers, Brussels, 10pp.

Wilson, T. G. and Fabian, J. (1986) A *Drosophila melanogaster* mutant resistant to a chemical analog of juvenile hormone. *Dev. Biol.* **118**, 190–201.

Yadav, N., McDevitt, R. E., Benard, S. and Falco, S. C. (1986) Single amino acid substitutions in the enzyme acetolactate synthase confer resistance to the herbicide sulfometuron methyl. *Proc. Natl. Acad. Sci. USA* **83**, 4418–4422.

Zijlstra, J. A., Vogel, E. W. and Breimer, D. E. (1987) Pharmacological and toxicological aspects of mutagenicity research in *Drosophila melanogaster. Rev. Biochem. Toxicol.* **8**, 121–153.

16 Methods to Anticipate Effects of Biotechnology on Integrated Pest Management

C. HAGEDORN and G. LACY

Departments of Plant Pathology and Agronomy, Virginia Polytechnic Institute and State University, USA

16.1 INTRODUCTION

Integrated management of pests (IPM) or pathogens is an important part of crop production strategies. Integrated management strategies have as their goal providing maximum economic yields for the farmer, while improving and/or maintaining the production site and protecting adjacent habitats. IPM has as its goal, therefore, the protection of crops from pests and pathogens without producing negative environmental impacts. IPM differs from conventional control in that former deals with the long-range goal of maintaining or increasing productivity; whereas the latter protects the cropped environment and does not include site preservation or non-target effects on adjacent habitats and organisms. Consequently, as a component of integrated crop production strategies, IPM requires long-term investment at the production site and adjacent sites; thus, it mandates an investment in the future that can reduce short-term productivity and profits. However, production practices afforded by integrated crop management strategies can lead ultimately to enhanced productivity and minimal environmental impact. Certainly, producers will not apply IPM strategies if the short-term benefits do not result in profitable returns, since losing the farm because of financial losses is a powerful argument for short-term solutions. IPM must be used to develop more cost-effective methods for farming while protecting both production and adjacent environments for the future. Biotechnology has a significant role to play in contemporary IPM strategies and applications (Napoli and Staskawicz, 1985).

IPM requires coordination of biology, ecology, chemistry, and engineering for crop production; thus, biologists, ecologists, chemists, and agricultural

Methods to Assess Adverse Effects of Pesticides on Non-target Organisms
Edited by R. G. Tardiff
© 1992 SCOPE Published by John Wiley & Sons Ltd

engineers must work together to solve anticipated and unexpected problems. Biotechnology will accelerate the production of more vigorous, productive, and resistant crop plants less susceptible to environmental stresses. This advance includes microbes that contribute to plant productivity by causing more rapid plant development or by protecting plants from pathogens or pests. Engineered plants and beneficial microbes also have the potential to cause problems, since careless development or release may inadvertently lead to the introduction of environmental problems capable of self-replication (Tauber et al., 1985). This chapter deals with the methodologies for assessing the impact of organisms engineered for IPM applications, by examining possible strategies to evaluate and develop biotechnology methodologies related to IPM, describing organisms currently being developed that may impact IPM, and identifying research needs.

16.2   BIOLOGICAL CONTROL CONCEPTS

Historically, biological control has been an important part of IPM. Biological control is defined as the management of a pest or pathogen using a second organism, or biological control agent, and cultural methods directed towards reducing the impact of a specific pest. Biotechnology will have an impact on IPM in the near future (Mets et al., 1986). The first biotechnological successes related to IPM have already been achieved, with engineered microorganisms or genes of microbes engineered into plants (Lincoln et al., 1985). A stated goal of IPM projects is to reduce the levels and frequency of application of agricultural chemicals. This goal creates an expanded role for the use of biological control methods, including genetically engineered microorganisms (GEMs) designed as antagonists towards specific plant pathogens. The following sections will address recombinant DNA technology, including the introduction of microbial genes in plants, applied to microbes for biological control. Genetic engineering of animals and products designed for the improvement of animal health will not be covered.

16.3   BIOTECHNOLOGY CONCEPTS

Biotechnology has been difficult to define for both laymen and scientists. Simplistically stated, biotechnology is the application of biological principles to the technologies for production of food, fibre, fuel, or pharmaceuticals. Realistically, biotechnology has been utilized since the first human intentionally planted crop plants or husbanded animals. The addition of recombinant DNA techniques to biotechnology may provide a revolution as profound as the prehistoric discoveries that using seed from more productive plants or breeding animals with desirable characteristics increased the number or quality of agricultural products (Ouellette and Cheremisinoff, 1985).

In the United States, the consistent development of agricultural biotechnology began with the establishment of the first agricultural experiment station in 1887 in New Haven, Connecticut. Until that time, biotechnology had developed in a non-directed manner similar to initial developments in some other field of science or engineering and similar to the application of developments in agriculture. Within the current system of experiment stations, land-grant universities, federally supported research, and the Extension Service, the process of biotechnology development has accelerated at an extraordinary pace, with new scientific breakthroughs reported almost weekly. Biotechnology has evolved to include the application of the newest scientific methodologies to biological productivity. This situation means that, for agricultural biotechnology, those sciences related to genetic engineering will actually encompass recombinant DNA technologies along with the support disciplines for the regeneration of whole organisms, including plant regeneration, *in vitro* fertilization, and embryo implantation of animals.

16.4 SHORTCOMINGS OF BIOCONTROL AGENTS

16.4.1 DETECTION, RECOVERY, AND ENUMERATION

To monitor the fate of recombinant DNA in the environment, methods utilized for detection, recovery, and enumeration must be precise, accurate, and sensitive. An important concept is that the products of recombinant DNA may reside in the engineered organism, in other organisms, or in the inorganic or organic components of the habitat to which the organism was applied. Therefore, monitoring techniques should have enough flexibility to cover all these possibilities. Obviously, a combination of techniques is usually more effective than a single procedure (Milewski, 1985; Rissler, 1984).

16.4.1.1 Culture

Two limitations of culture techniques exist: the organism(s) must be able to grow on some selective medium in order to be detected at low population levels. If gene exchange has occurred, the recipient organism may not be detectable by these means. A final limitation is that viable counts, by definition, will only record actively growing cells. Stressed and hypobiotic cells or free DNA that are non-detectable may be important in the dissemination of recombinant DNA (Atlas, 1982; Roszak and Colwell, 1987).

16.4.1.2 Detection limits

Methodologies for assessing safety of engineered biological control agents are only useful if the limits of detection are clearly understood. By currently available methods, detection of viable or non-viable cells at population levels below 10^3 colony-forming units per gram of soil is usually inaccurate.

16.4.1.3   Direct counts

Direct counting procedures (e.g., acridine orange staining, immunofluorescence assays ELISA, serological staining, and monoclonal antibody procedures) usually reveal higher numbers in a population, and may be more sensitive than viable cell counts; but they are limited, since they are usually less accurate (i.e., acridine orange stains nucleic acids in all bacteria and fungi) and often count dead as well as living cells. Polyclonal serological systems recognize a battery of antigens that may occur in several organisms. Monoclonal serological systems may be specific enough to follow the presence of a gene product related to recombinant DNA. An attractive system would be to use a battery of monoclonals to recognize recombinant DNA gene products and the possible hosts of that DNA.

16.4.1.4   Genetic markers

Genetic markers, such as spontaneous indicators to antibiotic resistance, are useful in selecting strains that have been introduced into a habitat; and they often increase the levels of detection, especially if two or more markers are used in combination (Hagedorn, 1986). The limitations of this procedure are that only introduced strains—which are weak because they are mutants—can be followed, and that there are no markers to follow indigenous strains, such as the wild-type parent (Hagedorn, 1986). The use of genetic markers also hinges on the stability of the markers. For instance, ampicillin mutants occur at a frequency approximately 100 times higher than tetracycline-resistant mutants. At high population densities, spontaneous ampicillin mutants among indigenous bacteria will interfere with the interpretation of results before spontaneous tetracycline mutants would do so. Recently, there has been considerable discussion of the potential mobility of the mutant gene within the general microbial population. The issue is the transfer of the resistant element to other bacterial strains, thus dispersing into the environment resistance to clinically important antibiotics. There is also the possibility that such strains or genetic recipients might enter food chains and contribute to antibiotic resistance in microbes inhabiting the gastrointestinal tract of humans or animals. However, new technologies afforded by transposable elements have provided solutions to many of the problems, such as marker stability, that are inherent in selecting for spontaneous mutants. As an example, genes coded for lactose utilization (Monsanto LacZ) have bene introduced into a strain of *Pseudomonas aureofaciens* that has been introduced in a field test. This marker is selective and non-antibiotic and provides a specific identifying characteristic for the introduced strain.

16.4.1.5   Detection of DNA from soil

Perhaps the most sensitive method for detecting genetically engineered organisms in the soil is to detect the recombinant DNA itself in the environment. This method may be quite important, since it will detect cell-free DNA as well as DNA in non-viable and viable cells. Cell-free DNA and DNA in non-viable cells may be important in the dissemination of recombinant DNA through the process of transformation of competent recipient cells with naked DNA. DNA may persist for long periods adsorbed on mineral particles or in or on organic debris. Some of these sites may be relatively protected from soil nucleases (Kelman *et al.*, 1987). The analytical technique is based upon amplification of the DNA extracted from the environment, followed by detection using specific hybridization probes (Somerville *et al.* 1988). Simply, total DNA is isolated from soil using a variety of techniques, usually featuring polyvinyl polypyrrolidone to remove humic compounds, sodium dodecyl sulphate as a lysis detergent, and purification by buoyant density centrifugation in caesium chloride gradients. The DNA amplification cycle consist of rounds of denaturing the DNA to single strands, annealing a specific primer, and DNA polymerase-mediated manufacture of a complete second strand (Ou *et al.*, 1988; Saiki *et al.*, 1988). By repeating these three steps several times, DNA from as little as one bacterial cell per gram of soil may be detected. This is a significant increase in sensitivity and level of detection compared to viable-cell-count and immunofluorescence procedures described above.

16.4.1.6 Movement of genetic material

Genetic transfer by microorganisms has been recorded in aquatic and marine habitats (Morrison, *et al.*, 1978; Baross *et al.*, 1967), in soil (Graham and Istock, 1978; Weinberg and Stotzky, 1972), and in plants (Kerr *et al.*, 1977; Lacy, 1978; Lacy and Leary, 1975; Talbot *et al.*, 1980; Lacy *et al.*, 1984). Philosophically, some level of genetic exchange among microbes—engineered or not—must be expected, since they have so many useful exchange mechanisms, including conjugation, transformation, transduction, and cell fusion. The frequency of transfer may be expected to be lower than in the laboratory in soil and water, since the conditions may not be as optimal as on laboratory media. However, in plants, transfer frequencies have been recorded that are higher than laboratory frequencies, possibly due to the absence of microbial competitors, the presence of abundant nutrients, and support for mating pairs in plant tissue (Kerr *et al.*, 1977; Lacy, 1978; Lacy and Leary, 1975; Lacy *et al.*, 1984). Some tentative evidence has been collected indicating that engineered microbes may rearrange recombinant DNA *in vivo* and transfer DNA to indigenous organisms. Confirmation will be required for these results (Jansson and Tiedje, 1988; Orvos *et al.*, 1988).

Detection of transfer has been performed by conventional genetic procedures which require expression of a genetic trait and detection by viable counts of the bacterium acquiring the genetic trait. Dissemination of genetic elements below the limits of detection cannot be measured; likewise, unexpressed DNA, which may later be disseminated to a second organism in which expression may occur, cannot be detected. Enrichment culturing may increase the sensitivity of viable counting, but this technique assumes we know which organisms to culture and how to culture them. Using the new DNA amplification techniques, it should be possible to detect the continued presence of DNA in the environment below the limits of viable counts. If that DNA is contained in a living organism, it will be more difficult to determine.

16.4.2 HABITAT SIMULATION

Artificial habitats (i.e., microcosms) are an essential intermediate step to ecologically sound analyses leading to environmental release. The problem with microcosms is that they never adequately duplicate natural ecosystems (Klute, 1985; Morley et al., 1983; Page et al., 1982). Simplistic microcosms may be replicated, but they do not mimic environmental fluctuations in temperature, humidity, pH, light intensity, and other multitudinous variables. Complex microcosms simulate some, but not all, environmental parameters, and are difficult to replicate because of the cost and complexity (Roberge, 1978). Larger microcosms (mesocosms) circumvent some of the problems by increasing the number of samples taken within one mesocosm. Mesocosms are difficult and expensive to duplicate; hence, treatment numbers and replicates are limited (Brown, 1987). Research is needed to increase basic understanding of environmental interactions and cycles. Currently, our understanding of these phenomena is so scanty that our ability to engineer adequate microcosms and to interpret results derived from them is restricted (Armstrong et al., 1987; DeAngelis, 1973; Kool et al., 1987). Scientific understanding and appropriate methodologies are absent to examine the effects of GEMs on ecosystem structure and function. Studies that add a GEM to a natural ecosystem usually require extensive microcosm simulations. Three principal research approaches that appear to be useful include: expanded use of microcosms as representations of various ecosystems, including appropriate design features, characterization of the most critical parameters, calibration to the field, and standardization of protocols; establishment of ecosystem baseline data for any particular habitat to permit confident analysis of ecological effects (and the degree of change required to detect a significant effect); and the generation of positive controls to ensure that test systems are appropriate to assess ecosystem effects (Brezhnev et al., 1974; Hunter et al., 1986).

16.4.3 MODELLING FOR PREDICTIVE CAPACITY

Modelling procedures are suggested by any use of microcosms. Three types of models exist: descriptive, analytical, and predictive. To date, most models are descriptive, since our knowledge of microbial survival, movement, and colonization is very limited. Most models are reactive, since they are usually based on existing data. Active models are needed that indicate what data are required to satisfy the questions being posed. Evolution of modelling is related directly to the amount of accurate descriptive data available. At this time, modelling becomes more precise and analytical as the quality and amount of data improve. Eventually, models may develop predictive capacity based on the precision of the analytical forebears. Numerous modelling approaches are available to encompass habitat and organism inventories, population dynamics, nutrient flow and cycling, and interrelationships among environmental factors (Corapcioğlu and Haridas, 1984). Such simulation models are useful to characterize parameters, establish baseline data points, and identify and prioritize the most important processes for investigation (Brezhnev et al., 1974; King and DeAngelis, 1986). Research trends in modelling must include some element of experimental procedure that incorporates: the design of a microcosm to simulate some important aspects of the proposed release area; evaluation of the GEM by monitoring a set of parameters deemed 'most critical' for the particular microcosm; and development of a descriptive model of the microcosm that can account for process rates, perturbations, and analyses (Hicks and Newell, 1984; Minogue and Fry, 1983; Thingstad and Pengerud, 1985). Lastly, numerical analyses of data assume a uniquely important aspect in ecosystem studies because of the large variation inherent in the components of the system and the difficulty of establishing cause and effect relationships (Rouse, 1985). It will be necessary to define normal ranges of variability and function for specific ecological populations and/or processes and naturally occurring levels of change (Gladden and Ginzburg, 1982). Only then can perturbations be detected and the probability be determined that the alteration was associated with the presence and/or activities of a GEM.

16.4.4   ASSESSING ORGANISMAL FITNESS

Organismal fitness is a measure of an engineered biological control agent and its ability to enter into, survive, and colonize a particular habitat whether that habitat is the target or a non-target habitat. Fitness, therefore, is related to a complex assortment of traits for competitiveness, substrate utilization, rate of replication, optimum growth temperature of pH, and a myriad of other abilities. Since the components of fitness are so many and complex, testing them separately, although of academic interest, would be the least efficient method for determining fitness (Silver et al., 1986). Currently, direct evelution by competition of the engineered organism is the most efficient method for testing fitness. In this method, a series of mixed inocula are utilized so that the wild-type parent is the dominant population in some inocula, and the engineered strain progeny is dominant in others. By measuring relative changes in the ratios of colonization, the competitive ability of the engineered strain may be measured directly against the parental strain.

16.4.5   ESTIMATING RISK

Currently, risk assessment is an imprecise art that involves determining exposure combined with potential hazard to arrive at a level of relative risk or probability of a specific adverse effect. Risk assessment involves using available background data to design an effective artificial habitat that will generate enough additional data to construct a predictive model. This model can then be used to estimate the probability that a specific adverse effect might occur. The limitations of risk assessment are that non-specific effects are difficult to assess, the reliability of predictive systems is poor, and negative results (i.e., no adverse effect is detected) do not provide adequate statistical confidence (Cairns and Pratt, 1987).

16.5   ENGINEERED BIOCONTROL AGENTS

16.5.1   MICROBIAL INSECTICIDES

Bacillus thuringiensis produces a group of closely related potent polypeptide toxins (BT toxins) that are active against several chewing insects, including various beetles and moths (Bernhard, 1986). Some of these insects are serious pests of economically important crop plants. The activity spectrum of species against which the toxin is effective may be manipulated by selecting strains of *B. thuringiensis* that produce toxins with different activities (Krieg *et al.*, 1983). Since the gene responsible for the production of this toxin has been cloned and characterized at the molecular level, the possibility for genetic engineering to further restrict or extend the activity spectrum of the toxins is a distinct possibility (Hernstadt *et al.*, 1987). BT toxins have been utilized very successfully in biological control for many years. Their effectiveness is due in part to the ability of *B. thuringiensis* to produce very resistant structures called endospores, which contain protein crystals of the toxin (Bulla *et al.*, 1979; Whitely and Schnepf, 1986). Sprayed on aerial surfaces of plants, these spores are ingested by chewing insects, releasing the toxin into the gut of the insect. If the insect is susceptible to its toxic effects, it dies. Below ground applications of the endospores have not been effective due to the relatively low cost of treatment and to their rapid deterioration probably by microbial degradation (Hernstadt *et al.*, 1986).

Biotechnological research has indicated other ways to utilize BT toxins for the biological control of pests. For example, the genes mediating production of BT toxin have been moved into strains of fluorescent pseudomonads, bacteria that inhabit the rhizoplane and rhizosphere of plants. The biological control tactic was that the BT toxin, now produced by the pseudomonads, would be ingested by root-grazing insects, thus extending the use of BT toxins below the surface of the ground (Schroth and Hancock, 1985). The toxins were found to be effective in laboratory tests for controlling some root pests. The development of this method for biological control has apparently been suspended, since the system did not offer methods for controlling the movement of the root-inhabiting pseudomonads to other plants and possible environmental impacts on the distribution of non-target insects. A second tactic incorporates the genes for BT toxin production into the genome of a crop plant (Horsch *et al.*, 1984). Chewing insects feeding on the plant tissue ingest BT toxin. Ecologically, this is a better strategy, since the BT toxin will only be active against insects that are pests on that particular plant. However, the movement of the BT toxin gene from one plant to others through sexual exchanges may allow the gene to escape into weed plants affecting those insects that are pests on the weeds (Tomashow *et al.*, 1980).

Baculoviruses are among the most promising alternatives to chemical pesticide control of major agricultural and forest insect pests. These viruses are presently being genetically engineered by commercial companies to enhance their pathogenicity and for their expression in vector systems. Within the next five years, commercially desirable, genetically engineered baculovirus (GEV) pesticides will probably be available for release into many types of environmental settings. These GEVs will contain a variety of foreign genes (Biever *et al.* 1982; Falcon *et al.*, 1968).

Several strategies can be used for inserting 'pesticidal' genes into baculoviruses. The first calls for early insertion of the foreign gene under the control of a duplicated immediate or early viral promoter (Summers *et al.* 1980). The second calls for insertion of the foreign gene under the control of a very late viral promoter. The third strategy for construction of a GEV is to remove the polyhedron gene (poly-GEV) and to replace it with a 'pesticidal' gene. The polyhedron gene product is responsible for occlusion of virions within polyhedra, which is required for survival and transmission of baculoviruses in nature. For field application, the poly-GEV will need to be occluded by the polyhedron gene product provided by the wild type (poly + virus). This can be achieved by co-infection with both virus types. Accordingly, the poly-GEV can only persist following co-infection of larval cells, and will rapidly be lost from the environment. The only avenue available for persistence of the GEV is through illegitimate recombination (foreign gene insertion into the poly + genome without displacement or inactivation of viral genes).

Other microbial insecticides being actively investigated include both fungi and protozoa (Falcon, 1985), although these entomopathogens are at present of little importance compared to BT and the baculoviruses.

16.5.2 FROST CONTROL

Ice crystal formation in plant cells ruptures cell and organelle membranes, and often results in cell death. Plants, especially those that have evolved in temperate climates, have developed several methods to deal with ice formation. Among these are cytoplasm concentration to reduce the formation of ice and nucleation of ice at warmer temperatures, so that ice forms intercellularly rather than intracellularly. Many economically important crop species evolved in warmer climates and do not have obvious methods for protection from ice formation. However, a paradox exists; plants are often damaged by frost at temperatures of -2 to $-5\,°C$, yet plant tissue freezes at much lower temperatures of -7 to $-10\,°C$; because the cytoplasm is not pure water. This difference is attributed to the presence of ice-catalysing epiphytic bacteria such as members of the almost universally present genera of *Pseudomonas*, *Erwinia* and *Xanthomonas* (Kim *et al.*, 1987; Lindow, 1982). Molecular studies indicate that ice-nucleation-active bacteria contain a single gene coding for a protein that seems to be responsible for catalysing ice (Ou *et al.* 1988). Using natural strains of non-ice-nucleating bacteria or chemical mutants deficient in the ability to catalyse ice formation, it was discovered that plants may be protected to some extent from ice damage by manipulating their epiphytic flora to favour the non-ice-nucleating strains (Lindow, 1982; Orser *et al.*, 1985). Since strains of ice-nucleating bacteria demonstrate more or less host specificity in their epiphytic relationships with plants, greater protection is afforded by constructing non-ice-nucleating strains from the wild-type ice-nucleating strains by deleting the ice-nucleation gene (Lindow, 1985). Since chemical mutants usually have secondary mutations often affecting growth rate and nutrition, genetic engineering was selected as the technique of choice to modify wild-type, highly strain-specific bacteria into non-ice-nucleating biological control agents for protection from warm temperature frost damage (-2 to $-5\,°C$). One potential environmental impact would be that non-ice-nucleating engineered strains might affect weather patterns by perturbing any role ice nucleators might have in rain nucleation. Since natural non-ice-nucleation-active strains occur in nature, this seems unlikely. Limited field trials with engineered strains indicate that some control of warm temperature frost damage may be expected without apparent environmental impact.

16.5.3   RESISTANCE TO VIRUS-CAUSED DISEASES

Molecular biology of plant–viral interactions have provided much information about plant infection, viral replication within the plant, and recognition of viruses by plants. Based on this information, several strategies have been developed to make plants more resistant to viral diseases (Ponz and Bruening, 1986). For the first strategy, plants resistant to virus-caused diseases often recognize some component of the virion, thus triggering a resistant response (Nelson *et al.*, 1988). To construct plants resistant to virus-caused diseases, genetic engineers have introduced a gene for viral coat proteins into the plant genome. In this manner, the plant produces a coat protein that triggers a plant's own defences, so that it is already in the resistant mode before contact with the virus.

The second tactic is to inactivate replicons of the viral genome as they are produced. Many plant viruses are single-stranded RNA replicated from a complementary strand of RNA that is in much lower concentration than the single-stranded virus itself. Observations indicate that the virus could actually be inactivated if the complementary strand were in higher concentration than the virus, perhaps by binding the complementary strand to the virus, thereby blocking the translocation of viral products required for disease initiation (Palukaitis and Zaitlin, 1984).

The third tactic is to engineer plants with a DNA copy of a satellite virus genome that causes attenuation of viral-caused disease. This system has an added advantage in that it is induced only when complementary viral particles are present; that is, resistance is 'turned on' only when needed and does not form a continuous energy drag on the host plant. Tolerance, rather than complete resistance, is mediated by this form of disease control (Harrison *et al.*, 1987).

The fourth tactic takes advantage of the newly discovered class of enzymatic nucleic acids—ribozymes, or catalytic RNAs. In this system, a sequence of DNA containing an inserted template for a ribozyme produces an mRNA complementary to the viral genome and is introduced into the plant genome. Upon complementation of the viral genome, the ribozyme catalytically cleaves the viral genome in such a manner as to prevent further viral replication (Gerlach, 1988; Gerlach *et al.*, 1987).

16.5.4 HERBICIDE RESISTANCE

Genetic improvement of crop tolerance to herbicides would provide the possibility for weed control using fewer herbicides, since crop plants now susceptible to those herbicides would be resistant to commonly employed herbicides (Cocking *et al.*, 1981; Hatzios, 1987).

16.5.4.1 Triazine resistance

Triazines are photosynthesis-inhibiting herbicides known to act on the pastoquinone-binding chloroplast-membrane Q_b protein encoded by the *psbA* gene. Genes from triazine-resistant and sensitive weeds are found to differ by as little as a single nucleotide base in their sequences (Arntzen, 1986; Mets *et al.*, 1986). Triazine-resistant plants have been constructed by moving a gene from bacteria into plants using the molecular vectors developed from the plant pathogenic bacterium *Agrobacterium tumefaciens* and its plasmid (*pTi*) which is the vector of oncogenicity genes.

16.5.4.2 Glyphosate resistance

Glyphosate inhibits 5-enolpyruvyl-shikimate-ε-phosphate synthetase (EPSP) in the shikimate pathway for biosynthesis of amino acids, plant growth hormones, phytoalexins, and other phenolic compounds (Amrhein *et al.*, 1983). Alleles of the *aroA* gene encoding EPSP that provide a resistant phenotype have been described for species of bacteria. An *aroA* gene from the human pathogen

Salmonella typhimurium was moved using the *Agrobacterium-pTi* system into plants and conferred some tolerance to the herbicide (Comai *et al.*, 1986; Shah *et al.*, 1986).

16.5.4.3 Sulphonylurea and imidazolinone resistance

Susceptibility to the structurally unrelated sulphonylurea and imidazolinone herbicides is due to inhibition of a single enzyme, acetolactate synthase (ALS) (Chaleff and Mauvais, 1984; Shaner *et al.*, 1984). This enzyme is the first specific one in the pathway to branched-chain amino acids such as valine, leucine, and isoleucine. Resistance to chlorsulphuron (a sulphonylurea herbicide) was engineered into tobacco by first fusing the open reading frame of a chlorsulphuron-resistant ALS gene from yeast to the sequence coding for the lead peptide of a small subunit gene for ribulose biphosphate carboxylase in tobacco, and then transferring it into the plant using a *pTi* vector (Falco *et al.*, 1985). The chimeric gene increased threefold the resistance to a herbicide, indicating that further refinement of the system will be necessary before field use is practicable (Fraley *et al.*, 1986).

16.5.4.4 Herbicide degradation

Biodegradation is an important factor affecting environmental persistence of most organic herbicides used in contemporary agriculture. Microbes are the chief agents of herbicide degradation, most probably through the action of selected constitutive or inducible enzyme systems (Hatzios, 1987). Often components of the herbicides may be used as microbial nutrients. The rate of microbial degradation is influenced by physicochemical characteristics of soils, rate and frequency of herbicide application, the cropping system, and the presence of other pesticides. Repeated applications of herbicides may lead to increased levels of microbial degradation to the point where succeeding applications are ineffective on target pests.

Currently, the mechanisms of biodegradation in soils are poorly understood. However, over thirteen genera of bacteria and five genera of fungi have been associated with biodegradation of herbicides to date. Elucidation of the mechanisms for biodegradation using molecular techniques will aid in the design of herbicides increasingly resistant to microbial degradation.

Environmental benefit may be hidden within the problem of herbicide biodegradation. Improved strain selection and biological engineering may provide strains to be used to ameliorate environmental damage due to pesticide spills or to detoxify pesticides in the soil column to protect groundwater from contamination.

16.5.4.5 Herbicide 'safeners'

A 'safener' is a term used to describe a compound that protects crop plants from herbicide injury. Antidote, protectant, and antagonist are synonyms.

Microbial strain selection and genetic engineering may result in the development of improved herbicide safeners. Safeners allow the extended use of herbicides on crops that would ordinarily be damaged by those herbicides. In IPM schemes, safeners simplify crop protection by reducing the numbers of pesticides in the environment.

Microbial safeners may be developed by using herbicide-biodegrading microbial strains to protect susceptible crop plants from these herbicides. Microbial safeners will probably be most effective against soil-applied herbicides (Hatzios, 1987). The crop plants may be specifically protected by applying the microbial safeners directly to roots of transplants or to seeds before sowing.

16.5.5 BIOLOGICAL CONTROL

Specific strains of *Pseudomonas fluorescens* and *Pseudomonas putida* provide biological control of fungal plant pathogens and deleterious rhizobacteria with concomitant positive growth responses above and beyond simple amelioration of disease. The ability of these strains to act as biological control agents has been attributed to their ability to rapidly and competitively colonize roots and to produce siderophores (iron-binding compounds) and antibiotics. The first of these biological control formulations based on *Pseudomonas* has been placed into the field for commercial control of damping-off fungi on cotton by Ecogen Inc. (Makulowich, 1988). Not much is understood about the competitive ability to colonize plant roots or the host plant specificity demonstrated by some of the bacterial strains. However, some information is known about siderophore and antibiotic production and is discussed below.

16.5.5.1 Siderophores

Most microorganisms respond to low-iron stress by producing extracellular, low-molecular-weight (500–1000 Daltons), iron transport compounds (or siderophones) which bind iron selectively and with great binding power. These compounds are bound with iron for microbial metabolism. For instance, oxidative phosphorylation—probably the most important energy-producing process in a cell—requires iron-containing proteins for electron capture and transfer. Among fluorescent pseudomonads, such as *P. fluorescens* and *P. putida*, yellow-green fluorescent pyoverdines act as siderophores. The best known of these is pseudobactin, a hexapeptide cyclized through a fluorescent quinoline derivative with a hydroxamic iron-chelating group derived from moieties of ornithin, aspartic acid, and aniline residues (Leong, 1986). Pseudobactin requires several genes for its biosynthesis; at least five gene clusters and a minimum of seven genes are required for biosynthesis of pyoverdine siderophores (Marugg *et al.*, 1985; Weisbeek *et al.*, 1986).

Siderophores evidently have a role in disease control, since the incidence and severity of disease is reduced in soils containing either siderophore-producing microbes or deliberately added pyoverdine siderophores. Finally, in soils containing excess iron, neither siderophore-producing bacteria nor added pyoverdine siderophores were as effective in reducing disease incidence or severity (Leong, 1986). Unknown is whether siderophores act by chelating iron so that it is unavailable to fungal plant pathogens (Leong, 1986), act as antibiotics (Ahl *et al.*, 1986), or act by a combination of mechanisms. Genetic engineers may manipulate siderophore production to produce greater efficiency, higher levels of production, and constitutive variations of siderophores. Until these experimental constructions are made and tested, the role of siderophores in biological control and integrated pest management remains to be fully understood.

16.5.5.2 Antibiotics

Pseudomonads produce a host of antibiotics including phenazines, pyrroles, pseudomonic acid, pyo compounds, and amino acid-containing antibiotics (Leisinger and Margraff, 1979). By correlating the activity spectrum of each antibiotic *in vitro* with the control of target pathogens using purified antibiotics, the antibiotics pyrrolnitrin, pyoluteorin, and phenazine-1-carboxylate have been found to play roles in biological control (Gurusiddaiah *et al.*, 1986; Howell and Stipanovic, 1979, 1980). Like the pyoverdine siderophores, roles for the antibiotics in the biological control phenomonenon may be contributory or central, but have not been established firmly. Genetic engineers may manipulate antibiotic production to produce more efficient antibiotics and higher levels of production.

16.5.6 COPPER AND FUNGICIDE RESISTANCE

Manipulating copper and/or fungicide resistance in non-pathogenic bacteria to enhance biological control of pathogens is a unique scheme under consideration for IPM. Copper resistance was discovered on conjugal plasmids in *Pseudomonas syringae* pv. tomato, the causal agent of bacterial speck of tomato (Bender and Cooksey, 1987). The presence of copper resistance interferes with the control of bacterial speck using copper sprays; however, the use of copper sprays interferes with the saprophytic barrier to disease established by non-pathogenic bacteria on the surface of tomatoes. By moving copper-resistance plasmids into non-pathogenic epiphytic bacteria, glass-house experiments have demonstrated that a saprophytic barrier to the non-copper-resistant pathogen may be established in the presence of copper sprays, thus reducing disease incidence and severity to a greater extent than that with either the biological control strain or the copper treatment separately (Cooksey, 1988). Most likely, this combined control would reduce the incidence and severity of disease caused by the copper-resistant pathogen, since the epiphytic population of the biological control agent remains to provide the saprophytic barrier.

Similar studies have been conducted with benomyl (TeBeest, 1984) and other fungicidal compounds (Delp, 1980).

16.6 SUMMARY

The use of techniques developed for recombinant DNA in the biological control of plant pathogens is currently a very active area of research in both academic and industrial institutions. The application of molecular genetics to selected biocontrol systems can potentially provide an understanding of the genes involved in biological control phenomena. An establishment of a genetic basis for biological control is a prerequisite to further molecular studies that centre on the enhancement of biological control phenomena. It is not necessary to completely understand a biological control system to use it successfully in the field. However, this basic understanding is necessary to apply molecular genetics as a means to improve a biological control system. Initially, a model system that consistently works under field conditions should be exploited and genetically dissected. Biological control can be best approached by collaborations between molecular biologists and plant pathologists. Thus, the plant pathologist can provide the biological material and the practical experience, while the molecular biologist can manipulate the specific genes of interest.

An obstacle to the effective use of biocontrol agents is the complex microscopic ecosystem in which biological control agents for plant disease must survive, multiply, and decrease disease. Disease can be reduced by: a reduction in inoculum density of the pest, as with insects; protection of infection sites; or modification of the response of the host to the pathogen (i.e., induced resistance and cross protection). The latter two cases appear to be more common in plant pathology. Whether on leaves (Lindow, 1982; Blakeman, 1981) or roots (Schroth and Hancock, 1985), the control agent must be highly competitive.

The delivery of control agents is critical in plant disease control. The beneficial microorganisms must be placed in an environment where they can survive and interact with a pathogen or plant in such a manner as to reduce disease. Favourable environments are usually found where colonizaton by other microorganisms is reduced, such as young leaves (Lindow, 1982), fumigated soils (Martin et al., 1985), roots of transplants, or fresh wounds (Carroll, 1988; Schroth and Hancock, 1985).

Due to the difficulty of establishing organisms in complex communities it is important to consider the agroecosystem as a continuum: from relatively simple greenhouse systems, where large amounts of energy and chemical inputs are used to maintain a constant agroecosystem, to complex natural forest systems, where little or no inputs are available (Shikano and Kurihara, 1985). The simpler, more intensive greenhouse systems are more amenable to biological control, because control agents can be applied to steamed or fumigated soils, where competition from other microorganisms is low. The agroecosystem continuum can be extended to include annual crops transplanted to fumigated soils, annual crops seeded into fumigated soils, annual crops seeded into non-fumigated soils, perennial fruit and nut crops intensively managed, perennial crops that receive little or no management, and finally unmanaged natural systems. Due to the increase in complexity and decrease in areas available for introduction of control agents, the implementation of biological control is more difficult as one moves along the continuum (Cairns, 1986, 1987; Cairns and Pratt, 1987).

The release of engineered microorganisms into the environment has been the focus of much public and scientific concern (Rissler, 1984). Before a release is allowed, the construction of effective and safe biological control agents should be carefully analysed and the risks and benefits assessed. Collaboration among pathologists, molecular biologists and microbial ecologists is essential at this point. Such policies are already in place or are in the developmental stage in many countries throughout the world.

Lastly, to implement biological control programs based on biotechnology within IPM, the following need to be improved: understanding of total ecosystems; mass production and delivery of control agents; selection and enhancement of control agents; and the specificity of control agents to only one disease on the crop in a small geographic area. Those researching the biological control of insects share many of these same problems. The success rate of recently developed biocontrol agents (naturally occurring and genetically altered) is impressive, and demonstrates the potential that genetic engineering has on biocontrol systems. The future appears filled with exciting possibilities for applying effective biologicals to help reduce the chemical dependency of agricultural production systems.

16.7 REFERENCES

Ahl, P., Voisard, C. and Defago, G. (1986) Iron-bound siderophores, cyanic acid, and antibiotics involved in suppression of *Thielaviopsis basicola* by a *Pseudomonas fluorescens* strain. *J. Phytopathol.* **116**, 121–124.

Amrhein, N., Johanning, D., Schab, J. and Schultz, A. (1983) *FEBS Lett.* **157**, 191–196.

Armstrong, J. L., Knudsen, G. R. and Seider, R. J. (1987) Microcosm method to assess survival of recombinant bacteria associated with plants and herbivorous insects. *Curr. Microbiol.* **15**(4), 229–232.

Arntzen, C. J. (1986) Protein engineering of herbicide target sites. *Abstracts of the International Congress on Pesticide Chemistry*, 6th IUPAC, Ottawa 3S-04.

Atlas, R. M. (1982) Enumeration and estimation of biomass of components in the biosphere. In: Burns, R. G. and Slater, J. H. (Eds) *Experimental Microbial Ecology*, Blackwell Scientific, Oxford, UK, pp. 84–102.

Baross, J. H., Liston, J. and Morita, R. Y. (1967) Some implications of genetic exchange among marine vibrios, including *Vibrio parahaemolyticus*, naturally occurring in the Pacific oyster. In: Fujino, T., Sakaguchi, G., Sakazaki, R. and Takeda, Y. (Eds) *International Symposium on Vibrio parahaemolyticus*, Saikon Publishing, Tokyo, pp. 126–137.

Bender, C. L. and Cooksey, D. A. (1987) Molecular cloning of copper resistance genes from *Pseudomonas syringae* pv. tomato. *J. Bacteriol.* **169**, 470–474.

Bernhard, K. (1986) Studies on the delta-endotoxin of *Bacillus thuringiensis* var. tenebrionis. *FEMS Microbiol. Lett.* **3**, 261–265.

Biever, K. D., Andrews, P. L. and Andrews, P. A. (1982) Use of a predator, *Podusus maculiventris*, to distribute virus and initiate epizootics. *J. Econ. Entomol.* **75**, 150–152.

Blakeman, J. P. (Ed.) (1981) *Microbial Ecology of the Phylloplane*, Academic Press, New York.

Brezhnev, A. I., Ginzburg, L. R., Pluektov, R. A., and Poluektov, R. A. (1974) The structural optimization of exploited populations. *Econ. Math. Meth.* **4**, 808–811.

Brown, J. R. (Ed.) (1987) *Soil Testing: Sampling, Correlation, Calibration and Interpretation*, Special Publication No. 21, Soil Science Society of America, Madison, Wisconsin, 144pp.

Bulla, L. A., Davidson, L. I., Kramer, K. J. and Jones, B. L. (1979) Purification of the insecticidal toxin form the parasporal crystal of *Bacillus thuringiensis* subsp. Kurstaki. *Biochem. Biophys. Res. Commun.* **91**, 1121–1130.

Cairns, J. Jr (1986) The myth of the most sensitive species. *BioScience* **36**, 670–672.

Cairns, J. Jr (1987) Problems associated with selecting the most sensitive species for toxicity testing. *Hydrobiologia* **153**, 87–94.

Cairns, J. Jr and Pratt, J. R. (1987) Ecotoxial effect indices: a rapidly evolving system. *Water Sci. Tech.* **19**(11)1, 1–12.

Carroll, G. (1988) Fungal endophytes in stems and leaves: from latent pathogen to mutalistic symbiont. *Ecology* **69**, 2–9.

Chaleff, R. S. and Mauvais, C. J. (1984) Acetolactate synthase is the site of action of two sulfonylurea herbicides in higher plants. *Science* **224**, 1443–1445.

Cocking, E. C., Davey, M. R., Pental, D. and Power, J. B. (1981) Aspects of plant genetic manipulation. *Nature* **293**, 265–270.

Comai, L., Facciotti, D., Stalker, D. M., Thompson, G. A. and Hiatt, W. R. (1986) Expression in plants of a bacterial gene coding for glyphosate resistance. In: Zaitlin, M., Day, P. and Hollaender, A. (Eds) *Biotechnology in Plant Science: Relevance to Agriculture in the Eighties*, Academic Press, New York, pp. 329–338.

Cooksey, D. A. (1988) Reduction of infection by *Pseudomonas syringae* pb. tomato using a nonpathogenic, copper-resistant strain combined with a copper bactericide. *Phytopathology* **78**, 601–603.

Corapcioğlu, M. Y. and Haridas, A. (1984) Transport and fate of microorganisms in porous media: a theoretical investigation. *J. Hydrol. (Amsterdam)* **72**, 149–169.

DeAngelis, D. L. (1973) A general code for ecosystem models. *Gött Bodenkdl. Ber.* **29**, 55–92.

Delp, C. J. (1980) Coping with resistance to plant disease control agents. *Plant Dis.* **64**, 652–657.

Falco, S. C., Dumas, S. K. and McDevitt, R. (1985) Molecular genetic analysis of sulfonylurea herbicide action and resistance in yeast. In: van Vloten-Doting, L., Groot, G. S. P. and Hall, T. C. (Eds) *Molecular Form and Function of the Plant Genome*, NATO ASI Series A, Life Sciences Vol. 83, Plenum, New York, pp. 467–478.

Falcon, L. A. (1985) Development and use of microbial insecticides. In: Hoy, M. A. and Herzog, D. C. (Eds) *Biological Control in Agricultrual IPM Systems*, Academic Press, New York, pp. 229–242.

Falcon, L. A., Kane, W. R. and Bethell, R. S. (1968) Preliminary evaluation of a granulosis virus for control of the codling moth. *J. Econ. Entomol.* **61**, 1208–1213.

Fraley, R. T., Rogers, S. G. and Horsch, R. B. (1986) Genetic transformation on higher plants. *CRC Crit. Rev. Plant Sci.* **4**, 1–46.

Gerlach, W. (1988) Plant virus resistance based on the satellite RNA of tobacco ringspot virus. *J. Cell. Biochem.* **12C**, 239 (abstr.).

Gerlach, W. L., Llewellyn, D. and Haseloff, J. (1987) Construction of a plant disease resistance gene from the satellite RNA of tobacco ringspot virus. *Nature* **328**, 802–805.

Gladden, J. and Ginzburg, L. R. (1982) Variation and persistence in stochastic population models with differing age structures. *Bull. Ecol. Soc. Am.*, **63**, 139.

Graham, J. B. and Istock, C. A. (1978) Genetic exchange in *Bacillus subtillis* in soil. *Mol. Gen. Genet.* **166**, 287–290.

Gurusiddaiah, S., Weller, D. M., Sarkar, A. and Cook, R. J. (1986) Characterization of an antibiotic produced by a strain of *Pseudomonas fluorescens* inhibitory to *Gaeumannomyces graminis* var. tritici and Pythium spp. *Antimicrob. Agents Chemother.* **29**, 488–495.

Hagedorn, C. (1986) Role of genetic variants in autecological research. In: Tate, R. L. (Ed.) *Microbial Autecology: A Method for Environmental Studies*, John Wiley & Sons, New York, pp. 61–74.

Harrison, B. D., Mayo, M. A. and Baulcombe, D. C. (1987) Virus resistance in transgenic plants that express cucumber mosaic virus satellite RNA. *Nature* **328**, 799–802.

Hatzios, K. K. (1987) Biotechnology applications in weed management: now and in the future. *Adv. Agron.* **41**, 325–375.

Hernstadt, C., Soares, G., Wilcox, E. and Edward, D. (1986) A new strain of *Bacillus thuringiensis* with activity against coleopteran insects. *BioTechnology* **4**, 305–308.

Hernstadt, C., Gilroy, T. E., Sobieski, D. A., Bennett, B. D. and Gaertner, F. H. (1987) Nucleotide sequence and deduced amino acid sequence of a coleopteran active δ-endotoxin gene from *Bacillus thuringiensis* subsp. San Diego. *Gene* **57**, 37–46.

Hicks, R. E. and Newell, S. Y. (1984) The growth of bacteria and the fungus *Phaesphaeria-typharum Eumycota Ascomycotina* in salt marsh microcosms in the presence and absence of mercury. *J. Exp. Mar. Biol. Ecol.* **78**(1–2), 143–156.

Horsch, R. B., Fraley, R. T., Rogers, S. G., Sanders, P. R., Lloyd, A. and Hoffman, N. (1984) Inheritance of functional foreign genes in plants. Genetic engineering with T-DNA from *Agrobacterium tumefaciens, Nicotiana plumbaginifolia*. *Science* **223**, 496–498.

Howell, C. R. and Stipanovic, R. D. (1979) Control of *Rhizoctonia solani* on cotton seedlings with *Pseudomonas fluorescens* and with an antibiotic produced by the bacterium. *Phytopathology* **69**, 480–482.

Howell, C. R. and Stipanovic, R. D. (1980) Suppression of *Pythium ultimum*-induced damping-off of cotton seedlings by *Pseudomonas fluorescens* and its antibiotic, pyoluteorin. *Phytopathology* **70**, 712–715.

Hunter, M., Stephenson, T., Kirk, P. W. W., Perry, R. and Lester, J. N. (1986) Effect of salinity gradients and heterotrophic microbial activity on biodegradation of nitrilotriacetic-acid in laboratory simulations of the estuarine environment. *Appl. Environ. Microbiol.* **51**(5), 919–925.

Jansson, J. K. and Tiedje, J. M. (1988) Detection of gene rearrangement in soil using gene probes. In: M. Sussman *et al.* (Eds), *The Release of Genetically Engineered Microorganisms*, Academic Press, New York.

Kelman, A., Anderson, W., Falkow, S., Federoff, N. V. and Levin, S. (1987) *Introduction of Recombinant DNA-Engineered Organisms into the Environment: Key Issues*. Prepared for the National Research Council of the National Academy of Sciences by the Committee on the Introduction of Genetically Engineered Organisms into the Environment, National Research Council, Washington DC.

Kerr, A. Manigault, P. and Tempe, J. (1977) Transfer of virulence *in vitro* and *in vivo* in Agrobacterium. *Nature* **265**, 560–561.

of freeze thaw stress on bacterial populations in soil microcosms. *Microb. Ecol.* **9**(4), 329–340.

Morrison, W. D., Miller, R. V. and Saylor, G. S. (1978) Frequency of F-116 mediated transduction of *Pseudomonas aeruginosa* in a freshwater environment. *Appl. Environ. Microbiol.* **36**, 724–730.

Napoli, C. and Staskawicz, B. J. (1985) Molecular genetics of biological control agents of plant pathogens; status and prospects. In: Hoy, M. A. and Herzog, D. C. (Eds) *Biological Control in Agricultural IPM Systems*, Academic Press, New York, pp. 455–461.

Nelson, R. S., McCormick, S. H., Delannay, X., Dube, P., Layton, J., Anderson, E. J., Kaniewska, M., Proksch, R. K., Horsch, R. B., Rogers, S. G., Fraley, R. T. and Beachy, R. N. (1988) Virus tolerance, plant growth, and field performance of transgenic tomato plants expressing coat protein from tobacco mosaic virus. *Biotechnology* **6**, 403–409.

Orser, C., Staskawicz, B. J., Panopoulos, N. J., Dahlbeck, D. and Lindow, S. E. (1985) Cloning and expression of bacterial ice nucleation genes in *Escherichia coli*. *J. Bacteriol.* **164**, 359–366.

Orvos, D. R., Lacy, G. H. and Cairns, J. Jr (1988) Origin of antibiotic resistant strains isolated from microcosms contaminated with genetically-engineered microorganisms. In: M. Sussman *et al.* (Eds) *The Release of Genetically-engineered Microorganisms*, Academic Press, New York.

Ou, C. Y., Kwok, S., Mitchell, S. W., Mack, D. H., Sninsky, J. J., Krebs, J. W., Feorino, P., Warfield, D. and Schochetman, G. (1988) DNA amplification for direct detection of HIV-1 in DNA of peripheral blood mononuclear cells. *Science* **239**, 295–297.

Ouellette, R. P. and Cheremisinoff, P. N. (1985) *Applications of Biotechnology*, Technomic Publishing, Lancaster, Pennsylvania, 247pp.

Page, A. L., Miller, R. H. and Keeney, D. R. (Eds) (1982) *Methods of Soil Analysis, Part 2* (2nd edn), Special Publication No. 9, American Society of Agronomy, Madison, Wisconsin, 1159pp.

Palukaitis, P. and Zaitlin, M. (1984) A model to explain the 'cross-protection' phenomenon shown by plant viruses and viroids. In: Kosuge, T. and Nester, E. (Eds) *Plant–Microbe Interactions: Molecular and Genetic Perspectives*, Macmillan, New York, pp. 420–429.

Ponz, F. and Bruening, G. (1986) Mechanisms of resistance to plant viruses. *Annual Rev. Phytopathol.* **24**, 355–381.

Rissler, J. (1984) Research needs for detecting environmental effects of genetically engineered microorganisms. *Recomb. DNA Tech. Bull.* **7**, 20–30.

Roberge, M. R. (1978) Methodology of soil enzyme measurement and extraction. In: Burns, R. G. (Ed.) *Soil Enzymes*, Academic Press, New York, pp. 341–375.

zak, D. B. and Colwell, R. R. (1987) Survival strategies of bacteria in the natural ironment. *Microb. Rev.* **51**, 365–379.

D. I. (1985) Construction of temporal models: I. Disease progress of air-borne gens. *Adv. Plant Pathol.* **3**, 11–29.

K., Glenfand, D. H., Stoffel, S., Scharf, S. J., Higuchi, R., Horn, G. T., . B. and Erlich, H. A. (1988) Primer-directed enzymatic amplification of a thermostable DNA polymerase. *Science* **239**, 487–494.

V. and Hancock, J. G. (1985) Soil antagonists in IPM systems. In: Hoy, Ierzog, D. C. (Eds) *Biological Control in Agricultural IPM Systems*, ss, New York, pp. 415–432.

sch, R. B., Klee, H. J., Kishore, G. M., Winter, J. A., Tumer, N. M., Sanders, P. R., Glasser, C. S., Aykent, S., Siegel, N. R., Rogers, R. T. (1986) Engineering herbicide tolerance in transgenic plants. 1.

Shaner, D. L., Anderson, P. C. and Stidham, M. A. (1984) Imidazolinones: potent inhibitors of acetohydroxyacid synthase. *Plant Physiol.* **76**, 545–546.

Shikano, S. and Kurihara, Y. (1985) Community responses to organic loading in a microcosm. *Jpn. J. Ecol.* **35**(3), 297–306.

Silver, M., Ehrolich, H. L. and Ivarson, K. C. (1986) Soil mineral transformation mediated by soil microbes. In: Huang, P. M. and Schnitzer, M. (Eds) *Interactions of Soil Minerals with Natural Organics and Microbes*, Special Publication No. 17, Soil Science Society of America, Madison, Wisconsin, pp. 497–514.

Somerville, C. C., Knight, I. T., Straube, W. L. and Colwell, R. R. (1988) Probe-directed polymerization-enhanced detection of specific gene sequences in the environment. In: M. Sussman *et al.* (Eds), *The Release of Genetically Engineered Microorganisms*, Academic Press, New York.

Summers, M., Engler, R., Falcon, L. A. and Vail, P. V. (1980) Antibiotic resistance and its transfer among clinical and nonclinical *Klebsiella* strains in botanical environments. *Appl. Environ. Microbiol.* **39**, 97–104.

Talbot, H. W., Yamamoto, D. Y., Smith, M. W. and Seidler, R. J. (1980) Antibiotic resistance and its transfer among clinical and nonclinical Klebsiella strains in botannical environments. *Appl. Environ. Microbiol.* **39**, 97–104.

Tauber, H. J., Hoy, M. A. and Herzog, D. C. (1985) Biological control in agricultural IPM systems: a brief overview of the current status and future prospects. In: Hoy, M. A. and Herzog, D. C. (Eds) *Biological Control in Agricultural IPM Systems*, Academic Press, New York, pp. 3–12.

TeBeest, D. O. (1984) Induction of tolerance to benomyl in *Colletotrichum gloeosporioides* f. sp. aeschynomene by ethyl methanesulfonate. *Phytopathology* **7–4**, 864 (Abstract).

Thingstad, T. F. and Pengerud, B. (1985) Fate and effect of allochthonous organic material in aquatic microbial ecosystems: an analysis based on chemostat theory. *Mar. Ecol. Prog. Ser.* **21**(1–2), 47–62.

Tomashow, M. F., Nutter, R., Postle, K., Chilton, M. D., Blattner, F. R., Powell, A., Gordon, M. P. and Nester, E. W. (1980) Recombination between higher plant DNA and the Ti plasmid of *Agrobacterium tumefaciens*. *Proc. Nat. Acad. Sci. USA* **77**, 6448–6452.

Weinberg, S. R. and Stotzky, G. (1972) Conjugation and genetic recombination of *Escherichia coli* in soil. *Soil Biol. Biochem.* **4**, 171–180.

Weisbeek, P. I. J., Schippers, B., van der Hofstad, G. and Marugg, J. (1986) Molecular genetics of siderophore biosynthesis in *Pseudomonas putida* WCS358. In: Swinburne, T. R. (Ed.) *Iron, Siderophores and Plant Diseases*, NATO ASI Series A, Life Sciences Vol. 117, Plenum Press, New York.

Whitley, H. R. and Schnepf, H. E. (1986) The molecular biology of parasporal crystal body formation in *Bacillus thuringiensis*. *Ann. Rev. Microbiol.* **40**, 549–576.

Index

Index compiled by G. Jones